Speaking of Monsters

Speaking of Monsters

A Teratological Anthology

Edited by

Caroline Joan S. Picart and John Edgar Browning

palgrave
macmillan

First published in 2012 by
PALGRAVE MACMILLAN®
in the United States—a division of St. Martin's Press LLC,
175 Fifth Avenue, New York, NY 10010.

Where this book is distributed in the UK, Europe and the rest of the World, this is by Palgrave Macmillan, a division of Macmillan Publishers Limited, registered in England, company number 785998, of Houndmills, Basingstoke, Hampshire RG21 6XS.

Palgrave Macmillan is the global academic imprint of the above companies and has companies and representatives throughout the world.

Palgrave® and Macmillan® are registered trademarks in the United States, the United Kingdom, Europe and other countries.

ISBN: 978–0–230–11450–0

Library of Congress Cataloging-in-Publication Data

Speaking of monsters : a teratological anthology / edited by Caroline Joan S. Picart and John Edgar Browning.
p. cm.
Includes bibliographical references.
ISBN 978–0–230–11450–0 (alk. paper)
1. Monsters in motion pictures. 2. Horror films—History and criticism. 3. Teratology. I. Picart, Caroline Joan, 1966– II. Browning, John Edgar.
PN1995.9.M6S64 2012
791.43′6164—dc23 2011052891

A catalogue record of the book is available from the British Library.

Design by Integra Software Services

First edition: July 2012

10 9 8 7 6 5 4 3 2 1

Printed in the United States of America.

Contents

List of Figures and Tables

Figures

Table

Foreword

What We Talk About When We Talk About Monsters

David J. Skal

Monsters have long been stereotyped by a propensity for inarticulate grunts, when, in fact, they are often capable of expressing themselves quite eloquently. Most incarnations of Frankenstein's monster would scarcely be recognized by his literary progenitor, Mary Shelley, who originally gave him an excellent knowledge of French (rendered in English for her readers of 1818) and an impressive familiarity with translations of *Paradise Lost*, *Plutarch's Lives*, and *The Sorrows of Young Werther*. Yet, the monster's literacy and volubility have been of scant interest to stage and screen adaptors, who generally jettison most of Shelley's narrative and authorial intentions, along with all of Milton, Plutarch, and Goethe.

However, a constantly shifting conversation is the essence of survival when it comes to monsters. The single most iconic monster of the last century is unquestionably James Whale's and Boris Karloff's 1931 collaborative interpretation of Shelley's patchwork reanimatron, an image burned into the collective imagination throughout the world, even among people who have never seen the actual performance. It is ironic that one of the immortal roles of the early talkie era should be an exercise in pure pantomime, but it is precisely the lack of speech that makes the character and film impossible *not* to talk about. The mute Frankenstein monster is in essence a theatrical work-in-progress, incomplete without the added ingredient of the audience/beholder's reaction, projection, interpretation, and cultural assimilation. Karloff himself was wise in complaining about the even limited powers of speech given to the creature in the 1935 sequel *Bride of Frankenstein*, even if his objections were not based on critical theory but his own well-honed instincts as an actor.

Karloff was right: the less a monster explains itself, the more likely we are to get involved, start talking to ourselves and among ourselves, looking for our own meanings and explanations.

I've been personally talking about monsters on a professional stage for more than two decades, and, while I am not a career academic, I have done enough teaching, lecturing, and general lurking outside the schoolyard fence to know the utility of monsters in luring students to explore vast areas not directly associated with horror. Speak of monsters and you're soon speaking about all kinds of things. Shelley's *Frankenstein* can't be fully appreciated without a larger understanding of the tension between the self-satisfied Enlightenment and Romantic radicalism; *Dracula* doesn't start to make sense as a cultural document without at least a basic understanding of Darwinism's impact on Victorian thought and society. Movie monsters of the Great Depression similarly illuminate a complex social, economic, and political era with a renewed relevance to the present. Breadlines and underwater mortgages, it turns out, both provide excellent vantage points for our never-ending monster show.

The word "monster" in its present English form entered the language around the time of Shakespeare, whose characters find occasion to speak the word more than 80 times. The term descends from the Latin noun *monstrum* (divine portent) by way of the French verb *monere* (to warn) while yielding some quaint, discarded variations along the way, such as—a personal favorite—the archaic adjective "monstriferous."

Monsters are slippery, ever-adaptive metaphors, but above all, they are natural teachers and teaching tools. Monsters de*monstr*ate things, usually of a cautionary kind. As the title of this anthology indicates, monsters were originally the province of teratology. From antiquity onward, anomalous births were considered ominous, portents of disease and disaster. Birth defects were displayed for entertainment and profit at least from Elizabethan times, first for the rabble and later for the middle classes as "educational" diversion.

The first examples of American monster-speak were the excited spiels of carnival barkers in the heyday of P.T. Barnum, pitching their admixture of terror and wonder as they cajoled the public to behold "congresses of strange people." It should not be surprising that a rather direct line can be drawn between nineteenth-century sideshows and the rise of twentieth-century monstertainment. Significantly, the cinematograph itself was introduced as a carnival attraction. When the sideshow mountebank Dr. Caligari revealed his sleepwalking zombie to the world in 1919, he was also introducing the technology of motion pictures itself as a kind of somnambulist/golem—a creepy facsimile of living animation rendered from light, shadow, and celluloid, originally displayed in traveling tents and dime museums. The essential connection between sideshows and movie monsters is nowhere more clearly drawn than in the singular career of American film director Tod Browning, whose personal experience as a Caligari-esque carnie ("The Living Hypnotic Corpse") engendered a lifelong fascination with teratological

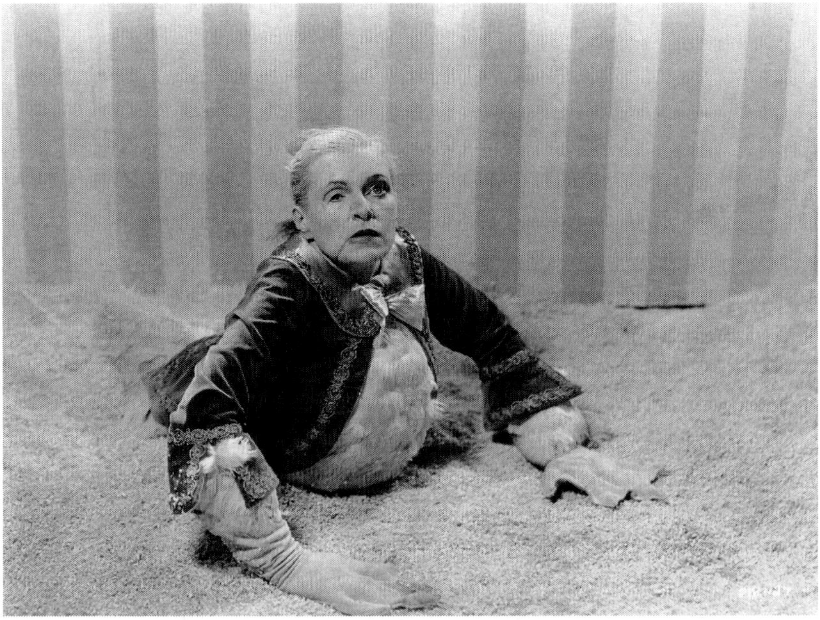

Figure 0.1 Olga Baclanova as Cleopatra in Tod Browning's *Freaks* (1932). (Courtesy of Metro-Goldwyn-Mayer.)

showmanship. It all culminated in the notorious *Freaks* (1932), which sounded a death knell to his previously charmed Hollywood tenure, but the monstrous outsider/other was a profitable component of his directorial bag of tricks and informed his noncircus films as well. Bela Lugosi, quoted from a publicity interview for Browning's *Dracula* (1931), speaks of "the feminine love of horror" in relation to sideshows and birth defects. "There is a profound biological reason," Lugosi opined. "Before a woman bears a child she goes through successive phases of horror, lest the fruit of her body be a monstrous thing."

Worry about misshapen things coming into being extends considerably beyond reproductive biology. While carnival monsters certainly serve the cathartic function of reinforcing one's own shaky sense of physical normalcy, and general good-standing membership in the tribe, they are also anxiety avatars for an age in which the familiar structures of society and identity are inexorably morphing.

It's hardly surprising, then, that monsters have eagerly entered the lingua franca of political discourse. Goya's dictum about the sleep of reason producing monsters is nowhere as evident as in today's debased and fact-free politicking, where demonization of all opposition has become the default strategy of the radical right. Monster metaphors are everywhere, with vituperative rhetoric seemingly informed by the populism of zombie and vampire narratives. Invading, economy-draining others, we are told, relentlessly, have our collective house under apocalyptic siege. Low-information voters (read: angry villagers) may not know much about history, science, or economics, but they know monster stories inside and out.

The sideshow has relocated from the dodgy periphery of town to Main Street. At one time, monster movies were low-budget programmers; today, misshapen creatures are central to the most prestigious and expensive motion pictures. An entire category of publishing—young adult fiction—is now thoroughly colonized by vampires. The exponential rise of cosmetic surgery tells us that more people see monsters in their own mirrors than ever before. The *doppelgänger*, or mirror-twin, is often the most terrifying monster of them all.

Monsters, ultimately, are supreme paradoxes, dreamlike constructions that attempt to reconcile the irreconcilable. Monsters always end up having it both ways, which is part of their enduring appeal. They're both living and dead, human and animal, or (in the case of cyborgs) organic and mechanical. These combinations don't happen in the real world, but monsterland is a place that helps us process and examine the nagging contradictions of modernity. Since it is in the nature of monsters to bridge divides, it should be no wonder that they offer an (un)natural tool for cross-disciplinary and cross-cultural studies, which almost, by definition, require some crucial encounter with some kind of Other.

Mary Shelley's monster craved nothing more fervently than a simple discourse with his maker, but was ultimately stifled and scorned. So, too, the myriad modern monsters of which we are all makers, co-creators, and cultural collaborators richly deserve a productive dialogue. A book called *Speaking of Monsters* is an excellent place to join the conversation.

Acknowledgments

Kay is indebted to Professors Berta Hernandez-Truyol, Danaya Wright, Michael Seigel, Kenneth Nunn, Katheryn Russell-Brown, Wentong Zheng, Charles Collier, Ulrich Loewenheim, Gaylin Soponis and Raymond Fleming for their mentorship, and Ms. Carol Huber and Deans Kari Mattox and Rachel Inman for their help with navigating administrative mazes. She also thanks Judge Richard Posner for encouraging her to pursue her interests in law. She dedicates this book to her loving and supportive husband, Jerry Rivera, as well as her two families—the Picart family in the Philippines and the Terrell family in Tallahassee, Florida. Kay views this book as a testament to her mother's life of courage and sacrifice because Kay has learned many things, including the love of literature, philosophy and the arts, from her mother; Dr. Anarose Santos Picart passed in March, 2012. In addition, Kay owes much to wonderfully helpful and intellectually curious colleagues, like Marlowe Fox, J.D., who found time to help out with indexing this book, despite his busy schedule as a practicing attorney. Furthermore, Kay owes much to devoted friends, such as Margaret Baker, whose loyalty, conscientiousness and attentiveness to detail were instrumental to helping generate the Index to this book, and especially John Edgar Browning, whose patience, collegiality, and intellectual acuity have helped make this book, in its entirety, possible. Kay also thanks all the contributors to this book for their professionalism and cordiality in helping bring this project to a successful close, and for their generous assistance in promoting the book; she is also grateful to the staff of Integra, especially Flora Kenson, and the editorial staff of Palgrave Macmillan, especially Robyn Curtis, for their professional and cordial assistance in seeing this book through the publication process. There are many, too numerous to document, whose kindness have made her life both rich and meaningful; to them, Kay will always be thankful.

John wishes especially to thank Michael Agan for his much appreciated, unyielding support. He also owes to Kay Picart more than can be expressed in words, for her confidence in him and her gift of teaching.

We would both like to thank the authors who have contributed to this anthology for their professionalism and brilliant insights. We are also indebted to the editorial staff at Palgrave, whose assistance helped to bring this book to completion.

The images reproduced in this book are from private collections and online databases and are used solely for educational purposes. The copyright for these images is most likely owned by either the individual party whose permission we obtained to reproduce the image or the publisher or distributor of the image.

Chapter 1. Jeffrey Jerome Cohen, "Monster Culture (Seven Theses)," excerpted by permission of the Publisher from *Monster Theory: Reading Culture*, ed. Jeffrey Jerome Cohen (Minneapolis, MN: University of Minnesota Press, 1997). Copyright © 1997.

Chapter 2. Stephen Prince, "Dread, Taboo, and *The Thing* (1982): Toward a Social Theory of the Horror Film," excerpted by permission of The Ohio University School of Film from *Wide Angle* 10, no. 3 (1988). Copyright © 1988.

Chapter 3. Noël Carroll, "Nightmare and the Horror Film: The Symbolic Biology of Fantastic Beings," excerpted by permission of The University of California Press from *Film Quarterly* 34, no. 3 (Spring 1981). Copyright © 1981.

Chapter 9. Caroline Joan (Kay) S. Picart and David Frank, "*Apt Pupil* (1998): The Hollywood Nazi-As-Monster Flick," excerpted by permission of the Publisher from *Frames of Evil: The Holocaust as Horror in American Film*, by Caroline Joan (Kay) S. Picart and David Frank (Carbondale, IL: Southern Illinois University Press, 2006). Copyright © 2006 by the Board of Trustees, Southern Illinois University.

Chapter 13. Judith (Jack) Halberstam, "*Seed of Chucky*: Transbiology and the Horror Flick," in which is included a portion excerpted by permission of the Publishers from "Animating Revolt/Revolting Animation: Penguin Love, Doll Sex and the Spectacle of the Queer Non-Human," in *Queering the Non/Human*, ed. Noreen Giffney and Myra J. Hird (Farnham etc.: Ashgate, 2008). Copyright © 2008.

Chapter 14. Lonnie H. Athens, "Stage Four: Virulency," excerpted by permission of the Publisher from *Creation of Dangerous Violent Criminals*, by Lonnie H. Athens (Champaign, IL: University of Illinois Press, 1992). Copyright © 1992 by the Board of Trustees, the University of Illinois Press.

Chapter 15. Caroline Joan (Kay) S. Picart and Cecil E. Greek, "Profiling the Terrorist as a Mass Murderer," excerpted by permission of the Publisher from *Monsters in and Among Us*, by Caroline Joan (Kay) S. Picart and Cecil E. Greek (Madison, NJ: Fairleigh Dickinson University Press, 2008). Copyright © 2008.

Chapter 23. Dominick LaCapra, "Reopening the Question of the Human and the Animal," excerpted by permission of the Publisher from *History and its Limits: Human, Animal, Violence*, by Dominick LaCapra (Ithaca, NY: Cornell University Press, 2009). Copyright © 2009 by Cornell University.

INTRODUCTION: MONSTROSITY AND MULTICULTURALISM

CAROLINE JOAN (KAY) S. PICART AND JOHN EDGAR BROWNING

WHAT IS "TERATOLOGY"?

The word "teratology" has multiple meanings, depending on the field or discourse in which it is deployed. Etymologically, "teratology" comes from the Greek word *teras,* meaning "monster," and the Latin *logy,* which in turn is derived from the Greek *logia,* meaning "a speaking, discourse, treatise, doctrine, theory, science."[1]

Despite its apparently monolithic etymology, at least denotatively, "teratology" seems almost infinitely malleable and is capable of crossing disciplinary boundaries, flourishing in and adapting to various rhetorical environments into which it is grafted. Medicine allocates to the term the domain of "studying the development of physical abnormalities during the fetal or early embryonic stage," while biology characterizes the term as the study of "abnormal formations in animals or plants."[2] *The American Heritage Science Dictionary* chooses a more generalized scientific umbrella characterization: "the scientific study of birth defects."[3] And literature defines this term as "a type of mythmaking or storytelling in which monsters and marvels are featured."[4]

Despite their differences, the definitions above have the following elements in common: (1) the "monstrous," understood as synonymous with the "abnormal" or "defective"; and (2) the genesis and development, growth, or genealogy of something "other" than "normal."

Above all, this *Teratological Anthology* simply maps what, in many ways, has already been occurring across several fields, as it tracks the expansion of this term, creating lacunae that form connections across multiple interpretive communities. Not surprisingly, teratologies stretch across science and the "sacred," the public and the private, the "real" and the "fantastic."

Though much of this book deals with the "disciplinary" function of the "monstrous"—that is, the function of policing the boundaries separating the "normal," "rational," and the "citizen" from the "abnormal," "irrational," and the "criminal"—what also emerges is that the site of the "other-than-normal" is also the nexus upon which, potentially, brave new worlds may be reimagined and forged.

Teratologies are more than simply a bestiary: a catalogue of "freaks" designed, implicitly, to celebrate the "normal" even as it flirts with a voyeuristic peep at the tabooed. Rather, as several chapters of this book show, teratologies potentially illustrate how humor, horror, fantasy, and the "real" cross-fertilize each other, resulting in the possibility of new worlds, new ethics, and new narratives coming into being.

Why Create a Book on the Monstrous?

As a general anthology of teratologies, this book aspires to perform several tasks. It distills literature crucial to the genesis and development of central questions that continue to spur further inquiry; it charts crucial, definitive, and authoritative discourses or texts while remaining reflexive, dialogical, accessible, and open to revision. It is more than a review of literature, though it documents seminal texts, without becoming slave to the archiving process or the obsession with finding the "perfect" canon of texts. It aims to communicate with a plurality of communities: from undergraduate and graduate students to established scholars, as well as scholars who desire to explore the field. Nevertheless, while it has a generally shared framework, it respects the integrity of different disciplinary and paradigmatic perspectives and does not seek to impose a "master narrative."

This book is envisaged as a "one-stop shop" of sorts for students, whether undergraduate or graduate, employing various approaches and media in the study of "teratologies," or discourses/symbolics/rhetorics of the "monstrous." For students, this book provides a ready-reference for studies they may encounter throughout their academic careers, both as scholars and teachers. The younger generation tends to be drawn to the evolution of new technologies; the nexus between film, graphic novels, and the Internet is only one result of such an evolution, and it is one this book aims to explore as it is important for ongoing research to not only stay on top of current technological and popular cultural developments but also cultivate its future scholars.

For instructors, this book could be a valuable teaching tool, written for multidisciplinary and international audiences. The book includes a mix of focused, theoretical studies to be used as foundations (such as pivotal studies by Cohen, Prince, and Carroll) for discussions tailored for different media (such as cinema, anime, and gaming), in addition to more concise case study–oriented frameworks. These frameworks also include a broad array of topics that move along a Gothic criminological model, implying a dynamic continuum across areas of fact and fiction (e.g., Picart and Greek's chapter on terrorists; Picart's chapter on the Atlanta youth murders). Such discussions would be a fruitful point from which to analyze the spectrum of issues related to the study of "monster talk," as Edward Ingebretsen[5] calls it, in the fields of, among others, sociology, psychology, political science, communication, anthropology, criminology, and critical studies. Another contributing aspect of this anthology is its expansion to global teratologies, using concrete case studies.

The Global Expansion of the Monstrous

As we have hinted earlier, "teratology," a term contemporary cultural critics have fashionably lifted from the biological sciences, refers to the study of the "monstrous" (which etymologically means both "to point to" and "to warn [against]").[6] One important building block of this study is to see that the term "monster" designates less of a "thing" than a category or class, and the task of an anthology like this one is to illustrate the multifariousness with which monsters are birthed. The chapters selected for this *Teratological Anthology* point less to some kind of primal psychological fear than they do to what Zakiya Hanafi calls an "ideological cluster"—one whose form and features are conceived from a "contextualized, localized set of characteristics, defined and accepted by the community."[7]

Unlike the Gothic, whose tropes developed principally in the West and then cross-culturally pollinated elsewhere, "monstrosity" is always already global, constructed from within a culture against the backdrop of a broader historical sketch, a product of an organized society's attempt to classify what it deems "normal" or "monstrous." The point is not so much that discourses on the "monstrous" function, as Wood points out, with an emphasis on the psychoanalytic and social aspects of these phenomena, as "collective nightmares,"[8] but rather that they function analogously, as in the way in which Joshua David Bellin characterizes fantasy films as "dominant social fantasies." Though Bellin limits his critique to selected fantasy films, such as *King Kong,* some elements of his analysis can be safely transplanted to a genealogy of teratologies. That is, rhetorics of the "monstrous" are not simply "constructed *by* their social contexts" but that they are also "constructive *of* their contexts: that they both *produce* and *reproduce* social discourse and practice."[9]

In this sense, discourses on monstrosity serve as global currencies. As such, "monster talk" may function as a means to inquire into the sociopolitics of given cultures and reflect much about how porous, and resistant, its boundaries are. In either case, teratologies, if conceived as a *global affair,* are neither limited purely to national borders nor subject to universalistic assumptions. And therein lies the monster's strength: both in its unwillingness to be pinned down by rules and in the regularity with which societies continue to adapt and hybridize its rhetorics.

Speaking of the Monstrous from Different Perspectives

This anthology employs several approaches in visualizing the monstrous as a critical tool. Section I, "General Theories of Monstrosity," is composed of five seminal chapters. Chapter 1, Jeffrey Jerome Cohen's "Monster Culture (Seven Theses)" (Chapter 1 from *Monster Theory: Reading Culture,* University of Minnesota Press, 1997: 3–25), provides many key recurring ideas in teratologies. Cohen begins with a sketch of what he calls "a new *modus legendi:* a method of reading cultures from the monsters they engender." He recognizes that previous criticism in cultural studies had the "compulsion to historical specificity and the insistence that all knowledge is local." However, in lieu of arguing a "theory of teratology," Cohen proposes "a set of breakable postulates in search of specific cultural moments," that is, "seven theses toward understanding cultures through the monsters they bear." They include : (1) *Thesis I: The Monster's Body Is a Cultural Body,* in which Cohen states that "Monsters are the embodiment of a cultural moment"; (2) *Thesis II: The Monster Always Escapes,* in which he notes that "The monster itself turns immaterial and vanishes, to reappear somewhere else," and that "Monsters must be examined within the intricate matrix of relations (social, cultural, and literary-historical) that generate them"; (3) *Thesis III: The Monster Is the Harbinger of Category Crisis,* wherein he claims that monsters "are disturbing hybrids whose externally incoherent bodies resist attempts to include them in any systematic structuration . . . a form suspended between forms that threatens to smash distinctions"; (4) in *Thesis IV: The Monster Dwells at the Gates of Difference,* Cohen argues that "The monster is an incorporation of the Outside, the Beyond," and that "For the most part monstrous difference tends to be cultural, political, racial, economic, sexual"; (5) *Thesis V: The Monster Polices the Borders of the Possible,* in which Cohen states that "The monster prevents mobility (intellectual, geographic, or sexual) delimiting the social spaces through which private bodies may move. To step outside this official geography is to risk attack by some monstrous border patrol or (worse) to become monstrous oneself," in which case "Every monster is . . . a double narrative, two living stories: one that describes how the monster came to be and another, its testimony, detailing what cultural use the monster serves"; (6) *Thesis VI: Fear of the Monster Is Really a Kind of Desire,* in which Cohen finds that "the same creatures who terrify and interdict can evoke potent escapist fantasies," wherein the "simultaneous repulsion and attraction at the core of the monster's composition accounts greatly for its cultural popularity," and that "[t]he habitations of the monsters (Africa, Scandinavia, America, Venus, the Delta Quadrant—whatever land is sufficiently distant to be exoticized) are more than dark regions of uncertain danger: they are also realms of happy fantasy, horizons of liberation. Their monsters serve as secondary bodies through which the possibilities of other genders, other sexual practices, and other social customs can be explored"; and lastly, (7) *Thesis VII: The Monster Stands at the Threshold... of Becoming,* in which Cohen adds that monsters "can be pushed to the farthest margins of geography and discourse... but they always return. And when they come back, they bring not just a fuller knowledge of our place in history and the history of knowing our place, but they bear self-knowledge, human knowledge—and a discourse all the more sacred as it arises from the Outside."

Similarly, Stephen Prince's "Dread, Taboo, and *The Thing:* Toward a Social Theory of the Horror Film" (originally published in *Wide Angle* 10, no. 3 [1988]: 19–29) forgoes the psychological model of reading horror films in favor of a sociologically driven one, focusing instead on the significance of language to construct an environment that attempts to minimize or remove any trace of ambiguity and create systems of "clearly delineated order." Social prohibitions are perceived as dangerous because their existence, and their lack of obvious categorization, threatens the socially constructed order. It is this ambiguity that arouses the greatest fear and that horror films exploit, by manipulating the boundary relation of the self and the world. The monster, Prince argues, represents the unmapped areas bordering the outline of our social structure. Prince reads the alien creature in *The Thing* as:

> a horribly anomalous animal... represent[ing] a form of cosmic pollution, an entity existing outside the accepted categories that give shape to human life and knowledge. Its very existence challenges the ontology separating human from non-human, solid from liquid, edible from inedible. It threatens to erase the distinctions and, in doing so, to erase the bounded human world.

Prince relies on anthropological theory to "articulate the horror film along social rather than psychological lines." Unlocking the nature of horror films and their appeal "entails using theories that preserve the category of the social without reducing it exclusively to the realm of the psychological." Given these goals, taboos—and monsters—are perceived as dangerous because their very existence and their lack of clear categorization threaten the socially constructed order. Chapter 3, Noël Carroll's "Nightmare and the Horror Film: The Symbolic Biology of Fantastic Beings" (originally published in *Film Quarterly* 34, no. 3 [Spring 1981]: 16–25), examines how the imagery of horror/science fiction film, especially those of "horrific creatures" is envisaged in ways that correspond with the nightmare imagery, as "symbolic biologies." The creatures of horror and science fiction can be viewed as "symbolic formations that organize conflicting themes into figures" that stir primordial ambivalences because they are visualized as simultaneously attractive and repulsive. "Two major symbolic figures appear most prominent...: fusion, in which the conflicting themes are yoked together in one, spatio-temporally unified figure; and fission, in which the conflicting genres are distributed—over space or time—among more than one figure." Dracula and the Frankensteinian Monster are creatures of fusion, while *doppelgangers,* alter egos, and werewolves are monsters of fission. Although fusion and fission generate a huge diversity of symbolic biologies in horror films, there are other ways of visualizing the monstrous, such as through the magnification of power or size, as in the case of giant insects or "other exaggerated animalcules." Chapter 4, Ken Gelder's "Our Vampires, Our Neighbors," uses the key metaphor of genres of cinema being similar to neighborhoods—simultaneously formulaic, but also distinct, much like its cinematic visualizations of the monstrous. Gelder chooses two Swedish vampire films as the particular iteration of the monstrous to illustrate his approach of moving across the familiar and the strange, and weaves metaphor within metaphor: much as vampire films always entail porousness and promiscuity, genres are always shifting and slippery; hybrid; never antiseptically "pure"—which is precisely what makes them "fertile." Finally,

Mark Jancovich's " 'Psychological Thriller': *Dead of Night,* British Film Culture, and the 1940s Horror Cycle," argues that *Dead of Night* (1945) has acquired a privileged place in the history of the British horror films, and is often claimed to represent the "origin" of British horror cinema despite its seeming "aberration." As an illustration of a historically attuned methodology, Jancovich demonstrates that *Dead of Night* was fully consistent with British production trends at the time it was released. Consequently, the chapter argues that "the category of horror is not fixed and that its contents continually change from one historical moment to another as definitions of the monstrous change." Thus, Jancovich observes that "many of the films identified with horror in the 1940s were excluded from this category in the 1960s, and one of the key ways in which historical definitions of horror and the monstrous can be explored is through the study of film reviews and other extra-textual materials." Thus, he argues that film reviews should not be viewed as "failed criticism" but as "types of social discourse which . . . can aid the researcher in ascertaining the material conditions in forming the relation between the film and spectator at given moments."[10] Ultimately, Jancovich's project is "not to assert that *Black Narcissus* or any other film is really a horror film but rather to examine how it was related to historically specific definitions of horror and of the monstrous [that had] . . . significantly changed by the late 1960s and early 1970s, when academic canons of the genre began to be constructed."

Section II, on "Teratologies of Nationality and Race," brings together three chapters, all of which play upon the specific cultural milieu of particular monsters while studying their global crosscurrents. Chapter 6, "Monsters in the Literary Traditions of Asia: A Critical Appraisal," dives straight into complex connections binding teratologies, nationalities, gender, and power. As Andrew Hock-Soon Ng points out, the idea of the "nation," as Benedict Anderson conceives of it, is largely "imagined"; nevertheless, blood is continuously shed and lives needlessly lost to ensure "nationhood's" perpetuation and purity. Not surprisingly, nations are often appended with a feminine configuration (e.g., motherland, countries being referred to as "she") because the idea of national purity—a largely male imaginary—has to be iconized "through" the woman. For Ng, this patriarchal formation partly suggests the reason why women suffer greater levels of policing and limitations compared to their male counterparts, justifying in turn a greater degree of their transgressive potentialities. However, literature has often probed the dangers of "nationalism" on subjectivities. When the idea of the nation requires that women's bodies be offered in service of masculine pride, this augurs not only ideological confinement for women but also surprising opportunities to challenge the status quo. Ultimately, the specific goal of Ng's "Monstrosity and Asia" is to "analyse precisely the way in which writers such as Salman Rushdie (*Shame*), Michael Ondaatje (*Anil's Ghost*) and Lloyd Fernando (*Scorpion Orchid* and *Green Is the Color*) deploy the 'monstrous feminine' to challenge the restrictive codes of nationalism (and religion as well—the two being often symbiotically linked), and in the process deconstruct interlinked notions of purity, patriotism and of course, masculinity." Chapter 7, Margaret L. Carter's "Slayer as Monster in *Blood+* (2005–2006) and *Buffy the Vampire Slayer* (1997–2003)", begins with the observation that Japanese *anime* and *manga,* using motifs of supernatural horror, have cross-fertilized with American media for decades. Carter chooses to focus on *Buffy the Vampire Slayer* and *Blood+* because of the many similarities between the two central characters. However, there is one crucial difference, which Carter eventually arrives at: In *Blood+*, unlike *Buffy the Vampire Slayer,* the enemy is not an absolute Other, but instead Saya's twin sister Diva. Hence, the contrasting endings of these two narratives: (1) The final episode of *Buffy the Vampire Slayer* climaxes in the cataclysmic destruction of the Hellmouth and the town built over it; (2) By contrast, the climax of *Blood+* allows for a reconciliation with the Other, when Saya and her allies save Diva's twin children. For Carter, then, "the Japanese world-view, in contrast to the dominant dualism of Western culture, allows space for this kind of reconciliation rather than absolute annihilation of the 'evil' Other." Finally, Daniel Novak's "'Shapeless

Deformity': Monstrosity, Gender, and Racial Masquerade in Thomas Grattan's *The Cagot's Hut* (1823)" continues this trend of problematizing stereotypic depictions of "whiteness" in relation to nonwhiteness. Novak's chapter analyzes an early nineteenth-century novel entitled *The Cagot's Hut* (1823) in the context of British racial discourse. Like other colonial subjects, in a rhetorical pattern characteristic of teratologies, the Cagots were described as "animalistic, mentally and physically inferior, and even deformed." Yet one of Novak's conclusions is particularly startling and groundbreaking: "The Cagots were associated with an excessive whiteness, a trait which in this case was often (falsely) connected to leprosy.... If... the white race was increasingly equated with 'civilization' and racial superiority, the case of the Cagots suggests that one can be too white to be white; that is, their white color only confirmed their status as a racial Other."

Section III, "In Between Fear and Desire," collates chapters that examine the refractory and ambivalent reactions we display in response to monsters, to whom we react with a complex combination of fascination, disgust, horror, intrigue, repulsion, among others. Caroline Joan (Kay) S. Picart and David Frank's "*Apt Pupil:* The Hollywood Nazi-As-Monster Flick" (Chapter 5 from *Frames of Evil: The Holocaust as Horror in American Film,* Southern Illinois University Press, 2006: 98–125) explores the ambivalences in Bryan Singer's cinematic rendition of the Nazi-as-bogeyman theme. The film, derived from Stephen King's short story, replaced the story's misogyny with an equally ambivalent homoerotic–homophobic depictions of the relationship between Todd (the young American boy-man) and Dussander (the aging Nazi in hiding). A key visual leitmotif in this film is of shower scenes, as moments of vulnerability and erotic potential, which reference both *Psycho* and *Schindler's List.* On a parallel track, Jason C. Bivins in his chapter, "Demons Driven: Religious Teratologies," notes that the "fearful qualities" of religions are well known. This chapter analyzes the ways in which specifically Christian expressions of fear-talk and teratologies have not simply influenced public perceptions about specific classes of humans (such as religious Others from Catholics to Muslims) and behaviors (e.g., homosexuality) but "have also generated complex religious identities simultaneously by rhetorics of embattlement and privilege, by apocalypticism and amelioration, by attraction to and distance from the reviled." Finally, Ian Conrich's chapter, "An Age of Mechanical Destruction: Power Tools and the Monstrous in *The Texas Chain Saw Massacre* Films," returns us to the iconic *Texas Chain Saw Massacre* films to reflect upon the continuing fascination with this particular contemporary example of the monstrous in film, which again moves in between the real (Ed Gein) and the reel (fictional adaptations of Gein's character and crimes)—a theme that foreshadows Section V. Conrich argues that the original *Texas Chain Saw Massacre* was partly based on the activities of the Wisconsin serial killer Ed Gein. From Gein, a mask fashioned out of skin from human victims—as we observe in the *Texas Chain Saw Massacre* film worn by the iconic figure of Leatherface—was sourced. Conrich's chapter examines the recurring "cycle of themes, images and icons that have passed from Gein through the Texas Chain Saw films and into the imitators that have been drawn to a chain saw cult." By studying fanzines and fan cultures, and contextualizing the productions within the cinema industry, this chapter genealogizes how a body of films have "adapted, transferred, and reimagined specific icons of the modern monstrous—the mask made of human skin, moreover the power saw popularized in the title of an infamous movie."

Section IV, "Queer Theory and Boundary Crossings," brings together three chapters. Harry Benshoff's chapter, "Way Too Gay to Be Ignored?: The Production and Reception of Queer Horror Cinema in the Twenty-First Century," is an extension/revision of his book *Monsters in the Closet: Homosexuality and the Horror Film* (Manchester University Press, 1997), which is built upon the view, popularized by Robin Wood, that "monstrous figures in American cinema were and are informed by their given era's social understanding of homosexuality, or more broadly queerness." This chapter examines the production and reception of recent horror films that make the genre's latent queer concerns much more manifest. For example, writer-director David DeCoteau (*The Brotherhood* [2000], *Voodoo Academy* [2000], *Leeches!* [2003]) makes low-budget, straight-to-DVD films that campily recycle the tropes of earlier horror films with casts of sexy young men; Victor Salva (*Powder* [1995], *Jeepers Creepers* [2001]) has produced more mainstream films that face backlash from fans because of Salva's previous conviction for having had sex with an underage male. For Benshoff, while the production of DeCoteau's films represents a growing market for what might be termed "gay niche horror," the reception of his films (as well as Salva's) by straight horror fans reveals persistent homophobia among the general population, and also a tentative willingness among some fan communities to examine the horror genre's more heterosexist tropes and assumptions. Finally, Judith (Jack) Halberstam's "*Seed of Chucky*: Transbiology and the Horror Flick" employs a more theoretical mode of analyzing the nexus between queerness and teratology, influenced by scholars like Donna Haraway and Sarah Franklin. In her chapter, Halberstam's project is to examine the "narrative and visual transbiological leaps that we have made in our understandings of terms like 'heterosexuality' and 'homosexuality', male and female, individual and community, in an age of artificial insemination, transsexuality and cloning." Ultimately, for Halberstam, using *Seed of Chucky* as a witty, humor-filled example, brave new worlds beyond these binaries can already be glimpsed: "popular culture has already imagined multiple alternatives to male and female, masculine and feminine, family and individuality and, that contemporary popular culture, specifically horror film and animation, can provide a rich archive for an alternative politics of embodiment, reproduction and non-reproduction."

Section V, "Criminology, Law, and Teratologies: Between the Real and the Reel," moves across the interstices of documentary and docudramatic modes, refusing a pat distinction between "reality" and "fiction." The point of this section is not to show that there is no such thing as "reality" but that "reality" is complex, often involving irreducible but traceable cross-currents with "fiction" through the interactions flowing through popular culture, public policy, and law. Chapter 14, "Virulency," is excerpted from Lonnie H. Athens's *Creation of Dangerous Violent Criminals* (University of Illinois Press, 1992). For Athens, a "dangerous violent criminal" is someone "who will seriously injure or kill someone with little or no apparent provocation." To become such a "monster," a person must undergo three critical social experiences: "violent notoriety, social trepidation, and malevolency." Nevertheless, Athens refuses a socially deterministic lens: despite how "advanced" they become, these victim–victimizers can, at any point, still choose to "opt out of becoming a dangerous violent criminal by rejecting rather than accepting this designation of themselves." Following Athens's lead, Chapter 15, "Profiling the Terrorist as a Mass Murderer," by Caroline Joan (Kay) S. Picart and Cecil E. Greek is derived from an earlier book *Monsters In and Among Us: Toward a Gothic Criminology* (Fairleigh Dickinson University Press, 2008). In a preceding chapter from *Monsters In and Among Us,* Picart and Greek describe and explain the significance of a "Gothic criminology":

> What prompts this anthology is an explosion of books and films that link violence, fear, images of "monstrosity," and Gothic modes of narration and visualization in American popular culture, academia and even public policy. As Mark Edmundson (1997, xii) notes: "Gothic conventions have slipped over into ostensibly nonfictional realms. Gothic is alive not just in Stephen King's novels and Quentin Tarantino's films, but in the media renderings of the O.J. Simpson case, in our political discourse, in modes of therapy, on TV news, on talk shows like *Oprah,* in our discussions of AIDS and of the environment. American culture at large has become suffused with Gothic assumptions, with Gothic characters and plots." . . . The ongoing fascination with evil, as simultaneously repellant and irresistibly attractive, both in the Hollywood film, criminological case studies, popular culture and even public policy,

> points to the emergence of "Gothic criminology," with its focus on themes such as blood lust, compulsion, fear, godlike vengeance, and power and domination. Rather than assuming that film and the media tell us little about the reality of criminological phenomena, "Gothic criminology" . . . recognizes the complementarity of critical academic and aesthetic accounts of deviant behavior as intersecting with public policy in complex, nonreductive ways.[11]

What makes this chapter particularly significant is its focus on what has become arguably the most "monstrous" of all contemporary criminals: the mass-murdering terrorist against the backdrop of a series of pre- and post-9/11 Hollywood films, comparing their perspectives to the response of the Bush administration and its depiction of global monsters who must be defeated in a "war on terrorism." If Athens's chapter is about how real-life "monsters" can become what they are through a series of social processes constituting a rite of passage into virulence, Chapter 16, Ôrît Kāmîr's "What Makes Stalking Monsters So Monstrous, and How to Survive Them?" shows how cultural myths about "monsters" find their way into law and public policy. To Kāmîr, stories of stalking have always been inseparable from monstrous creatures such as Dracula, Frankenstein's Monster, and Michael of the paradigmatic horror film *Halloween.* For Kāmîr, the legislation prohibiting stalking, which started in California in the 1990s, is ripe with rhetorical references to these creatures. Consequently, Kāmîr argues that when applied to specific cases, these laws on stalking influence authorities as well as the public and press to compare human aggressors with the larger-than-life shadows of stalking monsters, like "Lilit" (or "Lilith") and "The Wandering Jew." The rhetorical weight to prosecute effectively is thus very difficult: if a defendant is not "monstrous" enough, then Kāmîr cautions, "he may be found 'inadequate' to be found guilty." Finally, Caroline Joan (Kay) S. Picart's "Race and Serial Killing in the Media: The Case of Wayne Williams" is about analyzing monstrous media myths and remembering the principal lesson from the Atlanta youth murders case: that racially stereotyping serial killers can have dangerous consequences, especially for a group vulnerable to victimization. One of the well-known myths, as illustrated in a scene from a film about serial killers, *Copycat,* is that "nearly all serial killers are white males; yet the reality is that one in every five serial killers is black, and nearly 16% of all serial killers are female." Wayne Williams, popularly dubbed by the mainstream media as "America's first black serial killer," was arrested as the killer of over twenty black children, though he was formally charged and convicted of murdering just two of his victims. The case of Wayne Williams was different from the general media pattern of ignoring black serial killers partly because of the prevalence and severity of monstrous metaphors in the coverage and reactions to the story, as evidenced in the rhetoric used by the predominantly white prosecution and the predominantly black civil rights community in relation to a mysterious fairer skinned black man. Yet there were other factors as well that contributed to the "newsworthiness" of the story: the initial suspicion that the killings were associated with a KKK-inspired plot to spark a race war; the political activism of the victims' mothers who ignited a grassroots movement; the detrimental effect of the stories on Atlanta's economy; the spectacle of a progressive city with a black mayor and a black police chief pitted against poor black constituents, in a city where racial tensions were rampant and the balance of power was tenuous. Finally, to illustrate the power of monster-talk, and how these discourses are perspectivally framed, for the most part, whites tended to identify with the prosecution's narrative concerning Wayne Williams, while blacks tended to be skeptical. Both sides engaged in a battle of warring monstrous metaphors. For the prosecution/predominantly white community, Wayne Williams was the same kind of creature as Attila the Hun, Adolf Hitler, and Idi Amin. For the predominantly black civil rights community, the monsters were the racist criminal justice and legal systems that produced the lies of the one-drop rule; the "half-breeds" who could hope to be treated as white; and the mentality of complicity with these institutional structures and cultural myths.

Section VI, on "The Biological Monstrous and Gender: The Human-Animal-Machine Divides," examines the often porous "human–animal–machine divides." Chapter 18, Kathleen Long's " 'Nature Abhors Normality': Theories of the Monstrous from Aristotle to *The X-Files,*" begins with an *X-Files* episode, "Humbug," as a starting-point to review the Aristotelian/Augustinian debate that ran throughout the Middle Ages and into the Early Modern Period, concerning the status of the monstrous. Simply sketched, for Aristotelians, monstrosity represents a defect of nature, either of excess or lack. Ultimately, Long threads this discussion through the Early Modern Period by examining texts such as Ambroise Pare's *On Monsters and Marvels,* in order to intersect with recent discussions of disability that focus on the social demand for "normalized" (meaning idealized) bodies (following the lines of inquiry established by Lennard Davis and Alice Dreger, among others). In the second essay, "Monster Spawn of Animal Experimentation in the Early Work of H. G. Wells: On the Containment of Psychopathic Violence as Preliminary to the Onset of the Capacity for Mourning," Rickels tracks as basic to science fiction the development—even in the case of H. G. Wells—of the ability to mourn, "out of the limit state of psychopathic unidentification." Before mourning can emerge in *The War of the Worlds,* for Rickels, "Wells [must reclaim] for identification the animal relation as the life-supporting early relation with the mother. In early childhood his mother had deposited inside him the melancholic assignment of mourning her dead daughter in lieu of his own continuing support." Thus, in *The Time Machine,* which foreshadows the process leading to Wells's identification as author of *The War of the Worlds,* the protagonist is able to shed, like the memory of a dream, the girl Weena, who can be interpreted as the stand-in for his undead sister, Fanny. For Rickels, "the theme of humankind treated as the livestock of uncanny heirs to technological progress introduces the problem of food and death on the basis of identification between humans and animals." Thus, in *The Island of Dr. Moreau* and *The Invisible Man*—two science fiction works that anticipated the composition of *The War of the Worlds*—the "identificatory relationship" between humans and animals is "tested under conditions of animal experimentation, even vivisection." Ultimately, as Rickels notes,

> Toward the end of *The War of the Worlds,* the narrator notes that the relationship to our animals had changed following our subjugation to the Martian need for our blood. But in the very last sentence, the narrator proclaims the change that has come over his marriage, in which each partner to the coupling or pairing has believed the other already dead. The integration of loss following in the tracks of animal identification concludes Wells's apprenticeship. The Martians succumb to their own evolutionary advances in denial of basic mortality. The invisible force of utter decay that human life postpones unto death thus besets the Martian conquerors while yet alive who decay away as live corpses. The end of the Martian invaders is the *vanitas* spread against which the narrator-protagonist as well as the author of *The War of the Worlds* can start over in the mode of integration rather than one of mere substitution.

In keeping with prior essays' emphases on the transgressive power of the monstrous, the third essay, Dejan Ognjanović's "Why Is the *Tension* So *High*? The Monstrous Feminine in (Post)Modern Slasher Films?" focuses on the instability of the killer's gender in those slasher-horror films in which an apparently male killer is unveiled in the end to have been female. Ultimately, for Ognjanović, gender reversal common to this subgenre is used for two different but closely associated purposes: (1) to invoke instability, suspense, and fear (necessary constituents of the horror genre) through the breakdown of established genre and gender-based expectations; and (2) to question those very conventions, usually rendering them merely "partial," unable to address a reality much more complex than the binary opposition of male–female. Finally, the last essay of this section is June Pulliam's "Blood and Bitches: Sexual Politics and the

Female Lycanthrope in Young Adult Fiction." For Pulliam, the teenaged female werewolf represents a "liberated female subjectivity that is often at odds with hegemonic culture because she visibly erupts the boundaries of normative femininity." For her, young adult fiction about adolescent female werewolves emphasizes the pressure that teen girls feel to embody a normative femininity that requires they repress their appetites for both sex and food "while stifling the justifiable anger they experience as a result of being required to suppress these drives so greatly."

Finally, Section VII, titled "Teratologies and Ethics," is comprised of three essays, all of which engage the issue of "ethics" in relation to the "monstrous" in different ways. The first, Patricia MacCormack's "The Queer Ethics of Monstrosity," tackles the question head-on. MacCormack begins with the observation that "teratology is increasingly informing theories of alterity, such as feminism, post-structuralism, anti-speciesism and queer theory." MacCormack's eventual conclusion is that "all monstrous relations are queer and all queer relations, when taken to their limits, are monstrous." To strengthen her arguments, MacCormack uses a preponderance of examples, such as Deleuze and Guattari's demonological, werewolf, and vampire philosophy; extreme body modification read through Lyotard; Serres's parasitic and Venusian contracts; and Braidotti's transpositional pleasures. It may seem strange to follow up MacCormack's chapter on queer theory with a chapter from Dominick LaCapra's *History and Its Limits: Human, Animal, Violence* (Cornell University Press, 2009). However, since so much of teratology's field of study is an attempt to explore boundaries separating the human from the nonhuman or animal (as in the case of werewolves or serial killers, or as illustrated in Rickels and Pulliam's essays), it seems only appropriate to begin with LaCapra's premise that "violence and victimization are prominent in the relation between the human and the animal." LaCapra questions the prevalent anthropocentrism (evident even in theorists of the "posthuman") and the ongoing search for a "decisive criterion separating or dividing the human from the animal." LaCapra ultimately regards this attempt to "fix the difference" as not only misguided but also potentially dangerous because "it renders insufficiently problematic the manner in which humans treat other animals and interact with the environment." Finally, the last essay, "Where Reality and Fantasy Meet and Bifurcate: Holocaust Themes in *Pan's Labyrinth* (2006), the *X-Men* (2000), and *V* (1983)," co-authored by Caroline Joan (Kay) S. Picart, John Edgar Browning, and Carla María Thomas, begins by referring back to Picart and Frank's *Frames of Evil: The Holocaust as Horror in American Film,* referenced in Section III.[12] Picart and Frank discuss the cross-fertilizations that have evolved, binding Holocaust films—usually shot in a documentary or docudramatic mode—and horror films—usually visually coded as drawing from the Gothic fictional tradition. Such cross-fertilizations call into question whose point of view we adopt as we view these films. "Realistic" documentary modes actually draw from "fictional" Gothic modes, which themselves have a complex relationship with the real. Yet the appropriation of fictional Gothic modes into factual documentary or docudramatic modes are acceptable or convincing as "true" only if these cinematic footnotes masquerade as partaking of the look of the "real," which immediately brings to the fore the question of how we locate ourselves as consumers of these films, which allude to and imaginatively re-create a very real historical trauma, the Holocaust.

The issue becomes more complex when one analyzes cinematic genres that reference the Holocaust, but defy privileging the documentary mode and choose more fantastic modes of narrativizing. In other words, what do the cinematic modes of fantasy and science fiction, for example, tell us about how the legacy of the Holocaust has seeped into the way that we collectively imagine and tell stories about heroes and monsters and "good" and "evil"? What do, for example, *Pan's Labyrinth,* the *X-Men* trilogy, and *V* tell us about how we cope with the trauma of the Holocaust through more fantastic, rather than documentary films?

A crucial tool in tackling this set of questions is derived from Isabel Christina Pinedo.[13] This tool lies in the distinctions drawn between a "classic horror frame" and a "conflicted horror frame."[14] The classic horror frame, more characteristic of Hollywood horror films of the 1930s and 1940s, demands the creation of a monster so utterly Other that only his or her killing/sacrifice can render closure, and with that, the restoration of normalcy to the story. As Pinedo writes, "the boundary between good and evil, normal and abnormal, human and alien is as firmly drawn as the imperative that good must conquer evil, thus producing a secure Manichean worldview in which the threats to the social order are largely external and (hu)man agency prevails, largely in the figure of the masterful male subject."[15] In contrast to the classic horror frame, the conflicted horror frame views evil as residing within the "normal." Whereas classic horror monsters "breach the norms of ontological propriety,"[16] such as the classic Hollywood Frankenstein monsters, monsters of the conflicted horror frame seem "ordinary" at a first glance, much like Norman Bates. While the classic horror frame breaches the ontology of "normal time," the conflicted horror frame, as Steffen Hantke observes, "violates the integrity and separateness of the two spheres"—the normal and the fantastic.[17]

Whereas the focus in *Holocaust as Horror* was in showing the differences between the two frames, the focus of this chapter is in mapping how the classic and conflicted frames, in fantasy and science fiction modes, are less diametrically opposed, than paired, in mirror-imaging ways, like Siamese twins. The resulting narratives, because they are not as constrained by "documentary" or "moral" binaries, are much more complex, and have much to tell us about the teratological reimagination of the Holocaust and its iconic monster, the Nazi. It is by examining these complexities and ambivalences, in which our deepest fears and hopes are reflected and refracted, that perhaps a new ethics of spectatorship, reminiscent of LaCapra's "ethic of response"—one not built upon simplistic binaries—may be glimpsed, as through a mirror darkly.

NOTES

1. "Logy," *Online Etymology Dictionary,* accessed August 16, 2011, http://www.etymonline.com/index.php?term= -logy.
2. "Teratologies-Definition," *The Free Dictionary,* accessed August 16, 2011, http://www.thefreedictionary.com/teratology.
3. The American Heritage® Science Dictionary Copyright © 2005 by Houghton Mifflin Company. Published by Houghton Mifflin Company. "Teratologies-Definition," *The Free Dictionary.*
4. "Teratologies-Definition," *The Free Dictionary.*
5. Edward J. Ingebretsen, *At Stake: Monsters and the Rhetoric of Fear in Public Culture* (Chicago, IL: University of Chicago Press, 2003).
6. See Caroline Joan S. Picart, *Remaking the Frankensteinian Myth on Film: Between Laughter and Horror* (Albany, NY: State University of New York Press, 2003) and Caroline Joan S. Picart, *The Cinematic Rebirths of Frankenstein: Universal, Hammer, and Beyond* (Westport, CT and London: Praeger, 2001).
7. Zakiya Hanafi, *The Monster in the Machine: Magic, Medicine, and the Marvelous in the Time of the Scientific Revolution* (Durham and London: Duke University Press, 2000), 14.
8. Robin Wood, "The American Nightmare: Horror in the '70's," in *Hollywood from Vietnam to Reagan* (New York: Columbia University Press, 1986), 78.
9. Joshua David Bellin, *Framing Monsters: Fantasy Film and Social Alienation* (Carbondale, IL: Southern Illinois University Press, 2005), 8.
10. Barbara Klinger, *Melodrama and Meaning: History, Culture, and the Films of Douglas Sirk* (Bloomington, IN: Indiana University Press, 1994), 69.
11. Caroline Joan (Kay) Picart and Cecil Greek, "Introduction: Toward a Gothic Criminology," *Monsters In and Among Us: Toward a Gothic Criminology* (Madison and Teaneck, NJ: Fairleigh Dickinson University Press, 2007), 11–12.

12. Caroline Joan (Kay) S. Picart and David A. Frank, *Frames of Evil: The Holocaust as Horror in American Film,* foreword Dominick LaCapra, introduction Edward J. Ingebretsen (Carbondale, IL: Southern Illinois University Press, 2006).
13. Isabel Christina Pinedo, "Postmodern Elements of the Contemporary Horror Film," in *The Horror Film,* ed. Steven Prince (New Brunswick, NJ: Rutgers University Press, 2004), 85–117.
14. Pinedo contrasts "postmodern" to "classic," but given the many rhetorical valences that freight the word "postmodern," we prefer to use "conflicted."
15. Pinedo, "Postmodern Elements of the Contemporary Horror Film," 89.
16. Noél Carroll, *Philosophy of Horror, or Paradoxes of the Heart* (New York: Routledge, 1990), 16.
17. Steffen Hantke, "The Kingdom of the Unimaginable: The Construction of Social Space and the Fantasy of Privacy in Serial Killer Narratives," *Literature/Film Quarterly* 26 (1998): 179–195.

Section I

General Theories of Monstrosity

CHAPTER 1

MONSTER CULTURE (SEVEN THESES)(EXTRACT)

JEFFREY JEROME COHEN

WHAT I WILL PROPOSE HERE BY WAY OF A FIRST FORAY, as entrance into this book of monstrous content, is a sketch of a new *modus legendi*: a method of reading cultures from the monsters they engender. In doing so, I will partially violate two of the sacred dicta of recent cultural studies: the compulsion to historical specificity and the insistence that all knowledge (and hence all cartographies of that knowledge) is local. Of the first I will say only that in cultural studies today history (disguised perhaps as "culture") tends to be fetishized as a *telos,* as a final determinant of meaning; post de Man, post Foucault, post Hayden White, one must bear in mind that history is just another text in a procession of texts, and not a guarantor of any singular signification. A movement away from the *longue durée* and toward micro economies (of capital or of gender) is associated most often with Foucauldian criticism; yet recent critics have found that where Foucault went wrong was mainly in his details, in his minute specifics. Nonetheless, his methodology—his archaeology of ideas, his histories of unthought—remains with good reason the chosen route of inquiry for most cultural critics today, whether they work in postmodern cyberculture or in the Middle Ages.

And so I would like to make some grand gestures. We live in an age that has rightly given up on Unified Theory, an age when we realize that history (like "individuality," "subjectivity," "gender," and "culture") is composed of a multitude of fragments, rather than of smooth epistemological wholes. Some fragments will be collected here and bound temporarily together to form a loosely integrated net—or, better, an unassimilated hybrid, a monstrous body. Rather than argue a "theory of teratology," I offer . . . a set of breakable postulates in search of specific cultural moments. I offer seven theses toward understanding cultures through the monsters they bear.

THESIS I: THE MONSTER'S BODY IS A CULTURAL BODY

[. . .]

The monster is born only at this metaphoric crossroads, as an embodiment of a certain cultural moment—of a time, a feeling, and a place.[1] The monster's body quite literally incorporates fear, desire, anxiety, and fantasy (ataractic or incendiary), giving them life and an uncanny independence. The monstrous body is pure culture. A construct and a projection, the monster exists only to be read: the *monstrum* is etymologically "that which reveals," "that which warns," a glyph that seeks a hierophant. Like a letter on the page, the monster signifies something other than itself: it is always a displacement, always inhabits the gap between the time of upheaval that created it and the moment into which it is received, to be born again. [. . .]

THESIS II: THE MONSTER ALWAYS ESCAPES

We see the damage that the monster wreaks, the material remains (the footprints of the yeti across Tibetan snow, the bones of the giant stranded on a rocky cliff), but the monster itself turns immaterial and vanishes, to reappear someplace else. [. . .]

Each time the grave opens and the unquiet slumberer strides forth ("come from the dead,/Come back to tell you all"), the message proclaimed is transformed by the air that gives its speaker new life. Monsters must be examined within the intricate matrix of relations (social, cultural, and literary-historical) that generate them. In speaking of the new kind of vampire. invented by Bram Stoker, we might explore the foreign count's transgressive but compelling sexuality, as subtly alluring to Jonathan Harker as Henry Irving, Stoker's mentor, was to Stoker.[2] Or we might analyze Murnau's self-loathing appropriation of the same demon in *Nosferatu,* where in the face of nascent fascism the undercurrent of desire surfaces in plague and bodily corruption. Anne Rice has given the myth a modern rewriting in which homosexuality and vampirism have been conjoined, apotheosized; that she has created a pop culture phenomenon in the process is not insignificant, especially at a time when gender as a construct has been scrutinized at almost every social register. In Francis Coppola's recent blockbuster, *Bram Stoker's Dracula,* the homosexual subtext present at least since the appearance of Sheridan Le Fanu's lesbian lamia (*Carmilla,* 1872) has, like the red corpuscles that serve as the film's leitmotif, risen to the surface, primarily as an AIDS awareness that transforms the disease of vampirism into a sadistic (and very medieval) form of redemption through the torments of the body in pain. No coincidence, then, that Coppola was putting together a documentary on AIDS at the same time he was working on *Dracula.*

In each of these vampire stories, the undead returns in slightly different clothing, each time to be read against contemporary social movements or a specific, determining event: *la décadence* and its new possibilities, homophobia and its hateful imperatives, the acceptance of new subjectivities unfixed by binary gender, a fin de siècle social activism paternalistic in its embrace. [. . .]

THESIS III: THE MONSTER IS THE HARBINGER OF CATEGORY CRISIS

The monster always escapes because it refuses easy categorization . . . . This refusal to participate in the classificatory "order of things" is true of Monsters generally: they are disturbing hybrids whose externally incoherent bodies resist attempts to include them in any systematic structuration. And so the monster is dangerous, a form suspended between forms that threatens to smash distinctions.

[. . .]

The horizon where the monsters dwell might well be imagined as the visible edge of the hermeneutic circle itself: the monstrous offers an escape from its hermetic path, an invitation to explore new spirals, new and interconnected methods of perceiving the world.[3] In the face of the monster, scientific inquiry and its ordered rationality crumble. The monstrous is a genus too large to be encapsulated in any conceptual system; the monster's very existence is a rebuke to boundary and enclosure. [. . .]

[. . .]

Thesis IV: The Monster Dwells at the Gates of Difference

The monster is difference made flesh, come to dwell among us. In its function as dialectical Other or third-term supplement, the monster is an incorporation of the Outside, the Beyond—of all those loci that are rhetorically placed as distant and distinct but originate Within. Any kind of alterity can be inscribed across (constructed through) the monstrous body, but for the most part monstrous difference tends to be cultural, political, racial, economic, sexual.

[. . .]

By revealing that difference is arbitrary and potentially free-floating, mutable rather than essential, the monster threatens to destroy not just individual members of a society, but the very cultural apparatus through which individuality is constituted and allowed. Because it is a body across which difference has been repeatedly written, the monster (like Frankenstein's creature, that combination of odd somatic pieces stitched together from a community of cadavers) seeks out its author to demand its *raison d'etre*—and to bear witness to the fact that it could have been constructed Otherwise. Godzilla trampled Tokyo; Girard frees him here to fragment the delicate matrix of relational systems that unite every private body to the public world.

Thesis V: The Monster Polices the Borders of the Possible

The monster resists capture in the epistemological nets of the erudite, but it is something more than a Bakhtinian ally of the popular. From its position at the limits of knowing, the monster stands as a warning against exploration of its uncertain demesnes. The giants of Patagonia, the dragons of the Orient, and the dinosaurs of Jurassic Park together declare that curiosity is more often punished than rewarded, that one is better off safely contained within one's own domestic sphere than abroad, away from the watchful eyes of the state. The monster prevents mobility (intellectual, geographic, or sexual), delimiting the social spaces through which private bodies may move. To step outside this official geography is to risk attack by some monstrous border patrol or (worse) to become monstrous oneself.

[. . .]

Whereas monsters born of political expedience and self-justifying nationalism function as living invitations to action, usually military (invasions, usurpations, colonizations), the monster of prohibition polices the borders of the possible, interdicting through its grotesque body some behaviors and actions, envaluing others. . . . Every monster is in this way a double narrative, two living stories: one that describes how the monster came to be and another, its testimony, detailing what cultural use the monster serves. The monster of prohibition exists to demarcate the bonds that hold together that system of relations we call culture, to call horrid attention to the borders that cannot—*must* not—be crossed.

[. . .]

Thesis VI: Fear of the Monster Is Really a Kind of Desire

The monster is continually linked to forbidden practices, in order to normalize and to enforce. The monster also attracts. The same creatures who terrify and interdict can evoke potent escapist fantasies; the linking of monstrosity with the forbidden makes the monster all the more appealing as a temporary egress from constraint. This simultaneous repulsion and attraction at the core of the monster's composition accounts greatly for its continued cultural popularity, for the fact that the monster seldom can be contained in a simple, binary dialectic (thesis, antithesis . . . no synthesis). We distrust and loathe the monster at the same time we envy its freedom, and perhaps its sublime despair.

[. . .]

The habitations of the monsters (Africa, Scandinavia, America, Venus, the Delta Quadrant—whatever land is sufficiently distant to be exoticized) are more than dark regions of uncertain danger: they are also realms of happy fantasy, horizons of liberation. Their monsters serve as secondary bodies through which the possibilities of other genders, other sexual practices and other social customs can be explored. [. . .]

[. . .]

Thesis VII: The Monster Stands at the Threshold . . . of Becoming

"This thing of darkness I acknowledge mine."

Monsters are our children. They can be pushed to the farthest margins of geography and discourse, hidden away at the edges of the world and in the forbidden recesses of our mind, but they always return. And when they come back, they bring not just a fuller knowledge of our place in history and the history of knowing our place, but they bear self-knowledge, *human* knowledge—and a discourse all the more sacred as it arises from the Outside. These monsters ask us how we perceive the world, and how we have misrepresented what we have attempted to place. They ask us to reevaluate our cultural assumptions about race, gender, sexuality, our perception of difference, our tolerance toward its expression. They ask us why we have created them.

Notes

1. Literally, here, *Zeitgeist*: Time Ghost, the bodiless spirit that uncannily incorporates a "place" that is a series of places, the crossroads that is a point in a *movement* toward an uncertain elsewhere. Bury the Zeitgeist by the crossroads: it is confused as it awakens, it is not going anywhere, it intersects everyplace; all roads lead back to the monster.
2. I realize that this is an interpretative biographical maneuver Barthes would surely have called "the living death of the author."
3. "The hermeneutic circle does not permit access or escape to an uninterpreted reality; but we do not [have to] keep going around in the same path." See Barbara Herrnstein Smith, "Belief and Resistance: A Symmetrical Account," *Critical Inquiry* 18 (Autumn 1991): 137–138.

CHAPTER 2

DREAD, TABOO, AND *THE THING* (1982): TOWARD A SOCIAL THEORY OF THE HORROR FILM (EXTRACT)

STEPHEN PRINCE

BEASTS, DEMONS, AND OTHER NEFARIOUS CREATURES that stalk through horror films are legion, as are the diverse critical interpretations they call forth. For example, monsters, and the films in which they figure, have been regarded as excavating "archaic fears . . . and deeply buried wishes,"[1] anxieties connected with sexuality and death are masochistic pleasures generated through the imagery of suffering, violence, and death, "and fears of ideological collapse and breakdown." Despite the apparently disparate nature of such interpretations, however, a common, connecting logic unifies them. This is the logic of a psychological model, in which horror films are interpreted as the manifestation of psychic processes. [. . .]

[. . .]

However suggestive such a psychoanalytic account may be in its application to horror films, the model has certain lacunae that prevent it from coming to terms with the films as social products. Can this genre be satisfactorily theorized by relying on mechanisms of individual or group psychology? This essay will suggest that it cannot and will advance an alternate model, drawn from anthropological theory, which may usefully articulate the horror film along social rather than psychological lines. After the model is described and briefly developed, it will be tested through close examination of John Carpenter's remake of *The Thing* (1982). The structure of this film illustrates the model's relevance with exceptional clarity.

The aim here is not to remove psychological accounts from the terrain of the horror film, but merely to restrict the scope of their explanatory sweep. Freud tended to move too quickly from the individual to the social, attempting explanations of such collective phenomena as group dynamics, art, or religion in relation to the operation of laws of the psyche, writ large. By collapsing the social into the psychic life of the individual, Freud risked losing the social, and a similar problem exists with regard to our theoretical understanding of horror films. These films, after all, are the mass-produced products of popular culture. Unlocking the nature of their appeal entails using theories that preserve the category of the social without reducing it exclusively to the realm of psychology.

[. . .]

Anthropologists distinguish a category of beliefs known as taboo, a set of explicit prohibitions governing speech or behavior that are surrounded by powerful social or supernatural sanctions, the violation of which is accompanied by a sense of sin or defilement. These theories of taboo are very useful in understanding the horror film, so I shall describe them in some detail, drawing primarily upon the work of Mary Douglas and Edmund Leach.

Both Douglas and Leach see the task of language and society, of culture, as one of creating distinctions by projecting categories on an unbounded natural world such that a human order may emerge. Douglas writes that "ideas about separating, purifying, demarcating and punishing transgressions have as their main function to impose system on an inherently untidy experience."[2] Creating systems of order based on a network of culturally constructed classifications—human and nonhuman, female and male, edible and inedible, holy and profane—is a fundamental prerequisite of social experience.

Leach describes the manner in which language imposes discriminations on the world and how a child, making entrance into the language system of its culture, is endowed with the perception of a world filled with discrete objects, each labeled with a name.[3] The child, learning the language of its culture, is taught to impose a classifying grid upon its environment, resulting in the appearance of a stable, orderly world filled with identifiable things. Of central importance to the language system's ability to construct such an environment is the elimination of Ambiguity . . . . Language centers individuals in a social space "which is ordered in a logical and reassuring way."[4]

The symbolic system operates to construct differences, but, inevitably, the process of classifying will generate intermediate categories, items that mediate between binary distinctions to the extent that they exhibit both sets of characteristics. The linguistic and social creation of order, realized through an elaborate classifying activity in which male is sorted from female, and so on, creates at the same time a system of disorder, whose categories are regarded by members of the social community as dirt, pollution, taboo. This is a concomitance of the ability to perceive the social world as filled with separate things: such things are separate only because "nonthings" fill the interstices. "Language gives us the names to distinguish the things, taboo inhibits the recognition of those parts of the continuum which separate the things."[5]

Douglas points out that the social perception of dirt entails a perception of danger because dirt is synonymous with disorder, because, that is, its existence threatens the network of socially constructed discriminations: "Dirt is never a unique, isolated event. Where there is dirt there is system. Dirt is the by-product of a systematic ordering and classification of matter, in so far as ordering involves rejecting inappropriate elements."[6] Beliefs about dirt in the industrial world are dominated by the awareness of pathogenic organisms, but, Douglas maintains, the structure of these beliefs is not fundamentally different from the pollution beliefs of nonindustrial societies.

The precise shape and location of a perception of danger or disorder depends on socially structured factors, Douglas suggests. Where social roles are clearly bounded and noncontradictory, beneficent powers tend to be vested in centralized authorities, such as priests. However, where the social order dictates a contradictory or ambiguous status for some of its members, those members may be perceived as covert or unconscious sources of danger (e.g., as witches). [. . .]

Perceptions of malevolent and antisocial powers, then, may emerge from the ill-defined, contradictory lines of the social structure where networks of authority and allegiance are unclear, and the categories that arouse the greatest fear, interest, and sense of mystery are the ambiguous ones. These are the categories that become taboo because they play on the distinction between form and formlessness.

Such ambiguous terms are the stuff of horror films, which base their appeal on portraying the intermediate categories whose anomalies elicit horror and anxiety to the extent that they escape established social classifications. The creatures of horror films are far worse than the abominations of Leviticus. Werewolves violate the separation of human and animal, as do witches, who may assume the form of a familiar animal. The monsters from the *Alien* movies (1979 and 1986) are neither human, animal, nor insect, but a compendium of all three. In addition to such disturbing creatures, horror films routinely feature other sources of disquietude. For example, bodily orifices and their products generate extraordinary attention and interest in these films. The vomiting in *The Exorcist* (1973), the vomit, spittle, and semen in Cronenberg's *The Fly* (1986), the menstrual blood in *Carrie* (1976), the blood drawn by vampires—all play upon ambiguities of the body. As Leach points out, feces, urine, semen, and other bodily products are universally tabooed because they "are both me and not me," confounding the initial boundary relation of self and world.

[. . .]

The horror film may be regarded as a visualization of the dialectic between linguistic and socially imposed systems of order and the breakdown of those systems through their own internal contradictions. This view does not necessitate reliance upon mechanisms of projection or reaction formation. Rather than signifying the projection of repressed sexuality or some other psychological process, the monster represents those unmapped areas bordering the familiar configurations of the social world. [. . .]

[. . .]

John Carpenter's *The Thing* is far more than a remake of the 1951 film. Carpenter's version draws more closely on its original source in the short story by John Campbell Jr. (published in 1938 in *Astounding Science Fiction*) to provide, not a monster in human form as in the earlier film, but a shape-altering, formshifting monster whose threat lies in the very unpredictability of its appearance. Evil and malevolence are everywhere in the Carpenter film, and are more profoundly visualized. In describing the results of contact by a team of researchers in the Antarctic with an alien organism, *The Thing* details the breakdown of the team's networks of authority, friendship, and trust as the social order is infiltrated by the ambiguous "thing," a pathogenic organism whose spread is portrayed in epidemiological terms.[7] The members of National Science Institute Station 4 attempt to contain and isolate the danger, to barricade themselves within zones of safety, but, like the abominations of Leviticus, the thing's very existence threatens the meaning of the community, and the film relentlessly documents its disintegration.

In doing so, the film marks itself off from the 1951 version, which emphasized the resourcefulness of the human community, its solidarity and efficiency, in defeating the intruder. Since direction of the earlier version is often credited to Howard Hawks, Carpenter's version may be seen as a reply and as a definitively anti-Hawksian movie. Not only does the group not prevail, but such Hawksian qualities as teamwork and camaraderie are nowhere in evidence. Even before the appearance of the thing, the community of NSI Station 4 is dysfunctional and riddled with tension. Unlike the community of scientists in the earlier film, which has a female member, the research team in Carpenter's film is entirely male and is portrayed as an artificial, pathological group. Lacking a basic, differentiating term—the female—the male social order is dangerously skewed and vulnerable to threat, which is soon forthcoming.

[. . .]

They take the monstrous body back to camp and Blair (Wilford Brimley) begins an autopsy, uncovering what appears to be a normal set of internal organs. However, this thing has two human faces, which seem to have melted together. The faces grimace in agony, connected by a common tongue, an insane Janus. The creature is neither human nor nonhuman, but occupies a disturbing, unclear intermediate place. As such, it cannot be classified, but can only be identified as a "thing." In an additional, repellent detail, the creature is covered with a slimy, amniotic-like fluid, which, in later scenes, it will shoot onto its victims and use to digest them. Invading the boundary of the human body—the skin—the viscous fluid will affix itself to the human and transform it.

[. . .] For Sartre, experience of the slimy is one of dissolution, of what he terms "Antivalue." As MacReady, Copper, and the other men face the dripping, twisted, asymmetrical thing brought back from the Norwegian camp, they confront the shadow side of their human order. As the creature thaws in the warmth of the compound, Antivalue is unleashed throughout the camp, attacking and altering both human organisms and their social structure. As a horribly anomalous animal, the thing represents a form of cosmic pollution, an entity existing outside the accepted categories that give shape to human life and knowledge. Its very existence challenges the ontology separating human from nonhuman, solid from liquid, edible from inedible. It threatens to erase the distinctions and, in doing so, to erase the bounded human world.

[. . .]

Notes

1. Morris Dickstein, "The Aesthetics of Fright," in *Planks of Reason: Essays on the Horror Film,* ed. Barry K. Grant (Metuchen, NJ: Scarecrow, 1984), 65–78.
2. Mary Douglas, *Purity and Danger: An Analysis of the Concepts of Pollution and Taboo* (Boston: Ark Paperbacks, 1966), 4.
3. Edmund Leach, "Anthropological Aspects of Language: Animal Categories and Verbal Abuse," in *New Directions in the Study of Language,* ed. Eric H. Lenneberg (Cambridge, MA: Massachusetts Institute of Technology Press, 1967), 34.
4. Leach, "Anthropological Aspects of Language," 36.
5. Leach, "Anthropological Aspects of Language," 35.
6. Douglas, *Purity and Danger,* 35.
7. The intruder organism attacks its victims at the cellular level, is capable of physiologically mutating, and spreads with a frightening relentlessness. Carpenter's film, therefore, may also be read as a parable about AIDS. In this respect, the film's hysteria about pollution and the disintegration of society manifests a particular urgency.

CHAPTER 3

NIGHTMARE AND THE HORROR FILM: THE SYMBOLIC BIOLOGY OF FANTASTIC BEINGS (EXTRACT)

NOËL CARROLL

[. . .]

THE PURPOSE OF THIS PAPER IS TO EXAMINE the basic structures and themes of [horror and science fiction] . . . by extending some of the points made in Ernest Jones's *On the Nightmare* . . . . I will consider the manner in which the imagery of the horror/science fiction film is constructed in ways that correspond to the construction of nightmare imagery. My special, though not exclusive, focus will be on the articulation of the imagery horrific creatures—on what I call their symbolic biologies. A less pretentious subtitle for this essay might have been "How to make a monster."

[. . .]

The fantastic beings of horror films can be seen as symbolic formations that organize conflicting themes into figures that are simultaneously attractive and repulsive. Two major symbolic structures appear most prominent in this regard: fusion, in which the conflicting themes are yoked together in one, spatio-temporally unified figure; and fission, in which the conflicting themes are distributed—over space or time—among more than one figure.

Dracula, one of the classic film monsters, falls into the category of fusion. In order to identify the symbolic import of this figure we can begin with Jones's account of vampires—since Dracula is a vampire—but we must also amplify that account since Dracula is a very special vampire. According to Jones, the vampires of superstition have two fundamental constituent attributes: revenance and blood sucking. The mythic, as opposed to movie, vampire first visits its relatives. For Jones, this stands for the relatives' longing for the loved one to return from the dead. But the figure is charged with terror. What is fearful is blood sucking, which Jones associates with seduction. In short, the desire for an incestuous encounter with the dead relative is transformed, through a form of denial, into an assault—attraction and love metamorphose into repulsion and sadism. At the same time, via projection, the living portray themselves as passive victims, imbuing the dead with a dimension of active agency that permits the "victim" pleasure without blame. Lastly, Jones not only connects blood sucking with the exhausting embrace of the incubus but with a regressive mixture of sucking and biting characteristic of the oral stage of psychosexual development. By negation—the transformation of love to hate, by projection—through which the desired dead become active, and the desiring living passive, and by regression—from genital to oral sexuality, the vampire legend gratifies incestuous and necrophiliac desires by amalgamating them in a fearsome iconography.

The vampire of lore and the Dracula figure of stage and screen have several points of tangency, but Dracula also has a number of distinctive attributes. Of necessity, Dracula is Count Dracula. He is an aristocrat; his bearing is noble; and, of course, through hypnosis, he is a paradigmatic authority figure. He is commanding in both senses of the word. Above all, Dracula demands *obedience* of his minions and mistresses. He is extremely old—associated with *ancient* castles—and possessed of incontestable strength. Dracula cannot be overcome by force—he can only be outsmarted or outmaneuvered; humans are typically described as puny in comparison to him. At times, Dracula is invested with omniscience, observing from afar the measures taken against him. He also hoards women and is a harem master. In brief, Dracula is a bad father figure, often balanced off against Van Helsing who defends virgins against the seemingly younger, more vibrant Count. The phallic symbolism of Dracula is hard to miss—he is aged, buried in a filthy place, impure, powerful, and aggressive.

The contrast with Van Helsing immediately suggests another cluster of Dracula's attributes. He does appear the younger of the two specifically because he represents the rebellious son at the same time that he is the violent father. This identification is achieved by means of the Satanic imagery that contributes to Dracula's persona. Dracula is the Devil—one film in fact refers to him in its title as the "Prince of Darkness." With few exceptions, Dracula is depicted as eternally uncontrite, bent on luring hapless souls. Most importantly, Dracula is a modern devil which, as Jones points out, means that he is a rival to God. Religiously, Dracula is presented as a force of unmitigated evil. Dramatically, this is translated into a quantum of awesome will or willfulness, often flexed in those mental duels with Van Helsing. Dracula, in part, exists as a rival to the father, as a figure of defiance and rebellion, fulfilling the oedipal wish via a hero of Miltonic proclivities. The Dracula image, then, is a fusion of conflicting attributes of the bad (primal) father and the rebellious son which is simultaneously appealing and forbidding because of the way it conjoins different dimensions of the oedipal fantasy.

The fusion of conflicting tendencies in the figure of the monster in horror films has the dream process of condensation as its approximate psychic prototype. In analyzing the symbolic meaning of these fusion figures our task is to individuate the conflicting themes that constitute the creature. Like Dracula, the Frankenstein monster is a fusion figure, one that is quite literally a composite. Mary Shelley first dreamed of the creature at a time in her life fraught with tragedies connected with childbirth.[1] Victor Frankenstein's creation—his "hideous progeny"—is a gruesome parody of birth; indeed, Shelley's description of the creature's appearance bears passing correspondences to that of a newborn—its waxen skin, misshapen head, and touch of jaundice. James Whale's *Frankenstein* also emphasizes the association of the monster with a child; its walk is unsteady and halting, its head is outsized and its eyes sleepy. And in the film, though not in the novel, the creature's basic cognitive skills are barely developed; it is mystified by fire and has difficulty differentiating between little girls and flowers. The monster in one respect is a child and its creation is a birth that is presented as ghastly. At the same time, the monster is made of waste, of dead things, in "Frankenstein's workshop of filthy creation." The excremental reference is hardly disguised. The association of the creature with waste implies that, in part, the story is underwritten by the infantile confusion over the processes of elimination and reproduction. The monster is reviled as heinous and as unwholesome filth, rejected by its creator—its father—perhaps in a way that reorchestrated Mary Shelley's feelings of rejection by her father William Godwin.

But these images of loathesomeness are fused with opposite qualities. In the film myth, the monster is all but omnipotent (it can function as a sparring partner for Godzilla), indomitable and, for all intents and purposes, immortal (perhaps partly for the intent and purpose of sequels). It is both helpless and powerful, worthless and god-like. Its rejection spurs rampaging vengeance, combining fury and strength in infantile orgies of rage and destruction. Interestingly, in the novel this ire is directed against Victor Frankenstein's family. And even in Whale's 1931 version of the myth the monster's definition as outside (excluded from a place in) the family is maintained in a number of ways: the killing of Maria; the juxtaposition of the monster's wandering over the countryside with wedding preparations; and the opposition of Frankenstein's preoccupation with affairs centered around the monster to the interest of propagating an heir to the family barony. The emotional logic of the tale proceeds from the initial loathesomeness of the monster, which triggers its rejection, which causes the monster to explode in omnipotent rage over its alienation from the family, which, in turn, confirms the earlier intimation of "badness," thereby justifying the parental rejection.[2] This scenario, moreover, is predicated on the inherently conflicting tendencies—of being waste and being god—that are condensed in the creature from the start. It is, therefore, a necessary condition for the success of the tale that the creature be repellent.

One method for composing fantastic beings is fusion. On the visual level, this often entails the construction of creatures that transgress categorical distinctions such as inside/outside, insect/human, flesh/machine, etc.[3] The particular affective significance of these admixtures depends to a large extent on the specific narrative context in which they are embedded. But apart from fusion, another means for articulating emotional conflicts in horror films is fission. That is, conflicts concerning sexuality, identity, aggressiveness, etc. can be mapped over different entities—each standing for a different facet of the conflict—which are nevertheless linked by some magical, supernatural, or sci-fi process. The type of creatures that I have in mind here include[s] doppelgängers, alter-egos, and werewolves.

Fission has two major modes in the horror film.[4] The first distributes the conflict over space through the creation of doubles, e.g., *The Portrait of Dorian Gray, The Student of Prague,* and *Warning Shadows.* Structurally, what is involved in spatial fission is a process of multiplication, i.e., a character or set of characters is multiplied into one or more new facets each standing for another aspect of the self, generally one that is either hidden, ignored, repressed, or denied by the character who has been cloned. These examples each employ some mechanism of reflection—a portrait, a mirror, shadows—as the pretext for doubling. But this sort of fission figure can appear without such devices. [. . .]

Fission occurs in horror films not only in terms of multiplication but also in terms of division. That is, a character can be divided in time as well as multiplied in space. *Dr. Jekyll and Mr. Hyde* (see Figure 3.1) and the various werewolves, cat people, gorgons, and other changelings of the genre are immediate examples. In the horror film, temporal fission—usually marked by shape changing—is often self-consciously concerned with repression. In *Curse of the Werewolf* one shot shows the prospective monster behind the bars of a wine cellar window holding a bottle; it is an icon of restrained delirium. The traditional conflict in these films is sexuality. Stevenson's *Jekyll and Hyde* is altered in screen variants so that the central theme of Hyde's brutality—which

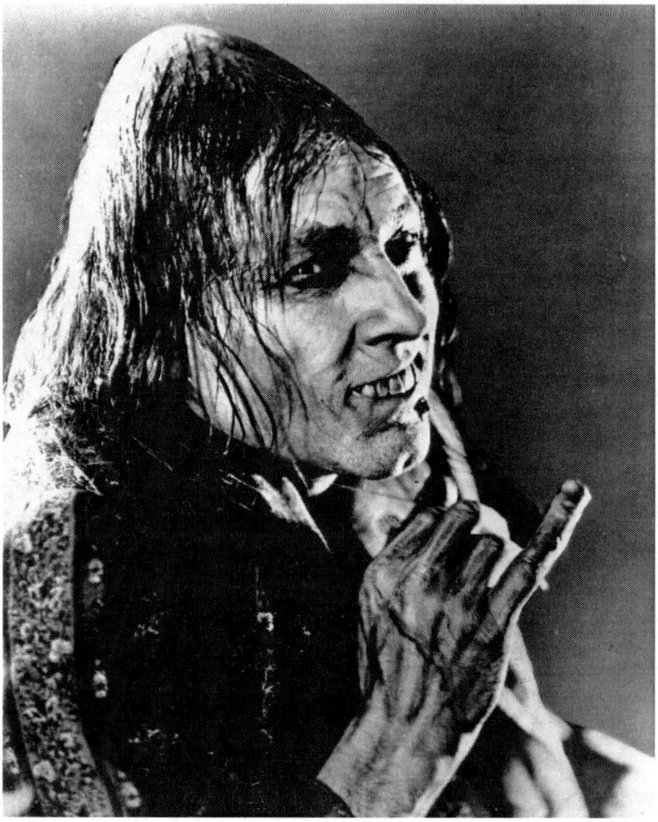

Figure 3.1 John Barrymore as Dr. Henry Jekyll/Mr. Edward Hyde in *Dr. Jekyll and Mr. Hyde* (1920). (Courtesy of Famous Players-Lasky Corporation/Paramount Pictures.)

I think is connected to an allegory against alcoholism in the text—becomes a preoccupation with lechery. Often changeling films, like *The Werewolf of London* or *The Cat People,* eventuate in the monster attacking its lover, suggesting that this subgenre begins in infantile confusions over sexuality and aggression. The imagery of werewolf films also has been associated with conflicts connected with the bodily changes of puberty and adolescence: unprecedented hair spreads over the body, accompanied by uncontrollable, vaguely understood urges leading to puzzlement and even to fear of madness.[5] This imagery becomes especially compelling in *The Wolfman,* where the tension between father and son mounts through anger and tyranny until at last the father beats the son to death with a silver cane in a paroxysm of oedipal anxiety.[6]

Fusion and fission generate a large number of the symbolic biologies of horror films, but not all. Magnification of power or size—e.g., giant insects (and other exaggerated animalcules)—is another mode of symbol formation. Often magnification takes a particular phobia as its subject. [. . .]

[. . .] The giant spider, for instance, appeared in silent film in John Barrymore's *Jekyll and Hyde* as an explicit symbol of desire. Perhaps insects, especially spiders, can perform this role not only because of their resemblance to hands—the hairy hands of masturbation—but also because of their cultural association with impurity.[7] At the same time, their identification as poisonous and predatory—devouring—can be mobilized to express anxious fantasies over sexuality . . . .

Like the fusion and fission figures of horror films, these nightmares are also explicable as effigies of deep-seated, archaic conflicts.

[. . .]

NOTES

1. Ellen Moers, *Literary Women* (Garden City, NY: Anchor, 1977), 140–151.
2. The use of mythic types of fantasies to justify the paternal behavior is discussed in Dorothy Block, "*So the Witch Won't Eat Me*" (Boston: Houghton Mifflin Co., 1978).
3. The slave creatures in *This Island Earth* are examples of the fusion of inside/outside and insect/human while the last appropriation of the monster in *Alien*—with its spring-mounted iron maw—is an example of the fusion of flesh and machine, as is the alien's stranded spaceship.
4. Robert Rogers, *A Psychoanalytic Study of the Double in Literature* (Detroit: Wayne State University Press, 1970).
5. Daniel Dervin, "The Primal Scene and the Technology of Perception in Theater and Films: A Historical Perspective with a Look at *Potemkin* and *Psycho*," *Psychoanalytic Review* 62, no. 2 (1975): 278.
6. In regard to shape-changing figures, like werewolves, it is important to note that metamorphosis in and of itself does not indicate a fission figure. Vampires readily shed human form to become bats and wolves; yet vampires are not fission figures. They are allotropic, varying their physical properties while remaining the same in substance. But with werewolves the change in shape betokens a change in its nature.

   Another, though connected, difference between werewolves and vampires hinges on the issue of will. Werewolves—most often futilely—resist their fate while vampires, especially Dracula, prefer theirs. This is a crucial reason for having the two myths.
7. The spider, of course, has polyvalent associations. It figures importantly as a phobic object because of its ruthlessness—i.e. its use of a trap, its oral sadism—it sucks its prey, and, for men, because of its sexual practices—some female spiders feast upon their mates. In much of the psychoanalytic literature the spider is correlated with the oral, sadistic mother; its body is associated with the vagina; its legs are sometimes glossed as the fantasized penis that the mother is believed to possess. Some references concerning spider imagery include: Karl Abraham, "The Spider as a Dream Symbol," in *Selected Papers,* trans. Douglas Bryand and Alix Strachey (London: Hogarth Press, 1927); Ralph Little, "Oral Aggression in Spider Legends," *American Imago* 23 (1966): 169–180; R. Little, "Umbilical Cord Symbolism of the Spider's Dropline," *Psychoanalytic Quarterly* 35 (1966): 587–590; Richard Sterba, "On Spiders, Hanging and Oral Sadism," *American Imago* 7 (1950): 21–28. There is also an influential reading of "Little Miss Muffet . . . .," in Ella Freeman Sharpe, "Cautionary Tales," *International Journal of Psychoanalysis* 24 (1945): 41–45. In the preceding text I have also connected spiders to masturbation. I have done this not simply because spiders somewhat resemble hands but because that resemblance itself is part of our literary culture. Recall the legend of Arachne who was punished by Minerva by being reduced to a hand which becomes a spider. Bulfinch writes that Minerva sprinkled Arachne "with the juices of aconite, and immediately her hair came off and ears likewise. Her form shrank up, and her head grew smaller yet; her fingers cleaved to her side and served for legs. All the rest of her is a body, out of which she spins her thread, often hanging suspended from it, in the same attitude as when Minerva touched her and transformed her into a spider." See Thomas Bulfinch, *Mythology* (New York: Dell Publishing Co., 1959), 93.

Chapter 4

Our Vampires, Our Neighbors

Ken Gelder

Genres of cinema are a bit like neighborhoods. From a distance, they might have an identifiable character, a set of recognizable, distinctive (formulaic) traits or components. But closer up, these components begin to change shape; different features emerge, different affiliations, different genealogies. Like neighborhoods, for example, genres are never actually "local." New arrivals—new traits or characteristics—move in, while older inhabitants move out; some stay for a long time, as residues or relics, while others are transient, fleeting, emergent, staying for a moment then leaving (with) barely a trace. We now mostly tend to think of genres in the following way: as simultaneously vertical and horizontal, pure and contaminated, monogamous (a genre has a certain loyalty to itself, inhabiting and often paying extensive tribute to its own traditions) and promiscuous (since genres are routinely inhabited by other genres, invoking an often arbitrary range of affiliations that runs the risk of undoing them—as genres—altogether). Naturally enough, Linda Ruth Williams sees cinematic genres precisely in the latter way in her study of the "erotic thriller." "There are very few entirely uncontentious genres," she suggests, "and for most recent writers the more promiscuous a genre term becomes, sliding into bed with any and perhaps all of its neighbors, the more interesting it is."[1] It is as if the genre itself provides the language through which all genres come to be understood: so that "sexual cinema genres" in Williams's study work just as other genres do, by balancing "the desire for familiar and repeated satisfaction with the excitement of experiment."[2] In cinema studies, this is itself a familiar position on genre, in particular, the implied link between levels of promiscuity and levels of interestingness. No one speaks up for "pure" genres any more, for a genre's monogamy or horizontality. Genre, Susan Hayward typically notes, is "a shifting and slippery term"; "generally speaking a film is rarely generically pure," she writes, and since "genres also produce sub-genres, so again clarity is proscribed."[3] In this account, genres are both promiscuous and fertile, destined to spread vertically across the cinematic world. Of course, genres also have their skeptics, their nonbelievers. In "The Idea of Genre in the American Cinema," Edward Buscombe wonders, "do genres in the cinema really exist?"[4] This is a reconfiguration of a question routinely posed in vampire films. "Do you want me to believe you're a vampire?" is what Annika asks Dr Beckert in the Swedish vampire film *Frostbitten* (2006). The answer is inevitably yes, as both Annika and Buscombe soon come to realise. At the end of his essay, Buscombe in fact makes the link between vampires and genres explicit, turning (unusually for a cinema critic) not to promiscuity at all but, almost defiantly, to purity: "a genre," he writes, "is not a mere collection of dead images waiting for a director to animate it, but a tradition with a life of its own."[5]

Genres have a life of their own, but they invoke or beget other lives, too: sometimes neighborly, sometimes not. Jacques Derrida captured exactly this notion when he suggested (although he was thinking of literature) that the law of genre—the thing that defines genre, that separates it and gives it its distinction—is always occupied by another law, or "clause," that undoes the norms of generic stability. The law of genre says that "one must respect a norm, one must not cross a line of demarcation, one must not risk impurity, anomaly, or monstrosity."[6] But texts do not *belong* to genres; they participate in and across genres, which is another way of seeing them as pure and contaminated simultaneously. This is exactly how Tim Lucas understands Guillermo Del Toro's film *Cronos* (1993), a vampire film (although it never mentions the word "vampire") that demonstrates "a remarkable repository of influences": Clive Barker's *Hellraiser,* "any number of David Cronenberg films," Paul Morrissey's *Blood for Dracula,* Terence Fisher's *Frankenstein Must Be Destroyed,* Dario Argento's *Inferno,* and "even Orson Welles' *The Stranger*" (p. 88).[7] In terms of the promiscuity of genre, however, the only remarkable influence on *Cronos* would be Welles's postwar noir thriller—since it reveals the occupation of one genre by another. The rest of these influences are indeed relatively "pure", that is, they situate this vampire film in the vertical traditions of the horror genre generally and the vampire film genre specifically (through Morrissey's *Blood for Dracula*). They work primarily by adding citations of monstrosity to a film that is already monstrous, which keeps the vampire film "local": preserving the neighborhood. Other vampire films, on the other hand, can seem almost indiscriminately promiscuous. Scott Stewart's action vampire film *Priest* (2011) presents what Adam Lee Davies calls "a heroically hopeless appropriation of Indiana Jones mysticism, Peter Jackson's monsters and Joseph Campbell's monomyths," adding a *Mad Max* landscape and some association with Sergio Leone's Italian westerns: what Davies summarizes as a "hodgepodge of lower-to-middle allusions and blasé copycatting," further compromised by an "ultimately unforgivably plagiaristic script."[8] This vampire film would seem to have no purity at all; the horizontal extent of its citational range runs the risk of doing away with its generic identity altogether. On the other hand, vampire films plagiarize as a matter of routine: far from being something unusual, the capacity to plagiarize (to copy, to "remake" or "remark," to simulate, to quote or to *cite*) is also one of the things that lends the vampire film its generic purity.

What might some of the generic features of the vampire film be? Perhaps most obviously, it puts new life (the young orphaned granddaughter Aurora in *Cronos,* for example) into proximity with ancient, degenerating life (her grandfather, Jesus Gris, and the cancer-ridden de la Guardia), bringing them together in a potentially catastrophic way. The proximity of these two otherwise distinct domains means at least two things here. First, it means that vampire films stage their own capacity to "cross a line of demarcation," risking and soliciting "impurity" and "monstrosity"—and plagiarism—along the way. That is, vampire films stage an essentially generic problem. Second, it means that new life has to recognize ancient life for what it is and, as it does so, it crosses the threshold, steps into the framework of that genre, and participates in it. New life has to gain vampiric cultural capital as soon as it can: it has to learn quickly about the thing it is proximate to, and the genre it occupies. One key problem in vampire films is always to do with being noticed, being recognized *as* a vampire; that is, being identified generically. But vampires can work against this imperative, too. The ancient, world-weary New York vampire Peina in Abel Ferrara's *The Addiction* (1995) tells the philosophy graduate student Kathy, "The point is to blend in, not to stand out like a sore thumb." Vampires here are supposed to *not* be generic, to disguise or disperse whatever purity they might have (which makes Peina "almost human," but not quite). Purity and impurity—infection, contamination, and so on—struggle with each other in these ways, and in others. It can seem as a consequence as if vampire films stand for both the law of genre and the "clause" of genre that brings it to an end. Inevitably, perhaps, Derrida invokes the fantasy realm of the vampire when he tries to give this "clause" of genre some sort of recognizable identity:

> The clause or floodgate of genre . . . tolls the knell of genealogy or of genericity, which it however also brings forth to the light of day. Putting to death the very thing that it engenders, it cuts a strange figure; a formless form, it remains nearly invisible, it neither sees the day nor brings itself to light. Without it, neither genre or literature come to light, but as soon as there is this blinking of an eye, this clause or this floodgate of genre, at the very moment that a genre or a literature is broached, at that very moment, degenerescence has begun, the end begins.[9]

A vampire film like *Cronos* plays this out almost to the very letter, working its theme of degenerescence through to a potentially catastrophic conclusion that plays itself out on a dark rooftop as Gris's body—his formless form—begins both to decay and to be reborn ("with a life of its own"). *Cronos* does indeed participate in the vampire film genre, turning away from the light of day as it occupies that genre more completely. But it returns to the light of day at the end when Gris refuses to drink the blood of his granddaughter and thus condemns himself to death. Or rather, he "puts to death the very thing" that the vampire film brings into being. The final moment of the film is a sentimental deathbed scene that significantly shifts away from the vampire genre altogether, as Gris dies peacefully, his granddaughter and the widow Mercedes sitting beside him.

These remarks on genre, neighbors and neighborhoods, standing out and blending in, purity and contamination, darkness and the light of day all help to provide a rudimentary preamble for the close analysis of two new millennium vampire films from Sweden: *Frostbitten* and *Let the Right One In* (2008). What most obviously holds these films together (outside of their snowbound winter landscapes) is the apparent "ordinariness" of their monsters, the unsettling fact that they could—and, indeed, often do—live next door. Anders Banke's *Frostbitten* was eclipsed by the global success of *Let the Right One In,* although they share some common features as Swedish "winter vampire" films set in satellite suburbs. It differs profoundly from that film, however, through its opening sequences, which give the contemporary setting of the rest of the film a peculiar history that seems for a moment to have nothing to do with vampire films at all. *Frostbitten* begins in the snowscaped forests of Ukraine in 1944, where a Scandinavian volunteer army division is fighting on the side of the Germans. Under fire from the Russians, the few remaining soldiers from the SS Panzer Division Viking run into the forest and lose themselves. They stumble across an old hut and go inside, cold and hungry. Later on, the soldiers wonder how the former inhabitants of the hut managed to escape, because the doors and windows are jammed with the deep snow outside. Something attacks them: a monstrous peasant woman, it seems. One of the soldiers, Gerhard Beckert, goes into a cellar and finds a number of mutilated corpses, along with a small box with the name "Maria" imprinted on it. The nails in each corner suddenly begin to push out and guttural growls are heard from inside. In a comic-horror scene, Beckert pushes the nails back in and the soldiers finally weight the box down and bury it. The camera then goes out of the hut and glides across the forest and up into the sky, to reveal a full moon—which introduces the opening titles and credits to the film.

Vampire films often carry deep histories within them, some of which merely work as signifiers of ancientness or age (like the Old World origins of the Cronos device in *Cronos*), others of which work profoundly to shape whatever modern events later unfold. *Frostbitten* takes a repressed or forgotten moment from Sweden's military past and brings it into proximity with the present day—in a town in Norrbotten County in the far north of Sweden—for reasons that can only seem perverse. A couple of years before the film was released, Thorolf Hillblad's account of the Swedish SS Panzer Division Vikings, *Twilight of the Gods,* was reprinted (it was first published in Buenos Aires just after World War II). This is a triumphalist, unapologetically partisan account of the Swedish-German wartime collaboration and its campaigns against the Russian army, "the barbaric masses from the east."[10] *Frostbitten* seems to draw directly on one of the opening descriptions of a New Year's Eve mission in 1944–1945 in German-occupied Courland:

> In the reflected whiteness of the cold, sparkling snow, all outlines appeared razor sharp. A group of trees, riddled by bullets and shells, with their splintered trunks and twisted network of branches, reminded me of grotesque figures in a fairy-tale about brownies and hobgoblins.[11]

The village, or small town, or what once had been something like that, looked more ghostlike than usual . . . . No life was visible in the ruins. But if the alarm should go, warning of an enemy attack, swarms of "creatures" would leap up among them, because under the ground, in the cellars of the damaged houses, there were soldiers everywhere.[12]

This is a remarkable passage to find in a book about Swedish-German collaboration: one that turns occupation into a vivid Gothic trope, displacing the war (and history itself) into a fantasy landscape. In the present day of *Frostbitten,* the collaborator Beckert is now a famous, aging genetic scientist who works in the local hospital. Annika and her daughter Saga are new arrivals in town as darkness falls: "No daylight for a month," Saga says, "I should have moved in with Dad instead." *Frostbitten's* scenario is the opposite to David Slade's film, *30 Days of Night* (2007)—another "winter vampire" film, set this time in northern Alaska—which sees feral vampires from outside invade a small town at the beginning of a similarly extended period of darkness. In *Frostbitten,* the vampires are already there, lying comatose and dormant in Beckert's hospital where Annika now works: rather like the tick Giorgio Agamben describes in *The Open: Man and Animal* (2004), which is kept alive without food in another kind of experiment for 18 years, in isolation, sinking into "a dreamlike state of waiting but, without time, a suspended moment."[13] Later, Beckert tells Annika about events at the end of the war. He had taken the dead peasant woman outside to burn her body, but she had risen up and bitten his leg. "That was my last night as a human being," he says, becoming—like the tick—a single-minded, blood-sucking creature. The hospital is full of tubes of vampire blood, as Beckert conducts his experiments like a crazed Nazi doctor. "I'm close to perfection," he tells Annika, who is also soon bitten. "When I'm done, our kind will rule over all of you!" *Frostbitten* takes its own peculiar form of revenge against Swedish war collaborators like Thorolf Hillblad, putting them into a vampire film and allowing this repressed historical moment to occupy (and finally overrun) the present day. In the process it plays out a version of the narrative in *Cronos,* but it veers away from that film's closing act of refusal by casually unleashing a series of infections right across the townscape. In the meantime, a Goth girl, Vega, invites Saga to a New Year's Eve party: "I'm inviting you now. There, you're invited!" The problem for new arrivals Annika and Saga is how to blend in. "It's great you got to know people already," Annika proudly tells her daughter. But the townspeople are rapidly changing as more of them become infected with vampire blood. The film literally degenerates into a pitched battle between blood-crazed teenage partygoers and the local police: "I can't sleep," complains a neighbor, "they're even climbing the walls!" Saga soon recognizes the vampires around her for what they are; when Vega becomes a vampire and attacks her, Saga kills the girl who had welcomed her to the neighborhood and invited her to the party. As she is carried out of town in an ambulance, Saga finds another, younger girl sitting beside her, occupying the same space. "My name's Maria," the girl tells her. "Mother says we'll be sisters and we will always be together. You'll never be alone."

In terms of the law of genre, *Frostbitten* is both familiar (vampires are recognized through their red eyes, there are fangs, a lot of biting and blood-letting, etc.) and almost incoherent. In particular, the connection between its opening (the Swedish SS Panzer Division in the Ukrainian forests in 1944) and its ending (a teenage party in an undistinguished satellite town in northern Sweden) remains opaque, or at least idiosyncratic. But the narrative of Annika and Saga—mother and daughter, part of a separated family that moves into a new neighborhood which then solicits and transforms them, finally bonding Saga to a kind of uncanny vampire kid "sister"—provides a trope that other vampire films have invested in and developed. In Tomas Alfredson's *Let the Right One In,* it seems as if a young girl and her father have just arrived outside a block of apartments in a dark, snow-covered satellite suburb of Stockholm called Blackeberg—secretly watched by a pale, blond boy, Oskar, who stands at the window. *Let the Right One In* is an adaptation of the novel of the same name by John Ajvide Lindqvist, who also wrote the screenplay. Lindqvist grew up in Blackeberg and his novel describes the suburb in the following way:

> When this story begins, Blackeberg the suburb had been in existence for thirty years. One can imagine that it had fostered a pioneer spirit. The *Mayflower*; an unknown land. Yes. One can imagine all those empty buildings waiting for their occupants [. . ..]
>
> Where the three-storied apartment buildings now stood there had been only forest before.
>
> You were beyond the grasp of the mysteries of the past; there wasn't even a church. Nine thousand inhabitants and no church.
>
> That tells you something about the modernity of the place, its rationality. It tells you something of how free they were from the ghosts of history and of terror.
>
> It explains in part how unprepared they were.[14]

It is worth contrasting this passage with the one quoted above, from *Twilight of the Gods*: whereas the space of the latter is both occulted and historical (and desecrated), the world of *Let the Right One In* is perpetually and optimistically tied to a secular present. Its scenario is therefore closer to Slade's *30 Days of Night* than *Frostbitten,* with vampires as the new arrivals this time, the things that bring a kind of occulted history into a modernized neighborhood. But there is only one vampire in *Let the Right One In*: Eli, who has moved with her elderly guardian Hakan into the apartment next door to Oskar and his mother.

Bullied by a group of boys at school, Oskar plays alone in a bleak, snow-covered space outside his apartment block. Even his mother doesn't watch him. The neighborhood in *Let the Right One In* is atomized and emptied of content: quite different in kind to the inhabited, active space that picturesquely unfolds under James Stewart's character's watchful gaze in Hitchcock's exemplary "neighborhood watch" film, *Rear Window* (1954). In *Let the Right One In,* the "modern neighbourhood" is not panoptic,[15] nor is it reassuringly familiar. There are no teenage parties in this film, only a displaced, tiny community of older men who drink together in a desolate café, the ironically titled "Sun Palace." Characters walk in the dark streets on their own; murders go unsolved; strange events go unnoticed. But Eli notices Oskar, and as he plays below the apartment block she comes down to join him. *Let the Right One In* puts a boy and a vampire into proximity with each other, as if for a moment they are the same: from broken families, equally friendless, and so on. They even seem to be the same age. But Oskar is twelve and knows his exact time of birth, while Eli is twelve "more or less," later telling him that "I've been twelve for a long time." She may in fact be around 200 years old. New life is once again proximate to old life in this vampire film, which also asks Oskar to come to recognize Eli for what she is. But what is she? When she says, "Oskar, I'm not a girl," one might think she means she is a vampire. But as John Calhoun notes, she may also mean she is literally not a girl. The novel is clearer about her human origins as a boy, but the film also offers some support to this by providing a fleeting glimpse of "a scar where presumably something else was,"[16] witnessed by Oskar as he looks into his mother's bedroom and watches Eli putting on his mother's dress. For Calhoun, *Let the Right One In* is not so much a vampire film, as a film about troubled, creepy children: this is the genre he privileges in his discussion. But Oskar's recognition of Eli as a vampire is crucial to his self-development and self-empowerment. Eli is both remote from him and intimate with him. Although she agrees to "go steady" and slips naked into his bed, their relationship is not sexual. They are not underage lovers—although in Matt Reeves's American remake *Let Me In* (2009), this is presented as a heightened possibility, shown through its several "horizontal" citations of Shakespeare's *Romeo and Juliet.* In a certain precise sense, the relationship between Eli and Oskar is neighborly. The title of the film resonates throughout their various exchanges (whereas "let me in" is more urgent, more of a command than an ethical direction). When he realizes that she is a vampire, Oskar goes to her apartment and knocks on the door. Later, he tells her, "I want to go home now. If you'll let me." Reversing this sequence, Eli then knocks on Oskar's front door. "You have to invite me in," she tells him, effectively staging the moment at which the genre crosses its own "line of demarcation." "What happens if I don't?" Oskar asks, skeptically. "What happens if you walk in anyway? Is there something in the way?" Eli walks in and suddenly begins to shake uncontrollably, bleeding from the ears and eyes, from her nose and forehead. Oskar is overcome with sympathy for her ("You can come in!"), and takes her into his arms. When he asks her once again who she is, Eli replies: "I'm like you . . . " The scene brings them together through their neighbourliness, as if their apartments are now interchangeable and they can move freely between them—as if the genre, having crossed its line of demarcation, has become "pure." "Be me for a while . . . Oskar . . . be me," Eli tells him, and it seems as if the differences between boy, girl, and vampire have, for a moment at least, evaporated.

But Oskar is never bitten: he never does actually become like Eli, a vampire. *Let the Right One In,* like *Cronos,* refuses to relish in the transformation of new life into something ancient, something that can live barely in suspended animation, like Agamben's tick. Or perhaps it defers that transformation. The relationship between Eli and Oskar is sympathetic, but not empathetic; they are intimate with each other but they are differentiated and sometimes coldly remote from one another as well. This is part of their neighborliness, shown through the way Oskar listens to the muffled noises from Eli's apartment through his bedroom wall, disturbed yet intrigued by them and not quite knowing what he is hearing—and the way he teaches her to communicate through the walls by using Morse code. But it is a relationship that is also uncannily reflected through the role of Eli's guardian, Hakan. John Calhoun wonders about this odd, unsettling couple: "What is their relationship, exactly?"[17] This couple who live next door and yet don't belong there (like Annika and Saga in *Frostbitten,* they have no furniture, etc.) seem also to share both the intimacy and the coldness already manifesting itself between Eli and Oskar. Hakan warns Eli to stay away from Oskar, as if he sees the boy as a rival for Eli's affections—or, as if he sees himself as he once was. As Hakan becomes less and less able to provide human blood for Eli, her attentions turn instead to her neighbor. Her bid for companionship is thus also predatory, a bid to secure her own survival. By the end of the film, Oskar has indeed taken Hakan's place, travelling with Eli on the train away from Blackeberg. For the moment, he seems secure and confident, even dominant, with Eli hidden in the large box beside on the train—almost exactly like Maria in the opening scenes of *Frostbitten*—depending on him for support. But if Oskar takes Hakan's place, his fate is also already apparent: to grow old, to fail, to cease to be loved, to have his identity literally effaced (as Hakan does when he pours acid over his face, fearing discovery), and to die unrecognized and unrecognizable. Eli visits Hakan as he lies alone in the hospital ward, entering through the outside window ("Can I come in?"), drinking his blood and then casually pulling him out of the window so that he falls to his death. In contrast to *Cronos,* there is thus no peaceful deathbed scene here: the vampire cycle of neighborliness, companionship, neglect, and death is condemned to be repeated over and over. One of the most touching scenes in the film therefore occurs when Oskar tearfully rejects his distraught mother, locking her out of his bedroom; earlier, the mother had in fact supplied Matt Reeves's American remake with its title, as she knocks on the apartment door and calls to Oskar, "Let me in!" In *Let the Right One In,* mother is replaced by vampire. As for the father, he has long since departed, his house in rural Sweden occupied by another unidentified male companion ("We have a guest") who effectively drives Oskar back to his neighbor-vampire.

In *Our Vampires, Ourselves* (1997), Nina Auerbach writes,

> as a species vampires have been our companions for so long that it is hard to imagine living without them. They promise escape from our dull lives and the pressure of our times, but they matter because when properly understood, they make us see that our lives are implicated in theirs and our times are inescapable.[18]

But it is just as hard to imagine living *with* vampires; perhaps neighborliness is about the best that can happen here. Can neighbors be lived with, or even loved? In *Civilisation and Its Discontents* (1930), Sigmund Freud certainly didn't think so. Rejecting the Christian imperative to "love thy neighbor," he suggests something utterly different: "Not merely is this stranger in general unworthy of my love; I must honestly confess that he has more claim to my hostility and even my hatred."[19] Emphasizing human aggression and instinct over "gentleness," Freud captures precisely the relationship between Oskar and the boys who bully him at school in *Let the Right One In,* one which Eli incites and encourages ("Hit them hard!"):

> men are not gentle creatures who want to be loved, and who at the most can defend themselves if they are attacked; they are, on the contrary, creatures among whose instinctual endowments is to be reckoned a powerful share of aggressiveness. As a result, their neighbour is for them not only a potential helper or sexual object, but also someone who tempts them to satisfy their aggressiveness on him, to exploit his capacity for work without compensation, to use him sexually without his consent, to seize his possessions, to humiliate him, to cause him pain, to torture and to kill him. *Homo homini lupus* [Man is a wolf to man].[20]

Some vampire films—like *Priest,* or *30 Days of Night*—do indeed reduce their vampires down to ciphers of pure aggression, pure instinct: bad neighbors, neighbors as wolves. But *Let the Right One In* is quite different to these Manichean vampire films. Of course, Eli is wolfish too as she climbs a tree, growling as Maria had growled in *Frostbitten,* waiting in the same way for someone in the neighborhood to walk past and feast upon. But the film puts the capacity for pure instinct into proximity with neighborliness, with the sheer fact of living next door to someone else: to the extent that the imperative to "love thy neighbor," in all its ambivalence, can for a moment cancel out even a child's love for his mother.

In these Swedish vampire films (and more obviously in the *Fright Night* films, for example), the "vampire next door" is different in kind to the ghost: it isn't the house itself that is occupied, or preoccupied, but the space adjacent to the house, which is then simultaneously close and remote. The "vampire next door" is the subtitle of Jules Zanger's essay "Metaphor into Metonymy" (1997), which complained that the modern vampire had lost its earlier "metaphysical" and "religious" features to become, "in our concerned awareness for multiculturalism, merely ethnic, a victim of heredity, like being Sicilian or Jewish."[21] "This new, demystified vampire," he writes, "might as well be our next door neighbor, as Dracula, by origin, appearance, caste, and speech, could never pretend to be."[22] It is worth noting that Dracula himself, as he migrates to London and buys property there, had also wanted to be neighborly: to blend in, to go through the streets unrecognized. But for Zanger, the modern vampire has lost its "otherness." It circulates outside of the Judeo-Christian tradition, a "diminished" secular creature that is now "socialized and humanized,"[23] although no less single-minded and ravenous. In *Let the Right One In*, there is no doubt that the vampire is in some respects an "ordinary" monster. But if the vampire really does live next door, then its otherness is perhaps more unsettling than it ever was. In the field of "political theology," there has been much recent interest in the figure of the neighbor, and in the Judeo-Christian imperative to love that figure unconditionally. The Slovenian Lacanian Slavoj Žižek naturally (for those who are familiar with the various inversions, ironies, etc. that constitute his work) turns the literalness of this imperative on its head, turning to the Danish philosopher Soren Kierkagaard. "Kierkegaard," he writes, "develops the claim that . . . the only good neighbour is a dead neighbor."[24] This is because, in order to be perfect, the object of one's love must be deprived of all distinctions, any hint of "annoying excess" that might make the act of love self-conscious: the "annoying excess" of ethnicity, for example. One must therefore be, in a certain precise sense, indifferent to the neighbor in order to love the neighbor. For Žižek, loving the neighbor in this "nonpathological" way thus leads to both purity and promiscuity, since these are merely different sides of the same coin: both forms of love wipe out the "idiosyncrasies" of the love object.

Is Eli's love for Oskar—and Oskar's love for Eli—pathological or nonpathological? Is it pure? Or—from Eli's perspective in particular—is it merely instrumental, one event in a promiscuous and arbitrary chain of events in which Oskar functions simply as a replacement for the casually-disposed-of Hakan? Of course, Eli is not exactly a "dead neighbor": she is *undead*. For the kind of Judeo-Christian political theology developed over the last few years by Žižek as well as the American critic Eric Santner, "undeadness" is a condition defined by lack, a form of psychic paralysis: death-in-life.[25] Their messianic vitalism, producing a series of links that put Walter Benjamin, Kafka, Sebald, and others into genealogical (generic, citational) proximity with St. Paul and revelationary Christianity, sees undeadness as a kind of "petrified unrest": which Santner, interestingly, has characterized as "creaturely life."[26] But "undeadness" is also unstable; it can be "reanimated," brought into life all over again through its unexpected encounters with otherness. Like Žižek, Santner's psychoanalytical version of political theology regards the encounter with otherness as both self-enlivening and self-alienating, a form of excess or *ex-citation*.[27] This last word is important to look at: it also links the encounter with otherness to the practice of citation itself, in so far as the citation/encounter occupies the self and at the same time takes it somewhere else altogether. The word "citation" comes from the Latin *citare,* which means to set in motion, to move. To cite is already to excite, to be aroused. Citation is a self-transforming process. It also carries another set of meanings: to summon (before a court of law). In *Let the Right One In,* it is hard to know whether Oskar summons Eli, or Eli summons Oskar: they let *each other* into their respective apartments, touching each other, moving away, touching again. The vampire thus both cites and ex-cites. We might say that the vampire is citational by nature: summoning and being summoned, setting things into motion, occupying and preoccupying, transforming, arousing, moving on, arriving somewhere else altogether. The kind of encounter with otherness that Santner talks about in the framework of political theology therefore also produces a crisis of legitimation. For someone who only mentions vampires once or twice in passing, he in fact gets pretty close to capturing a key generic feature of the vampire film, one that—contrary to Zanger—brings a certain kind of "metaphysical" monstrosity right back into the picture. It all depends on one's receptiveness to the proximity of otherness, it seems. "What I am calling 'undeadness,' " Santner writes, "is thus correlative to the encounter—above all in the life of the child—with the Other's desire and the seemingly endless drama of legitimation it inaugurates."[28] From one point of view, *Let the Right One In* is precisely a rehearsal of this kind of drama, turning as it does on the question of who a lonely child decides to open his or her front door to, and what is risked when whatever it is that enters (human or vampire) is allowed to cross that "line of demarcation" and come inside.

Notes

1. Linda Ruth Williams, *The Erotic Thriller in Contemporary Cinema* (Bloomington, IN: Indiana University Press, 2005), 22–23.
2. Williams, *The Erotic Thriller in Contemporary Cinema,* 17.
3. Susan Hayward, *Cinema Studies: The Key Concepts* (London: Taylor and Francis, 2006), 163–164.
4. Edward Buscombe, "The Idea of Genre in the American Cinema," in *Film Genre Reader III,* ed. Barry Keith Grant (Austin, TX: University of Texas Press, 2003), 12.
5. Buscombe, "The Idea of Genre in the American Cinema," 25.
6. Jacques Derrida and Derek Attridge, *Acts of Literature* (London: Routledge, 1992), 224–225.
7. Tim Lucas, "Under the Influence," *Sight and Sound* (February 2011): 88.
8. Adam Lee Davies, "Priest," *Sight and Sound* (July 2011): 74.
9. Derrida and Attridge, *Acts of Literature,* 231.
10. Thorolf Hillblad, *Twilight of the Gods: A Swedish Waffen-SS Volunteer's Experiences with the 11th Panzergrendier Division "Nordland", Eastern Front 1944–45* (Solihull, England: Helion & Company Limited, 2004), 11.
11. Hillblad, *Twilight of the Gods,* 10.
12. Hillblad, *Twilight of the Gods,* 10.
13. Jussi Parikka, *Insect Media: An Archaeology of Animals and Technology* (Minneapolis, MN: University of Minnesota Press, 2010), 66.
14. John Ajvide Lindqvist, *Let the Right One In* (Melbourne: Text Publishing Company, 2007), 1–2.
15. Bran Nicol, " 'Police Thy Neighbour': Crime Culture and the *Rear Window* Paradigm," in *Crime Culture: Figuring Criminality in Fiction and Film,* eds. Bran Nicol, Eugene McNulty, and Patricia Pulham (London: Continuum, 2011), 196.
16. John Calhoun, "Childhood's End: *Let the Right One In* and Other Deaths of Innocence," *Cineaste* (Winter 2009): 31.
17. Calhoun, "Childhood's End," 31.
18. Nina Auerbach, *Our Vampires, Ourselves* (Chicago: University of Chicago Press, 1995), 9.
19. Sigmund Freud, *Civilisation and Its Discontents,* trans. James Strachey (New York: W.W. Norton & Company, Inc., 1962), 57.
20. Freud, *Civilisation and Its Discontents,* 58.
21. Jules Zanger, "Metaphor into Metonymy: The Vampire Next Door," in *Blood Read: The Vampire as Metaphor in Contemporary Culture,* ed. Veronica Hollinger (Philadelphia: University of Pennsylvania Press, 1997), 19.
22. Zanger, "Metaphor into Metonymy," 19.
23. Zanger, "Metaphor into Metonymy," 22.
24. Slavoj Žižek, "Afterword: Lenin's Choice," in Vladimir Lenin, *Revolution at the Gates: A Selection of Writings from February to October 1917,* ed. Slavoj Žižek (London: Verso, 2004), 213.
25. Eric L. Santner, *On Creaturely Life: Rilke/Benjamin/Sebald* (Chicago: University of Chicago Press, 2006), 119.
26. Santner, *On Creaturely Life,* xx.
27. Eric L. Santner, "Miracles Happen: Benjamin, Rosenweig, Freud, and the Matter of the Neighbour," in Slavoj Žižek, Eric L. Santner, and Kenneth Reinhard, *The Neighbour: Three Inquiries in Political Theology* (Chicago: University of Chicago Press, 2005), 86.
28. Santner, "Miracles Happen," 86.

CHAPTER 5

"Psychological Thriller": *Dead of Night* (1945), British Film Culture, and the 1940s Horror Cycle

MARK JANCOVICH

Dead of Night (1945) has acquired a privileged place in the history of the British horror films, and this reputation was established early. In one of the first major histories of the horror film, Ivan Butler claimed not only that the film was "Britain's first significant entry into the sphere of the supernatural,"[1] but that it "is difficult to recollect anything in the *genre* during the silent period" and little of significance before the release of *Curse of Frankenstein* (1957), "save for *Dead of Night*."[2]

Although Butler's book is a general history, this assessment is also found six years later in David Pirie's *A Heritage of Horror,* a study that proclaims itself to be far more focused. Rather than a general history, Pirie's book is both *nationally* focused—it is not just a study of British but *English* film—and *generically* focused—it is not a study of the horror film more generally but the "Gothic cinema" in particular. Nonetheless, Pirie takes the position implied by Butler and states it explicitly. Again, he presents *Dead of Night* as a film with no significant precedent and as the only significant example of the English Gothic cinema before "the sudden proliferation of English horror films in the late 1950s."[3] Furthermore, while he claims that most critics find this "sudden proliferation" to be "a daunting and inexplicable phenomenon," he simultaneously suggests that *Dead of Night* reveals the subterranean currents of the Gothic imagination that lay beneath the surface of English culture, but that it is also a "remarkable and some ways prophetic film."[4] Thus, it is both a symptom of something much larger and a special and unique case that may even signify the "inception" of the "sudden proliferation" that would take place over a decade afterwards.

Peter Hutchings challenges this view to some extent. He stresses that *Dead of Night* was "not without its precursors" and that it is therefore "rather problematic" to "view *Dead of Night* as marking the 'birth' of British horror cinema."[5] However, he simply pays more attention to the "pale imitations of American product" in the 1930s,[6] the "series of gruesome melodramas starring Tod Slaughter" later in the decade,[7] and the censorship conditions that, he suggests, blocked the development of a more consistent strain of British horror films. Interestingly, although he accepts the often-cited claim that "throughout World War Two no horror films were produced in Britain, and, significantly, the censor declined in general to pass 'H'—that is horror—films between 1942 and 1945,"[8] he also notes the presence of horror materials in "disguised or submerged" form in two examples: *Tower of London* (1941) and *A Canterbury Tale* (1944). Unfortunately, he makes nothing of this observation. Nor does he look much further for other examples that might contribute to a revised picture of production trends within the period.

Jonathan Rigby's account of the "English Gothic" seems quite different. He identifies a number of silent films that can be understood as horror (or horror-related) items; he spends much more time on the films of the 1930s; he explores the "queer fascination with cruelty" in 1940s British cinema, from *Gaslight* (1940) through to the Gainsborough melodramas;[9] and he even discusses the way in which "horror . . . tended to get in by the back door" in films, such as David Lean adaptations of Dickens.[10] However, despite a far more detailed sense of the various types of horror-related material produced by the British film industry, he still presents *Dead of Night* as a fairly isolated, if important, film. It may not be an origin but its significance is clearly suggested by the extensive analysis that Rigby undertakes in comparison with other films, an analysis so extensive that virtually an entire section of the first chapter is dedicated to the film. Nonetheless, despite this implied significance, Rigby makes little attempt to relate the film to other traditions that came before or after it, but rather discusses the film as an "aberration" in the output of Michael Balcon and Ealing Studios, an aberration that is given little explanation.[11] He even comments that "As Britain emerged from the war, the distinguished example of *Dead of Night* failed to establish a consistent trend towards films of a similar vein."[12]

However, far from being without precedent, or springing from a repressed subterranean Gothic imagination, or simply an inexplicable "aberration," *Dead of Night* was fully consistent with British production trends at the time, in which horror was a highly significant, if problematic, genre. If *Dead of Night* looks strangely disconnected from its period, this is due to the ways in which the first histories of horror were written in the 1960s and early 1970s in response to another cycle of horror production. These studies were caught up in the struggle to criticize or defend a particular definition of horror that was historically specific and they therefore constructed the horror canon in particular ways. While some critics, like Butler, regarded the "sudden proliferation of English horror films" associated with Hammer as a sad corruption of the Universal horror films, other critics, such as Pirie, attempted to defend them by establishing their credentials as legitimate contributions to the heritage of Gothic cinema.

Both strategies, however, worked to prioritize the Gothic horror films of Universal and Hammer, and marginalize or exclude other studios, periods, and generic definitions. Most significantly, for the purposes of this chapter, horror had been defined very differently in the 1940s, the period within which *Dead of Night* was made and during which virtually all the key examples of the paranoid women's films and film noir were understood as horror. In other words, during the 1940s, horror was understood as being a far larger category that was not distinguishable from the thriller, while the thriller was understood as a category that was largely synonymous with the "chiller."[13]

Consequently, the purpose of this chapter is to demonstrate that the category of horror is not fixed and that its contents continually change from one historical moment to another as definitions of the monstrous change. Many of the films identified with horror in the 1940s were excluded from this category in the 1960s, and one of the key ways in which historical definitions of horror and the monstrous can be explored is through the study of film reviews and other extratextual materials. In such studies, film reviews are not to be seen as "failed criticism" but as "types of social discourse which ... can aid the researcher in ascertaining the material conditions informing the relation between the film and spectator at given moments."[14] However, it is also important to be clear here: the purpose of such explorations should not be to privilege one definition over another. If the critics of the 1960s displayed ignorance or disinterest about earlier definitions of horror, these earlier definitions are no more "original," "real," or "true." The purpose of this chapter is not to claim specific films for the category of horror; not to complete a new comprehensive list but rather to identify definitions and associations that enrich or alter our sense of how films were understood and related to one another in specific historical situations.

However, historical definitions were not always explicit. During the 1940s, when *Dead of Night* was made, the industry explicitly acknowledged a need to disguise horror films in order to get them past the censor. For example, in 1943, *Variety* reported, "To meet toning down requirements of the British, studios here [in the U.S.] are ... whodunit-ing horrors to permit their classification as mystery yarn."[15] Of course, this report deliberately evades the extent to which this strategy was as much an attempt to circumvent the U.S. censors, but it also demonstrates that, during the 1940s, the Hollywood studios clearly believed that the British market had an appetite for horror but one that needed to be handled with care. If British audiences were seen as being receptive to horror, the censors were not; and films had to be produced that would not alarm the censors but could still be marketed as appealing to a taste for horror.

If the Hollywood studios self-consciously operated according to this strategy, one might expect British studios to have responded in a similar fashion. Moreover, given the size and significance of the 1940s horror boom in the United States,[16] British studios with an eye on the U.S. market were likely to have developed films that not only could be sold to British audiences but might also address trends within the United States, particularly given that this was a period in which the British were actively targeting the American market.[17] *Dead of Night*'s U.S. Pressbook even presents the film as one that would introduce British film culture to American audiences, and it contained pieces with titles such as "Film Brings Players to US screens" and "British Productions Please Theatre Patrons." The former piece even claims that "American filmgoers will [soon] be as familiar with English stars as the British now are with our own."[18]

If the horror films of the 1940s were therefore significantly different from the definitions with which figures such as Butler and Pirie were working, their features enable us to see how a series of British production trends were associated with horror at the time and so provided a perfectly explicable context for the production of *Dead of Night*.

For example, in 1940s Hollywood, many horror films were explicitly addressed at women, and many examples of the woman's films were explicitly identified as horror films, such as *Rebecca* (1940), *Jane Eyre* (1944), and *Gaslight* (1944), the last of which was itself based on a British play that had been adapted for the screen in 1940 by British National Films and is noticeably absent from Butler, Pirie, and Hutchings's accounts of British horror. These associations with the woman's film were also related to another aspect of the 1940s horror films, many of which were claimed to be "dressed up in full Class 'A' paraphernalia, including million-dollar budgets and big-name casts."[19] Rather than low-budget productions, the films of this horror cycle often featured lavish production values and claims to cultural respectability. The Universal horror films were therefore far from being central to this cycle and while Universal did initiate a series of Mummy films, Wolf Man films and resurrected both Frankenstein and Dracula, it also made a series of other films more closely tailored to these trends. For example, it produced a lavish, color remake of *The Phantom of the Opera* that featured extravagant set pieces, in which Nelson Eddy and Susanna Foster performed light opera.[20]

Finally, many of the examples of the 1940s horror cycle were identified as "psychological efforts"[21] and reviews often used the terms "psychological film" and "horror film" interchangeably during the period, as can be seen in the *New York Times*'s review of Universal's female-centred horror film *Phantom Lady*.[22] The identification of many horror films as "psychological" was not simply due to the high number of films that featured psychologically disturbed killers but also due to the disposition of their victims. In films such as *Gaslight,* the disturbed husband does not simply want to murder his wife but plots to drive her mad: he is driven by a sadism that offers little or no benefit to his ostensible scheme but, as with many other films, the threat to his victim is also psychological. As Siegfried Kracauer claimed at the time, the cycle was distinguished by "the theme of psychological destruction" in which the villains "no longer shoot, strangle or poison the females that they want to do away with, but systematically try to drive them insane."[23] Consequently, these films usually displayed anxieties about perception and about the difficulty of distinguishing fantasy from reality, or sanity from insanity, so that "many a current melodrama suggests that normal and abnormal states of mind merge into each other imperceptibly and are hard to keep separate."[24]

It is therefore significant that the *Los Angeles Times* referred to *Dead of Night* as a "psychological thriller"[25] and that, in his recent revisions to *A Heritage of Horror,* Pirie places *Dead of Night* within the context of a speech by the young Harold Wilson in June 1948: "We are getting tired of some of the gangster, sadistic and psychological films of which we seem to have so many . . . I would like to see more films which genuinely show our way of life, and I am not aware . . . that amnesia and schizophrenia are stock parts of our social life."[26] Surprisingly, while Pirie acknowledges that this reference refers to "movies that border on noir and horror" (movies that would all have been identified as horror during the period), he can identify "only four candidates" that fit such description, at least in so "far as Britain [or British production] is concerned."[27] Nonetheless, both Pirie and Hutchings see this concern with the psychological as being central to *Dead of Night,* and even go so far as to identify this as one of its original and innovative features. For Pirie, "Wilson's speech provides some idea of how entrenched such attitudes were," and *Dead of Night* is precisely defended as a film that "deserves its reputation as the most important English supernatural thriller prior to the late 1950s" on the grounds that the film is profoundly psychological: "the whole action is finally revealed to be a nightmare"[28] and the episode on which he focuses his critical attention, *The Haunted Mirror,* is read precisely as a metaphor about the eruption of the repressed into the "artificial" reality of middle-class English normality.[29]

Similarly, while quite different in his approach, Hutchings also sees this concern with the psychological as central to the narrative, in which "a division between fantasy and waking reality becomes increasingly difficult to sustain."[30] More recently, Burton and O'Sullivan have also seen the film as revolving around an "ensuing serial conflict between Freudian psychoanalysis and the uncanny manifestation of the paranormal" and have claimed that the film is "superbly rich in interpretive potential with its dramatic fabric of dread, anxiety, foreknowledge, repression and oneiric metaphor."[31] Furthermore, this conflict raises a more fundamental question about the status of the image so that the film is seen operating on "the uncertain ground between the objective and the subjective."[32]

For Hutchings, however, this aspect of *Dead of Night* is specifically related to its historical context so that the film is claimed to emerge "as an intense and obsessive mediation on issues arising from the transition from wartime to post-war society."[33] Conversely, it should be stressed that this concern with psychology and the 'difficulty of sustaining' a distinction between fantasy and reality was central to the 1940s cycle of horror films long before the end of the war. These concerns were not only a feature of films such as *Rebecca* and *Suspicion* but also gained a particular insistence after the success of Val Lewton's *Cat People* in 1943, a film that is often praised for its hesitation between fantasy and reality, its refusal to decide on a realist or fantastic account of its events.

Furthermore, when compared to the Universal horrors, *Dead of Night* is very much a quality production and one that was released by Universal in the United States as part of a new arrangement with British producer J. Arthur Rank. In 1946, the year in which the film was released in the United States, Rank had been pivotal in securing a merger between Universal and International pictures, a specialist in prestige productions. This merger was therefore part of a more general strategy that shifted Universal into the prestige market, a strategy that was also integral to a complex international distribution deal that Universal established with Rank, the owner of *Dead of Night*'s producers, Ealing Studio.[34]

Dead of Night was also released in the United States at a time when Universal was losing ground in the horror market. Its horror series were coming to an end by 1945, and it seemed that the prestige horror films associated with figures such as David O. Selznick were far more profitable. Not only did British cinema have considerable cache in the United States at this time[35] but many of the quality U.S. horror films were either set in Britain or evoked notions of Britishness through other means such as their casts and directors.[36] It is therefore hardly surprising to find that the *New York Times* identified *Dead of Night* as a strong, quality production that was "tightly and graphically told" and therefore could be appreciated as "good heterodox thriller stuff,"[37] while *Variety* praised its "[t]ightly-woven script," in which "each individual episode" is "equally good" although Michael Redgrave is singled out for providing "a masterful piece of acting."[38] *Dead of Night* even received special mention in the *New York Times*'s assessment of the best films of 1946, where it was identified along with a number of other films that might not have achieved the very highest quality but could be commended for their "entertainment values."[39]

Nor did *Dead of Night,* the first British contribution to the cycle, and the Gainsborough melodramas begin to look very different in the context of their U.S. reception. Most of these films featured the Gothic setting and sadistic males that was common to the cycle, so that *The Man in Gray* was seen as an "ostentatious costume picture" that is only distinguished by James Mason who "plays the cold scowling marquis in a swaggering, villainous style."[40] Although this film was actually released in 1943 in the United Kingdom, it was not released in the United States until 1945, when the cycle was well established and Gainsborough began to release other Gothic melodramas with sadistic males and/or psychological themes. *The Wicked Lady* also featured a Gothic setting but one which *Variety* found to be "unconvincing," although it praised James Mason's "swaggering love-'em-and-leave-'em rascal."[41] The *New York Times* took a slightly different tack and while it acknowledged Mason's Captain Jack Jackson to be "a definite dastard" and "a fascinating brigand,"[42] it claimed that Mason "seems to have [had] a point" when he "publicly voiced disgust" about his role.[43]

However, it was not just Mason's sadism that associated this film with the 1940s horror cycle and it was clearly discussed in psychological terms so that its female lead was "a victim of... a bundle of psychoses."[44] Furthermore, she can also be directly associated with the cycle of female monster films that followed the release of *Cat People,* a cycle that would give rise to a series of more realist versions from 1944 onwards.[45] One of the key facets of this cycle was a central female protagonist with a divided personality and, therefore, in line with this cycle, the female lead of *The Wicked Lady* is described as "simultaneously Lady Skelton and doxy to a highwayman, [a woman who] dispatches three gents [and] causes others plenty of mental anguish."[46]

Similarly, *Madonna of the Seven Moons* was claimed to be "another one of the pseudo-psychological studies in which the heroine has a split personality,"[47] and hence clearly resonant with the horror cycle's psychological themes, particularly the female doubles that were a central feature of the female monster cycle. Certainly, the psychological themes were hardly taken seriously and it was claimed that Phyllis Calvert's performance had "a great deal more artistry and finesse than Roland Pertwee has displayed in his adaptation of the novel by Margery Lawrence."[48] Furthermore, it is claimed that his screenplay "piles one melodramatic incident on another" until the film "does not make much sense."[49] However, these criticisms of the psychological plot were fully consistent with those leveled at many other psychological films at the time, and the *New York Times* often accused films of using psychology to provide unconvincing explanations for implausible behavior. Furthermore, like Lady Skelton, Phyllis Calvert's Maddalena is not just psychologically disturbed but also a dual personality. If Lady Skelton "dons boots, mask, pistol and plumed hat and takes to the road," where she leads a double life as a highwaywoman,[50] it is "Maddalena's schizophrenia, which apparently brings out her evil nature" so that, "at intervals of six years," the "philanthropic" Maddalena "turns into a flashy and fiery temptress."[51]

However, the *New York Times*'s position in relation to psychological films was beginning to change. While most papers still associated psychological dramas with horror so that *The Lost Weekend* was described as a "realistic horror film,"[52] the film was also praised for its serious handling of a social problem, alcoholism.[53] Similarly, *The Seventh Veil* (1945, which was only released two weeks after *The Lost Weekend*) was singled out for its "adult" approach to the psychological film. As the *New York Times* observed, "Since Hollywood's movie makers have been fascinated lately by mental trauma, it is not surprising that British producers should also delve into the mysteries of the mind."[54] In this case, however, the response was not supposed to be preposterous but "an intelligent and engrossing case history" about "a concert pianist tortured by complexes" that proves to be "a suspenseful and unusual treatment of a challenging theme" and manages to achieve a "denouement [that] is, oddly enough, both surprising and sensible."[55]

It also stars James Mason as yet another sadistic male: a "grim bachelor guardian" who subjects his young female ward to "merciless discipline."[56] The *New York Times* even refers to him as "a Svengali like esthete" who acts as a "brooding, crippled mentor" to a young, female pianist who finds herself in a position of "strange subservience" to him.[57] Nor is it simply its status as a "meticulous dissertation of psychotherapy" or the presence of the dominating male that associates this film with the horror cycle of the 1940s. The *New York Times* explicitly associated the Svengali figure with horror. For example, in its review of *Jane Eyre,* the *New York Times* complained that the producers had "mainly gave way to the aspects of morbid horror" in their adaptation and, in so doing, had made "Jane a sort of bloodless Trilby" to Rochester so that she "becomes . . . a hypnotic under his Svengali spell, and exists in a world of shapeless horrors which are governed entirely by him."[58] *The Seventh Veil* even features a visual echo from *Rebecca*: a portrait of a dead woman that dominates the guardian's house when the ward first arrives. Nor was *The Seventh Veil* the only film to use such a device. *Rebecca* was the most requested release by women in the United States during this period,[59] and a number of films from 1944 to 1945 involved prominent portraits of dead or absent women: *Laura* (1944), *Phantom Lady* (1944), *The Uninvited* (1944), and, of course, *Woman in the Window* (1944).

Nor were the Gainsborough films the only productions that can be understood in this context. Powell and Pressburger's films are often identified as a key alternative to realism within British cinema, but despite often being described as visionary, imaginative, and even fantastic, these films are rarely associated with horror today. Sarah Street does acknowledge that in *The Red Shoes*: "Powell and Pressburger expose the horror that is latent if not explicit (as in Anderson) in fairytales."[60] But such observations are all too rare: even Hutchings, who identifies *A Canterbury Tale* as a horror-related item, makes no mention of other films from the team. However, *A Matter of Life and Death* (1946) was clearly seen as a "romantic fantasy with psychological tie-ins,"[61] which is "set in this world (graced with Technicolor), and the Other World (relegated to dye monochrome) as it exists in the mind of an airman whose imagination has been affected by concussion."[62]

Furthermore, it not only starred Kim Hunter, who had previously starred in *The Seventh Victim* (1943)—a film by one of the key figures of the 1940s psychological horror films, Val Lewton—but also its central narrative conflict is claimed to exist within the airman's "disordered mind,"[63] although like many of the psychological films, *A Matter of Life and Death* never actually resolves whether "the Other World" is simply "the world of his fantasies"[64] and hence whether it is "a brain operation" that finally resolves matters.[65]

Powell and Pressburger's next film, *Black Narcissus* (1947), is also "a curiously fascinating psychological study" but a far darker and more Gothic psychological.[66] If the *New York Times* concentrated on the film as a work of "rare pictorial beauty," in which "the whole chromatic scheme of the picture is marvelous to behold,"[67] it also acknowledged that the film "will disturb" some viewers, just as "the barbaric magnificence of the [Himalayas] . . . coupled with the high altitude and the constant, unnerving singing of the wind, produces deleterious physical and mental effects" in the group of nuns who are the film's central characters.[68] Furthermore, special mention is made of Kathleen Byron's role as "the unfortunate Sister Ruth," a figure who is "eventually overcome by her desire" and turns both mad and murderous.[69] For the *New York Times,* Byron's portrayal of Sister Ruth is "truly a magnificent performance,"[70] and *Variety* agreed, claiming that the "most effective acting comes from Kathleen Byron who has the picture's plum as the *neurotic half-crazed* Sister Ruth [emphasis added]."[71]

However, during this period, it is *The Red Shoes* (1948) that is the most insistently Gothic, psychological, and horror-related of Powell and Pressburger's films. The film features a sadistic male, the "ruthless Boris Lermontov" who is the "guiding genius" of the film's ballet company,[72] a part played by Anton Walbrook, who had played the viscous spouse in the British version of *Gaslight.* Furthermore, the story is explicitly one of psychological domination and virtually demonic possession. As the *New York Times* puts it, the film's story "about an English girl who devotes herself to a famous ballet company, becomes its star and then falls in love "is also" a symbolic realization of the principle ballet, which is based on Hans Christian Andersons's fable of the little girl who is bewitched by her red dancing shoes."[73] In this way, although it is not stated overtly, Lermontov, like Mason's musical mentor in *The Seventh Veil,* is clearly a Svengali figure, too.

David Lean adaptations of Dickens can also be seen in this context. For example, *Great Expectations* (1946) was one of the most revered British films of the period, of which it was claimed that "the British have done for Dickens what they did for Shakespeare with 'Henry V' "[74] and it was praised for its adaptation of the novel: the filmmakers had "caught it right down to the last shiver of a frightened youngster or the haughty flash in Estella's eye."[75] For the *New York Times,* then, the film was judged as a perfect adaptation but it was also described as a "thrilling" one that is filled with the elements of a Gothic nightmare.[76] If the reference to "the last shiver of a frightened youngster"[77] refers to the film's opening sequences in which Pip encounters the terrifying Magwitch in a cemetery and hears about Magwitch's dark nemesis, Lean's adaptations of Dickens are famous for their nightmarishly Gothic depiction of Victorian Britain, a depiction in which "mad Miss Havisham"[78] and her decaying Gothic mansion are a central element, so central that the film ends with the hero, Pip, overcoming Miss Havisham's possession of Estella and exorcising her presence from the house.

Oliver Twist (1948) is also claimed to have "an eerie atmosphere that immediately grips the imagination,"[79] although the *New York Times* spends much of its time defending the film from accusations of anti-Semitism.[80] In other words, it is argued that "the character of Fagin and the fact that he is a Jew . . . are mere part and parcel of the whole canvas of social injustice and degradation which is so brilliantly filled out in Charles Dickens' great work"[81] and that "it is this extraordinary canvas, this vast picture of poverty and greed which oppressed nineteenth century England, that has been magnificently reproduced in this film."[82] If the film is therefore praised for its "somber mood" and "visual elaboration of the underworld,"[83] in which "there is an extraordinary richness of flavor, suggestion and atmosphere,"[84] the film's portrayal of Fagin is justified on the grounds that it "is society that is indicated as the real villain,"[85] not Fagin: Fagin, it is argued, is simply presented as a product of his environment rather than his ethnicity. Consequently, the film receives outstanding praise as "one of the finest screen translations of a literary classic ever made."[86]

As we have seen, however, the standard against which the Lean adaptations were judged was Olivier's film of *Henry V* (1944), which remained a touchstone of quality for the *New York Times* for decades after,[87] as did Olivier's film version of *Hamlet* (1948) a few years later. Furthermore, this second adaptation clearly operated in relation to the 1940s horror cycle and interpreted the play as a Gothic psychological. Not only does it open with Olivier's voice informing the audience that Hamlet is "a man who could not make up his mind" but the film was seen as one that concerns the "dark and troubled workings of [Hamlet's] mind."[88] It was even directly associated with Freudian analysis. If his character is "difficult, even for Freudians,"[89] Olivier's Hamlet was claimed to be motivated more by "his wretched dismay at the treachery of his mother than the death of his father," while Ophelia is "a victim . . . of parent's deceit."[90]

Consequently, the story was seen as one in which the central character was "tormented by the anguish and the horror of a double shock,"[91] while the setting was described in Gothic terms as a "vast and gloomy palace,"[92] with "misty battlements" through which the "quietly-moving camera . . . wanders intently around . . . a silent observer of great events . . . and anxious not to miss any of them."[93] The camera was therefore seen as contributing to the spectral features of the plot, and the *New York Times* was referring to more than the Ghost of Hamlet's father when it observes: "the palace conceived for this 'Hamlet' is a dark and haunted palace. It is the grim and majestic setting for an uncommon galvanic film."[94] Sarah Street even notes that Universal gave it a general release in the United States, during which it was described as "The Greatest Ghost Story of Them All" and was "advertised with an accompanying caption: 'Shrouded mist, clad in rusty armor, a horrifying spectre stalks the great stone battlements of the ancient castle. Its one command is . . . kill . . . kill . . . KILL!' "[95]

To conclude, *Dead of Night,* then, was hardly an isolated British contribution to the 1940s horror cycle, although critics have since reclassified many of the other British films and so obscured their association with the cycle. However, an analysis of the reception context of these films during the 1940s not only demonstrates their association with the cycle at the time but also identifies themes within the film and relationships between them that have since been lost or ignored over the intervening period. The point here is not to assert that *Black Narcissus* or any other film is *really* a horror film but rather to examine how it was related to historically specific definitions of horror and of the monstrous, definitions that are historically contingent and had therefore significantly changed by the late 1960s and early 1970s, when academic canons of the genre began to be constructed.

NOTES

1. Ivan Butler, *The Horror Film* (London: Zwemmer, 1967), 73.
2. Butler, *The Horror Film,* 59.
3. David Pirie, *A Heritage of Horror: The English Gothic Cinema, 1946–1972* (London: Equinox, 1973), 22. Pirie's position does not significantly change by the time of the new edition in 2008 (London: I. B. Tarius).
4. Pirie, *A Heritage of Horror,* 24. See also Julian Petley, "The Lost Continent," in *All Our Yesterdays: 90 Years of British Cinema,* ed. Charles Barr (London: British Film Institute, 1986), 98–119.

5. Peter Hutchings, *Hammer and Beyond: The British Horror Film* (Manchester: Manchester University Press, 1993), 25.
6. Hutchings, *Hammer and Beyond,* 24.
7. Hutchings, *Hammer and Beyond,* 25.
8. Hutchings, *Hammer and Beyond,* 25.
9. Jonathan Rigby, *English Gothic: A Century of Horror Cinema* (London: Reynolds and Hearn, 2000), 24–26.
10. Rigby, *English Gothic,* 29.
11. It is worth noting that Rigby even provides evidence that it was *not* an aberration, and he mentions not only *The Ghost of St. Michael,* a horror-themed Will Hay comedy that Ealing made in 1941, but also "two ghoulish black comedies, Robert Hamer's *Kind Hearts and Coronets* (1949) and Alexander Mackendrick's *The Ladykillers* (1955)." See Rigby, *English Gothic,* 28.
12. Rigby, *English Gothic,* 28.
13. See Mark Jancovich, " 'Thrills and Chills': Horror, the Woman's Film and the Origins of Film Noir," *The New Review of Film and Television* 7, no. 2 (June 2009): 157–171.
14. Barbara Klinger, *Melodrama and Meaning: History, Culture, and the Films of Douglas Sirk* (Bloomington, IL: Indiana University Press, 1994), 69.
15. Jim Cunningham, "Creepy Pix Cleaning Up: Studios Cash in on Cycle," *Variety,* March 31, 1943, 46.
16. The size of this boom is quite astonishing, and in 1944–1946, about one-third of the feature films reviewed by *Variety* and the *New York Times* were associated with horror.
17. See Sarah Street, *Transatlantic Crossings: British Feature Films in the USA* (London: Continuum, 2002).
18. Anon, "*Dead of Night* Pressbook" (Universal, 1946): no pagination.
19. Fred Stanley, "Hollywood Shivers: The Studios Are Busily Stirring Up a Grade A Witches Brew—Other Items," *New York Times* 48, May 1944, X3.
20. See Mark Jancovich, " 'An Italianmade Spectacle Film Dubbed in English': Cultural Distinctions, National Cinema and the Critical Reception of the Postwar Historical Epic," in *The Epic Film in World Culture,* ed. Robert Burgoyne (New York: Routledge/American Film Institute, 2012), 161–175.
21. Stanley, "Hollywood Shivers," X3.
22. Bosley Crowther, " 'Phantom Lady,' a Melodrama of Weird Effects, with Ella Raines and Franchot Tone, Has Premiere at Loew's State," *New York Times,* February 18, 1944, 15.
23. Siegfried Kracauer, "Hollywood's Terror Films: Do They Reflect an American State of Mind," *New German Critique* 89 (2003): 107.
24. Kracauer, "Hollywood's Terror Films," 107.
25. E. Schallert, "New British Psycho Opus Fantastic," *Los Angeles Times,* August 8, 1946, A3.
26. Quoted in David Pirie, *A New Heritage of Horror: The English Gothic Cinema, Revised and Updated Edition* (London: I. B. Tauris, 2008), 16.
27. Pirie, *A New Heritage of Horror* (2008), 16.
28. Pirie, *A Heritage of Horror,* 23.
29. Pirie, *A Heritage of Horror,* 24.
30. Hutchings, *Hammer and Beyond,* 26.
31. Alan Burton and Tim O'Sullivan, *The Cinema of Basil Dearden and Michael Relph* (Edinburgh: Edinburgh University Press, 2009), 74.
32. Burton and O'Sullivan, *The Cinema of Basil Dearden and Michael Relph,* 75.
33. Hutchings, *Hammer and Beyond,* 26.
34. See Geoffrey MacNab, *J. Arthur Rank and the British Film Industry* (London: Routledge, 1993); Robert Murphy, *Realism and Tinsel: Cinema and Society in Britain 1939–1949* (London: Routledge, 1989); Vincent Porter, "Methodism versus the Market-Place: The Rank Organisation and British Cinema," in *The British Cinema Book,* ed. Robert Murphy (London: British Film Institute, 1997), 122–132; and Street, *Transatlantic Crossings.*
35. See Mark Jancovich, " 'Two Ways of Looking': The Critical Reception of 1940s Horror," *Cinema Journal* 49, no. 3 (2010): 45–66; and Street, *Transatlantic Crossings.*
36. *Rebecca* was not only set in England and directed by Hitchcock but starred Lawrence Olivier, Joan Fontaine, George Sanders, and numerous other British actors; *Suspicion* was also set in England,

directed by Hitchcock and featured numerous British actors. The same was also true of many others.

37. Bosley Crowther, "THE SCREEN: 'Dead of Night,' a British-Made Film, Is Premiere at Winter Garden—Rialto Offers New Melodrama by Fox Studios," *New York Times,* June 29, 1946, 22.
38. Talb., "Dead of Night," *Variety,* September 19, 1945, 12.
39. Bosley Crowther, "The 'Ten Best'—Five Foreign Films Among the 1946 Leaders," *New York Times,* December 29, 1947, 11.
40. Bosley Crowther, "The Screen: A Costume Picture," *New York Times,* November 30, 1945, 18.
41. Talb., "The Wicked Lady," *Variety,* November 28, 1945, 10.
42. A.W., "At the Winter Garden," *New York Times,* December 23, 1946, 19.
43. A.W., "At the Winter Garden," 19.
44. A.W., "At the Winter Garden," 19.
45. See Mark Jancovich, "Female Monsters: Horror, the 'Femme Fatale' and World War II," *European Journal of American Culture* 27 (2008): 133–149.
46. A.W., "At the Winter Garden," 19.
47. T.M.P., " 'Madonna of the Seven Moons,' British Importation Starring Phyllis Calvert in Two Roles, Is New Bill at Winter Garden," *New York Times,* May 23, 1946, 18.
48. T.M.P., " 'Madonna of the Seven Moons,' " 18.
49. T.M.P., " 'Madonna of the Seven Moons,' " 18.
50. A.W., "At the Winter Garden," 19.
51. T.M.P., " 'Madonna of the Seven Moons,' " 18.
52. Kate Cameron, " 'Lost Weekend' Daring Film of Drunk's Orgy," in *New York Motion Picture Critics Reviews 1945* (New York: Critics' Theatre Reviews, Inc., 1945), 90.
53. Bosley Crowther, " 'The Lost Week-End,' in Which Ray Milland Presents a Study in Dipsomania, Makes Its Appearance at the Rivoli," *New York Times,* December 3, 1945, 28.
54. Bosley Crowther, "Screen in Review: Six New Films Arrive on the Holiday in Midtown Houses—Gene Tierney Appears in 'Leave Her to Heaven' at Roxy Cornered with Dick Powell, at Palace—'Seventh Veil,' a British Picture, Makes Its Debut at Winter Garden," *New York Times,* December 26, 1945, 15.
55. Crowther, "Screen in Review," 15.
56. Talb., "The Seventh Veil," *Variety,* October 31, 1945, 17.
57. Crowther, "Screen in Review," 15.
58. Bosley Crowther, " 'Jane Eyre,' A Sombre Version of the Bronte Novel, with Joan Fontaine and Orson Welles, Opens at the Music Hall," *New York Times,* February 4, 1944, 12.
59. See George Gallup and Associates, "ARI Report 163, Princeton 25th July," in *Gallup Looks at the Movies: Audience Research Reports 1940–1950* (Delaware: Scholarly Resources, 1979).
60. Sarah Street, *British National Cinema: 2* (London: Routledge, 2008), 201.
61. Bosley Crowther, "Screen in Review: 'Stairway to Heaven,' a British Production at Park Avenue, Proves Holiday Delight," *New York Times,* December 26, 1946, 28.
62. Cane, "Stairway to Heaven," *Variety,* November 13, 1946, 16.
63. Crowther, "Screen in Review," 28.
64. Crowther, "Screen in Review," 28.
65. Crowther, "Screen in Review," 28.
66. Thomas M. Pryor, "Black Narcissus," *New York Times,* August 14, 1947, 29.
67. Pryor, "Black Narcissus," 29.
68. Pryor, "Black Narcissus," 29.
69. Pryor, "Black Narcissus," 29.
70. Pryor, "Black Narcissus," 29.
71. Cane, "Black Narcissus," *Variety,* May 7, 1947, 18.
72. Anon, "The Red Shoes," *Variety,* August 4, 1948, 11.
73. Bosley Crowther, "The Screen in Review: 'The Red Shoes' a British Film About the Ballet, Stars Moira Shearer at Bijou," *New York Times,* October 23, 1948, 9.
74. Bosley Crowther, " 'Great Expectations,' in Which British Producers Do Very Well by Charles Dickens, Makes Its Bow at Radio City," *New York Times,* May 23, 1947, 31.

75. Crowther, "'Great Expectations,'" 31.
76. Crowther, "'Great Expectations,'" 31.
77. Crowther, "'Great Expectations,'" 31.
78. Crowther, "'Great Expectations,'" 31.
79. Anon, "Oliver Twist," *Variety,* June 30, 1948, 10.
80. Bosley Crowther, "The Screen in Review: 'Oliver Twist,' Rank Film Based on Charles Dickens Novel, at Park Avenue Theatre," *New York Times,* July 31, 1951, 17.
81. Crowther, "The Screen in Review," 17.
82. Crowther, "The Screen in Review," 17.
83. Crowther, "The Screen in Review," 17.
84. Crowther, "The Screen in Review," 17.
85. Crowther, "The Screen in Review," 17.
86. Crowther, "The Screen in Review," 17.
87. See Jancovich, "'An Italianmade Spectacle Film Dubbed in English.'"
88. Bosley Crowther, "Lawrence Olivier's 'Hamlet' Bows at the Park Avenue Theatre—'Saxon Charm' Seen," *New York Times,* September 30, 1948, 32.
89. Crowther, "Lawrence Olivier's 'Hamlet' Bows at the Park Avenue Theatre," 32.
90. Crowther, "Lawrence Olivier's 'Hamlet' Bows at the Park Avenue Theatre," 32.
91. Crowther, "Lawrence Olivier's 'Hamlet' Bows at the Park Avenue Theatre," 32.
92. Crowther, "Lawrence Olivier's 'Hamlet' Bows at the Park Avenue Theatre," 32.
93. Crowther, "Lawrence Olivier's 'Hamlet' Bows at the Park Avenue Theatre," 32.
94. Crowther, "Lawrence Olivier's 'Hamlet' Bows at the Park Avenue Theatre," 32.
95. Street, *Transatlantic Crossings,* 108.

Section II

Teratologies of Nationality and Race

CHAPTER 6

MONSTERS IN THE LITERARY TRADITIONS OF ASIA: A CRITICAL APPRAISAL

ANDREW HOCK-SOON NG

INTRODUCTION

There are few texts that have become foundational in the literary and cultural traditions of Asia. They may have originated in a particular region at one point in ancient history, but through political infiltration, trade, and the spread of religion, these texts have entered and become incorporated into the cultural imaginations of the different regions throughout the continent. They are altered to become aligned to specific environments and audiences. And their influence continues unabated even into the twenty-first century. For example, the Indian epic *The Ramayana* of Valmiki (possibly fourth century B.C.) is also an integral part of Southeast Asian literature today. Wu Cheng-en's *Journey to the West* (sixteenth century) is an epic novel familiar throughout the Chinese diaspora, while *Tales from the Arabian Nights* (consolidated by the fifteenth century, with some tales dating to as early as the tenth century) remains the representative narrative of the Middle East. Interestingly, a fundamental feature in all these texts is the predominance of monsters.[1]

The aim of this chapter is to consider the typology, functions, and transformations of monsters in the literary traditions of Asia. The three texts mentioned earlier occupy much of my discussion, but I will also look at folk- and morality tales to supplement my analysis. These tales provide a glimpse into the richness of the monster's signifying properties, often in ironic and paradoxical ways. I begin my foray into monsters in the literary traditions of Asia by discussing the extent to which Asian literatures treat monsters rather differently from their Western counterparts. If Western narratives tend to construct the monster via a binary logic that subscribes it to a dangerous alterity that must, at best, be rehabilitated, or otherwise annihilated, Asian literatures, with their encompassing worldviews, are more nuanced in their treatment of monsters. In fact, monsters in Asian narratives are rarely evil in an absolute sense, and they become transgressive usually either because of their refusal to comply with their allotted responsibilities as prescribed by the dominant structuring order (almost always religion) or because they harbor forbidden desires. In fact, Asian literatures often distinguish an *evil* monster by identifying it as a demon. This pattern seems consistent throughout the continent, whatever the literary traditions may be. It is this transition to the demonic that marks the monster's divergence from its predetermined place and function in the order of things. It is quite clear, therefore, that monsters are not a menace to, but form part of, religio-ideological structures. In fact, as I will demonstrate in my discussion of various narratives, the monster is sometimes the principal instrument necessary to reinforce these structures. Monsters in Asian literary traditions play varied functions, and as such, possess a wider significance than those of the West. Reading selected Asian narratives against the religio-ideological traditions from which they are derived and juxtaposing their monsters against Western perspectives of monstrosity, I demonstrate in the first part of this chapter how Asian monsters are more representative of what the term "monster," as implied in its Latin root, means: an "omen from God."[2]

One abiding characteristic of any monster is its paradoxical quality. Despite its alterity, the monster is also often an intimate stranger, whose proximity to "us" at once problematizes our notions of humanness and allegiance. If the monster is so much like "us," then what ultimately guarantees our difference from it? Moreover, if difference, as Deleuze asserts, is merely a "disguise" affected by the symbolic to reinforce repetition, sameness, and the self-same, then the monster, rather than the other, is actually a continuum or an extension of the self. The monster, following this view, is therefore not a "variation" that "come[s] from without," but a "differential [mechanism] which belong[s] to the essence and origin of that which is repeated."[3] In other words, rather than external to the status quo, monsters are actually produced by it, but in a way that also guarantees their otherness and danger to the status quo. Yet, monsters are ambiguous; even while they submit to the ideological status quo, they are also subtly subverting it. They are paradoxes that can simultaneously conform to and undermine the meanings imposed upon them at any given sociocultural and/or historical moment. The second part of my chapter discusses how monsters represent such a paradox by analyzing a tale from *Arabian Nights* and the short story "A Dream of Wolves," by the seventeenth-century master of macabre Chinese tales, Pu Songling. In the case of the latter, I further demonstrate how monstrosity is not merely a content of the story, but is, through formal techniques of self-reflexivity, the story itself.

The third part of my chapter wrestles with a conundrum: how is it that Asian writings today, despite their rich traditions in monster narratives, have made almost no significant innovations to these traditions? While ghost stories are currently undergoing a significant revival throughout Asia, most obviously in films that have gained international and critical acclaim, little has been done to promote the return of monsters apart from a few disparate works, such as the Godzilla films of Japan. One may argue that this is not necessarily the case, for many Asian films also feature beings that exhibit monstrous qualities. Yet such creatures are often more aligned with ghosts rather than monsters in any clear sense, as exemplified in the so-called monsters popular in contemporary Southeast Asian horror films. While it is arguable that creatures like the *pontianak,* the *kuntilanak,* and the *pocong* can be called monsters, the local term in Malaysia and Indonesia, for example, is the generic *hantu,* which means ghost. Undoubtedly, the historical developments experienced throughout the continent in the last century, although very different from country to country, have one thing in common: they have induced an effacement of monster texts from their cultural imaginary. Whether it is colonialism, aggressive Islamization, or Communism, these sociopolitical mechanisms have dealt a terrific blow to monsters in Asian literature. It is only recently that monster narratives have witnessed a return to Asia. I conclude this chapter by considering the handful of contemporary Asian narratives that feature monsters in prominent ways: Salman Rushdie's *Shame* (1983) and Ma Jian's novel *Beijing Coma* (2008). Like their literary predecessors, these texts continue to deploy monsters for "cultural work"[4] and retain their most powerful qualities—as paradox and ambiguity—to do this.

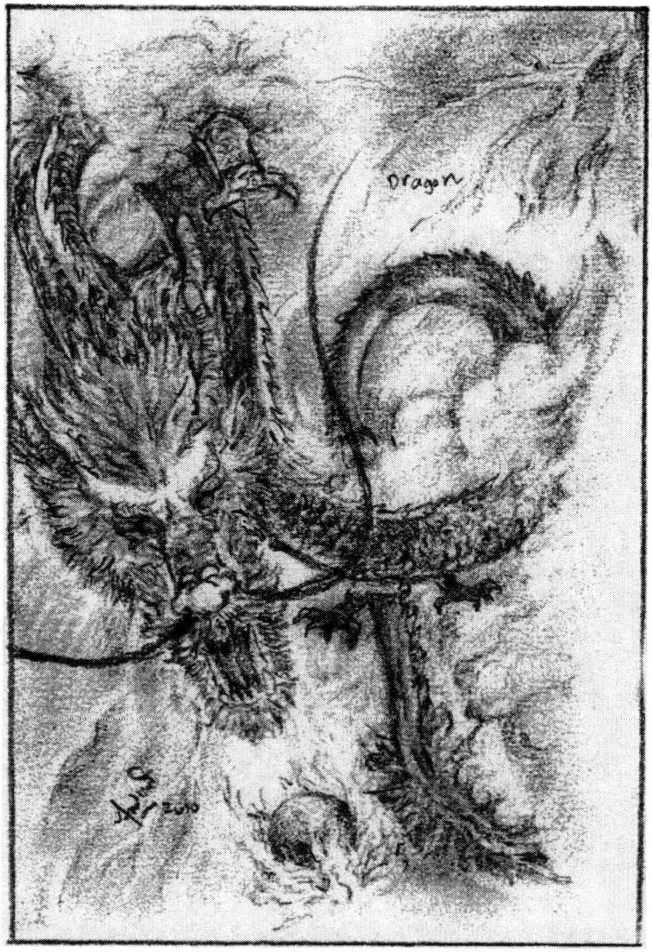

Figure 6.1 Pencil sketch of a mythological dragon. (Courtesy of Andrew Hock-Soon Ng.)

THE NECESSITY OF MONSTERS

There are features shared by both Eastern and Western conceptions of teratology that help delineate a monster. The first involves anomalies in measurement. The dragon (see Figure 6.1), for example, perhaps the most famous monster in Oriental myths, is a creature that began life as snake, but has, over an extended period of time, attained astronomical accentuation in both size and age. One classical Chinese text explains it this way: "A water snake after five hundred years changes into a *kiao* [a fish-like dragon], a *kiao* after a thousand years changes into a *lung* [dragon], a *lung* after five hundred years changes a *kioh lung* [horned dragon], and a *kioh lung* after another thousand years into a *ying lung* [winged dragon]."[5] Such anomalies result in a "confusion of categories"[6] and render familiar methods of measurement useless. Although exorbitant in age and size, the dragon remains snake-like in form; in this way, this creature simultaneously defies differentiation from, and similarity to, any known creature, and thus becomes by default a monster. Another aspect that characterizes both Western and Asian monsters is their association with the sublime. The dragon, according to anthropologist F. J. Daniels, owes much of its monstrous quality to its ability to elicit such "heightened emotion" that can sometimes culminate in a "fever."[7] Daniels equates this emotion with fear, but I am inclined to argue that it is more "awe," which is directly related to the sublime. In the West, the sublime as a philosophical category has long been associated with the monstrous. Merging otherwise contrasting emotions of dread and desire (or as Kearney puts it, an "admixture of horror and exuberance"[8]), the sublime occasions a heightening of the self to the point that the mind, or rationality, collapses, and the self is temporarily paralyzed. This view is not dissimilar to Daniels's reason for labeling the dragon a monster. As a sublime object, the dragon thus bears dualistic qualities that further reinforce the paradoxical nature embodied by monsters. Its presence may signal good fortune or divine retribution, good or ill omen. In Oriental myths, dragons manage the seasons and cure diseases,[9] and also cause eclipses, draughts, and protracted rainfalls that lead to floods.[10]

But unlike their Western counterparts, monsters in Asian literary traditions are rarely classified as an absolute alterity against which the self must guard. If monsters in the Western imagination, as Foucault argues, break the continuum in nature that guarantees transition from lower to higher life-forms, to instead "[ensure] the emergence of difference,"[11] monsters in Eastern narratives are actually part of the continuum and have a function in demonstrating, on the one hand, a hierarchy of beings, whereby the natural/supernatural, good/evil logic is rendered irrelevant, and, on the other, the panoply of beings possible in such a hierarchy, within which there is no "other," but only an assortment of levels, or facets, of "self." Foucault goes on to claim that transgressing "natural limits," "classification," and "the law of the table" is not enough to constitute the monstrous.[12] To qualify as true monstrosity, the being must ultimately:

> fall under, or at any rate challenge, an interdiction of civil and religious or divine law. There is monstrosity only when the confusion comes up against, overturns, or disturbs civil, canon, or religious law. The difference between disability and monstrosity is revealed at the meeting point, the point of friction, between a breach of the natural law-table and a breach of the law instituted by God or by society, at the point where these two breaches of law come together. Disability may well be something that upsets the natural order, but disability is not monstrosity because it has a place in civil or canon law.... Monstrosity, however, is the kind of natural irregularity that calls law into question and disables it.[13]

Clearly, the monster results in the breakdown of the classificatory discourse that is premised on the twin law of the civil and the divine. In fact, in the Judeo-Christian faith, the civil and divine are symbiotically related. With its strict definitions of limits, normalcy, and notions of self—all of which operate on the regulation of sameness—the law, as such, renders anomalous and alien anything that falls outside its rigid parameters; whatever is aberrant becomes, by logical extension, dangerous and a menace that must be countered and/or destroyed. It is not surprising therefore that the monster is eventually aligned with "evil." As Richard Kearney puts it, "Ever since early Western thought equated Good with notions of self-identity and sameness, the experience of evil has often been linked with notions of exteriority. Almost invariably, otherness was considered in terms of an estrangement which contaminates the pure unity of the soul."[14] Because the monster contravenes the neatness of the law of the table by calling into question its limitations and "irregularity," it directly challenges the supremacy of the latter and thus, invariably becomes an embodiment of otherness, a signifier of "estrangement" that must either be coerced and fitted back into the table or eliminated altogether so that the sanctity of the law is preserved.

Such a development of the monster in the Western imagination is ironic in view of the fact that the monster, as indicated by the term's Latin roots, actually means "omen from God," and whose presence serves as a warning to a community of its mounting sinfulness. The monster, as Alain Grosrichard notes, is "a divine sign of an impending threat or punishment."[15] Its function is to speak, or even embody, a truth that can only come from God, and if it is ignored will result in a divine judgment and catastrophe. The literary imagination of the West, at least since Christianity, has instead transformed the monster into a being that opposes the divine. While Greek and Nordic legends display a more varied representation of monsters, ranging from friend to foe, and constantly remind the readers that monsters are, in the end, part of the divine order and often render important services to it, monster narratives since Christianity's permeation of Europe seem to have forsaken this heritage. Instead, monsters are consistently cast as evil henceforth, and as the means by which the protagonist gains either ascendancy or ruin. In Gothic narratives popular in the eighteenth and nineteenth centuries, monsters that populate this genre—psychopaths (such as Stevenson's Mr. Hyde), vampires, and other unspeakable creatures—are beyond the pale of salvation. Their destruction (often via the mechanism of the Christian religion, or its philosophical handmaiden, scientific rationality) is ascertained so that "we" who are humans and aligned to the divine can survive and thrive. Even monsters that could gain the reader's sympathy, such as the creature in Shelley's *Frankenstein* (1818), must in the end be denied such a potential, thereby foreclosing whatever redemption that they may be afforded. Frankenstein's monster may be a metaphor for *hubris;* but he is ultimately Victor's unholy child, not God's messenger, which renders the creature an abomination before God (twice over, as an abominable creation and an extension of Victor's iniquity).

By contrast, monsters in Asian literary traditions rarely suffer such a fate. The ideological premises upon which these narratives stand are drawn from worldviews that eschew binary logic, promoting instead a more encompassing religio-ethical structure that can embrace an endless continuum of beings. As noted earlier, only monsters labeled as demons are considered evil, which suggests that there are good monsters as well—an oxymoron impossible in the Western religious and literary imaginations. For example, *Journey to the West,* one of the most beloved *bildungsroman* in Chinese literary history, is an epic narrative whose three principle protagonists are all monsters. Monkey, Piggy, and Sandy subscribe to William's definition of the monster in that they confuse categories and destabilize differentiation and similarity; for while all three resemble humans, they also manifest profoundly bestial (as evidenced by their names) and unnatural qualities (prior to their enlistment as monk Tripitaka's disciples, Sandy and Piggy were known to consume human flesh), and yet have an immense propensity for goodness, loyalty, and compassion despite their compromising histories. Along their journey to India to retrieve a valuable sutra, these three monsters must battle a host of demonic creatures to protect their master. But even their antagonists are never irredeemably evil. The underlying and controlling structure of *Journey* is Buddhism, and with its emphasis on compassion and regard for the sanctity of all life, including those of wicked beings, the many confrontations between a monkey and his brothers with the demons merely serve as fundamental occasions for the assertion of Buddhism's supremacy. The good gains merit, while evil is rehabilitated and assimilated back into an abiding, merciful structure.

Laurie Cozad postulates that the demons in *Journey* can be divided into three "types," with each successive type more powerful and therefore more threatening to the regulating structure than the preceding one. The first, of which the Green Buffalo demon is an example,[16] are lesser demons who have attained limited supernatural abilities through self-cultivation, and proceed to use them to vex the status quo. The second deliberately uses wayward alchemic practices to attain individual power and glory at the expense of Buddhist teachings and communal well-being. More than just monsters, such demons are also "god-like,"[17] in their capacity to substantially disrupt the cosmological structure. Examples include the Black Bear demon and the Red Boy.[18] The third type is the most threatening because it not only worries the structure but also has the potential to replace it with an alternative one. Interestingly, it is Monkey himself who, for Cozad, represents this final type. Utterly impervious to authority and almost impossible to subdue by even the most powerful deities, the only way he can be put to service is by permitting his pursuit of demonic activities, but in such a way that it helps reinforce the dominant structure. Thus, Tripitaka's purity is unsullied and his mission fulfilled because Monkey is present to perform the "necessary dirty deeds—killing monsters, fighting demons, stealing everything from food and drink to magical treasures, coercing intransigent gods, and engaging in trickery with all and sundry"[19]—that is, deeds expressively shunned by Buddhism because they imply submission to base desires. Monkey, in other words, must embody the necessary evil to guarantee Tripitaka's success.

Cozad's treatment of "demonic others" in *Journey* is particularly valuable because she demonstrates the way in which the abiding ideological structure informs the constructions and functions of monsters and demons in the narrative. Because the Buddhist cosmological order is vast and encompassing, there is no demon/monster type or embodiment that cannot, in the end, be integrated into the order again. All three types of monsters are, without exception, either rehabilitated or put in service of the divine order, or both, by the end of each episode. The first type will repent and resume its original form (usually an animal), while the second will, willingly (Black Bear demon) or through divine coercion (Red Boy), enter the service of a powerful Buddhist deity. Rob Campany, in his essay, wonders why demons in *Journey* "almost invariably [always] appear in the same, predictable way."[20] The answer is obvious: it is to depict the infinite structure that characterizes Buddhist cosmogony and, more importantly, the ethical imperatives that prohibit even demons from falling beyond the pale of the structure's compassion. In Buddhism, there is no "other," only a self that takes on a hierarchy of different guises before finally reaching enlightenment.

A somewhat similar ideology also operates in the Hindu epic, *The Ramayana.*[21] Like Buddhism, Hindu cosmogony also promotes a boundless structure that is inclusive of manifold creatures. Each creature birthed into existence is accompanied by *dharma,* or divine duty, for which he or she is responsible in his or her lifetime. The fulfillment of one's dharma sustains the rightness of the Hindu cosmic order; as such, to evade or refuse his or her preordained destiny is impossible because even such an act *is already constitutive* of the transgressor's dharma. This paradox is elegantly captured in the following passage from the Bhagavad-Gita: "One's own dharma, performed imperfectly, is better than another's dharma well performed. Destruction in one's own dharma is better, for to perform another's dharma leads to danger" (3.35).[22] In other words, so distinct is each creature's dharma that even if it means self-destruction, she must pursue it. The satisfactory execution of a creature's prescribed responsibility during her lifetime brings good karma, which guarantees better reincarnation, or even liberation (*moksha*) altogether from the cycle of rebirths (*samsara*). Understood in this perspective, that the ten-headed, twenty-armed demon-lord Ravana (see Figure 6.2) in *The Ramayana* is set on a course that will end with his destruction and the annihilation of his civilization is, in truth, the fulfillment of his dharma. Despite the many warnings by sages of the gravity of abducting Sita, Rama's wife, Ravana cannot waver from his divine destiny, but must pursue it valiantly to the end.

Notwithstanding the appellation of "demon-lord" prescribed to Ravana, and his role as a nearly indomitable arch-nemesis in one of Asia's most beloved and familiar epics, what is often missed or understated is the fact that Ravana is also a devout follower of Brahma, from whom a boon that sustains his mortality is obtained (but as with all boons in myths, there is a caveat that Rama will discover and exploit to his advantage). In R. K. Narayan's modern retelling of Ravana's story, for example, the reader is told that the demon "sat in *tapas* for a thousand years" in order to "acquire strength and merit through proper penance."[23] It is this tenacious display of piety that finally warmed Brahma to the monster, thus encouraging him to grant

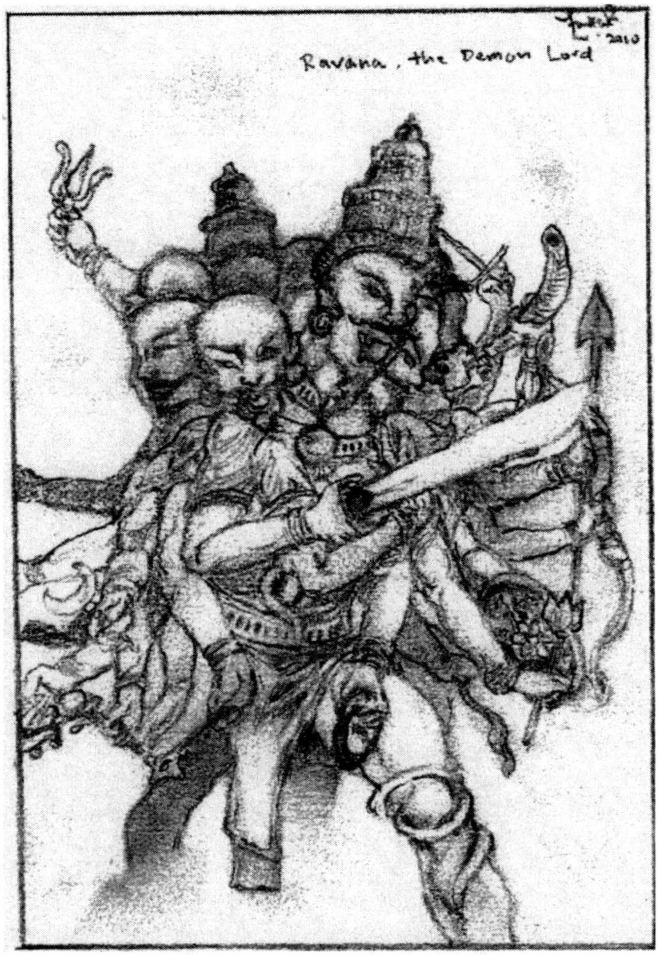

Figure 6.2 Pencil sketch of the mythological demon-lord Ravana. (Courtesy of Andrew Hock-Soon Ng.)

Ravana his request. Moreover, Ravana is also covered with the "grace of Shiva" that further endows him "with eminence and power."[24] Even after he has abducted Sita, Ravana never once devalues himself by asserting force on Sita; instead, he waits for and pleads with her patiently with the hope that she may eventually yield to his gentle persuasions. Such intermittent portrayals of Ravana show that the monster, rather than an embodiment of radical, unqualified evil, is actually a devout Hindu whose ascendance is an outcome of his religious practices. But dharma has ordained his self-destruction and the sacrifice of his kingdom (Lanka) and people, so that Rama can establish his renown. For this to happen, Ravana must necessarily assume malevolence.

Evident from the discussion is the fact that the textual construction of monsters is profoundly guided and influenced by the dominant ideological structure governing the narrative performance. In the West, the binary logic of the Christian faith can only allow otherness to be construed as aberrant and evil. Eastern worldview, in which philosophies advocating strict dichotomies are rare, incorporates monsters as part of the continuum of living creatures. If a monster is vicious, it is necessarily so because it sustains the correct order of things. In fact, as demonstrated in both *Journey* and *The Ramayana,* because the monster has willingly and faithfully performed his duties, he will receive his just reward. Rama commands his people to honor Ravana and to cherish his memory, "so that his spirit may go to heaven, where he has *his place* [my emphasis]."[25] With the fulfillment of his responsibility to be evil incarnate, Ravana, as Narayan euphemistically implies, attains moksha.[26] Monkey, at the end of the journey, becomes a Buddha, thus joining a host of other monsters who have, through religious acts and good deeds, achieved everlasting enlightenment.[27] Such a denouement, in which a monster becomes reinscribed as deity is consonant with Bernard Faure's evaluation of the trickster figure in Buddhism's literary tradition (more specifically Zen Buddhism); here, the prominence of Bodhisattvas "emphasizes both the monastic rule and social norms. The proximity of one of these poles, or the predominance of any one of these components, has permitted a heuristic classification of these ideal figures in the categories of the thaumaturge, the trickster, or the Bodhisattva—at the risk of creating another 'fraudulent narrative'."[28] Monkey (whom Faure does not discuss) is, as noted earlier, a "fraudulent" power able to subvert the existing status quo; to disallow this from occurring, he is transformed into another "ideal figure," one who

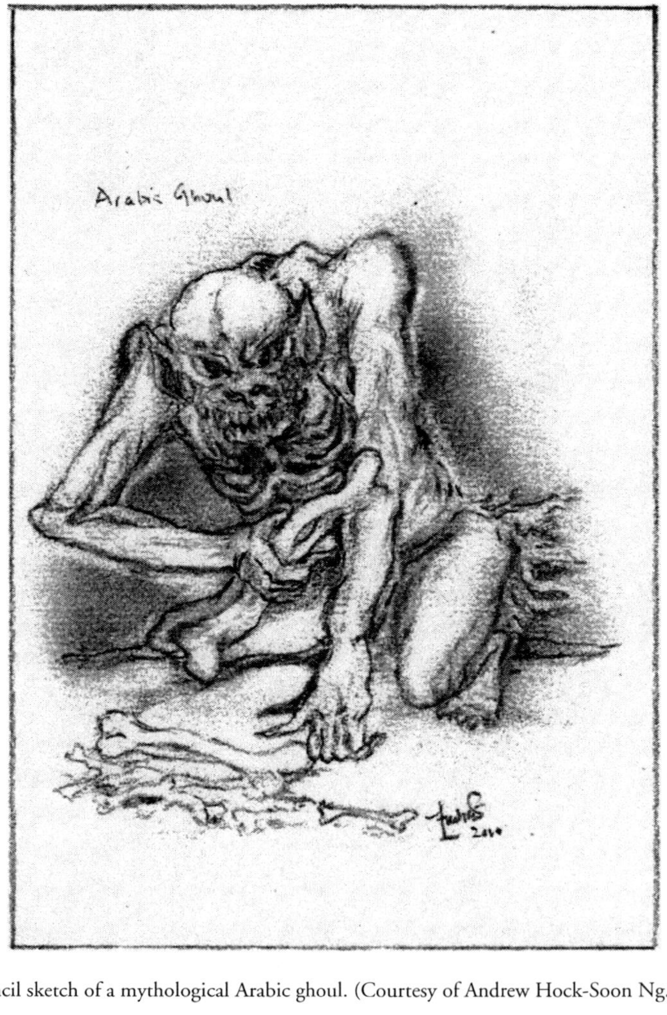

Figure 6.3 Pencil sketch of a mythological Arabic ghoul. (Courtesy of Andrew Hock-Soon Ng.)

surprisingly elevates the trickster to the Bodhisattva figure, thus suggesting the close proximity of both figures within Buddhism's heuristic classification.

Such nuanced treatments of monsters in Asian narratives cannot, however, be solely attributed to the fact that they hail from Buddhist or Hindu-influenced literary traditions. Even Arabic literature, heavily determined by Islam, is quite comprehensive in its representation of monsters, thus confounding the theory that monsters are absolutely evil only insofar when they operate within a theistic worldview. The ghoul (see Figure 6.3), a familiar monster in oral narratives throughout the Middle East—despite its etymological root (*ghāl,* "to kill"[29]) and penchant for human flesh—is rarely an evil creature in Arabic folklore. Stories such as "The Bird of the Golden Feather" (Syrian origin) and "A Tale within a Tale" (Iraqi origin) feature ghouls who aid the protagonist in his quest; others like "The Woodcutter's Wealthy Sister" foreground a ghoul whose evil is a form of divine retribution visited on a gluttonous man. Closer to *Journey* is "A Lost Shoe of Gold" (from Saudi Arabia),[30] in which the ghoul, reminiscent of the pantheon of monsters in the Chinese epic, reinforces the supremacy of the dominant ideological structure. In this story, the ghoul uses all manner of horrifying assaults (destruction of family, alleged infanticide) in order to coerce a woman into reneging on an oath. Nevertheless, she remains steadfast in her promise. The ghoul eventually reveals that he has been sent to test her faith in God and the story ends happily for the woman, whose wealth, family, and good name are all restored to her. Unlike Christianity, whose dominance in Europe beginning in the fifth century concurrently marked the monster as uncategorizable and therefore "other and evil", the spread of Islam (under the Ottoman Empire that began in the thirteenth century) in the Middle East and beyond actually provided monsters in the region's oral history with new significances and functions without divesting them of their former ones. Thus, like their Asian cousins, ghouls can be evil or benevolent and religious. If ghouls are primarily associated with iniquity today, it is, as I will argue later, because of the corrupting impact of colonialism.

MONSTER IN/AS TEXT

In an essay on monster theory, Jeffrey Jerome Cohen suggests that monsters are discursive products that must "be examined within the intricate matrix of relations (social, cultural, and literal historical) that generate them."[31] Monsters, in other words, reflect their historical moments; appreciation of the former's interpretive possibilities would entail an understanding of contemporary sociocultural contexts, without which the monster's variegated meanings cannot be fully apprehended. Take Bram Stoker's celebrated Gothic novel, for example. That *Dracula* can incorporate signifiers of anti-Semitic sentiments, homoeroticism, premodernity, and decadence (among others) is precisely because these were some of the issues confronting the nineteenth-century *fin-de-siècle.* Yet Dracula is a monster indistinguishable from its human victims, whose bloodlust and will-to-power could equally be interpreted (psychoanalytically) as the unconscious and destructive drives that belie our subjective formation, or, as Franco Moretti convincingly demonstrates in his Marxist reading of the novel, the motivation behind capitalism's rise and potency.[32] Dracula may be other, but he is also very much the mirror of the self as he exposes hidden levels of our identities, and our allegiance to a regulating system that operates on the premise of transforming the human into labor (the undead). Inhabiting the threshold that separates "us" from "them," and reflecting cultural anxieties while also deflecting their immediacy, Dracula clearly exemplifies that paradoxical characteristic peculiar to monsters, whose porosity defines, even as it exposes, the insecurity and instability of limits.[33]

In this respect, Asian monsters are no different from their Western cousins. To illustrate, I turn to a familiar, if little analyzed, tale from the *Arabian Nights.* This brief story of the monster called the "Old Man of the Sea" forms part of Sinbad's account of his fifth voyage.

Shipwrecked, Sinbad is marooned on an island where he encounters "an old man bent and feeble sitting upon the river bank,"[34] who implores Sinbad to carry him across the river. Sinbad complies out of pity, but soon realizes, to his horror, that his burden is not human at all, but a "terrible . . . creature"[35] who clings unyieldingly to his bearer until the latter dies of exhaustion. Sinbad, however, manages to trick the creature into consuming a fruit that induces inebriation, and while the "old monster"[36] is drunk and loosens his grip, Sinbad, "with one vigorous effort threw him to the ground from which he never moved again."[37] On one level, this story evidently reinforces the protagonist's heroism and resourcefulness in the face of adversity; yet, if the Sinbad tales are carefully examined in light of the ideological field (i.e., Islam) from which they originate, they will reveal that Molan's promotion, in fact, does not accord with what is implied in the narrative.[38] Molan's assertion, with which I am inclined to agree, is that Sinbad, now a wealthy and elderly merchant, tells his stories to any willing listener because he is trying to atone for his sinful and violent past, reminiscent of Coleridge's ancient mariner. But unlike the mariner, Sinbad's motivation behind repeatedly recounting his adventures is not a sign of being cursed, but his failure to confront his ghosts. Proud and with his reputation at stake, his accounts will always fall short of exposing the evil he has perpetrated on others in his quest (or greed) for wealth and fame. His stories, as such, are performances of self-justification that serve to accentuate his heroism, which then necessitate the transformation of his victims into enemies and monsters.[39]

Molan does not discuss the story of the Old Man in his essay, but his theory is a useful framework against which this monster's paradoxical quality can be demonstrated. As noted, monsters can serve as the self's metaphorical mirror, which must nevertheless be positioned as other to screen the self from confronting her own unacknowledgeable desires. Following this, it is therefore possible to read the Old Man as Sinbad's projection of his depravity onto an externalized, monstrous embodiment. Several clues support this interpretation. First, it is telling that the monster is cast as an "old" man. While a young, or disabled creature, could serve the plot equally well, the monster, as an emanation of Sinbad's unconscious, cannot be anything else except a figure imaged after him, but strategically differentiated so as to disguise any direct resemblance (Deleuze's concept of repetition is especially pertinent here). Since Sinbad is "noble," "venerable," and altogether magnificent,[40] the monster must be feeble, pitiable, and ultimately cruel. Second, the virulence of the monster lies in its greed (he eats endlessly) and enslavement or destruction of victims in order to satisfy this greed; however, these are traits that also characterize Sinbad, as evident in his sometimes brutal exploitation of others to attain what he wants. The account of his fourth voyage, in which he massacres countless innocent people (an act especially reprehensible to Islam[41]) in order to appropriate their valuables[42] is especially pronounced. Finally, that the monster is a burden Sinbad must carry until trickery exonerates him is perhaps the most telling, if subtle, parallel that links the two of them. If we replace old man/burden with sin and trickery with storytelling, it becomes clear that the very strategy Sinbad employs to gain spiritual reprieve, ironically, also undercuts that attempt. He may tell it to justify and aggrandize himself, but the story is also, unconsciously, his confession. Herein, then, is the ultimate paradox of the tale: it is not the Old Man that is the true monster, *but Sinbad himself.* His story may disguise this fact, but each repeated recounting only damns the storyteller further.

Sinbad's tale allows us to see how a monster can infiltrate a text to the extent that the latter ends up embodying the former. As excess, monsters not only defy any attempts to classify or circumscribe them (such as through storytelling), but radically render the mechanisms that seek to contain them monstrous as well in the process. Pu Songling's "A Dream of Wolves," on the other hand, suggests that the monster text is particularly effective when form and content are inseparable, thus dislodging any stable interpretation even as the text instigates them. Written during a politically and socially unstable climate (early Qing dynasty, ca. 1600–1700), Pu's stories are

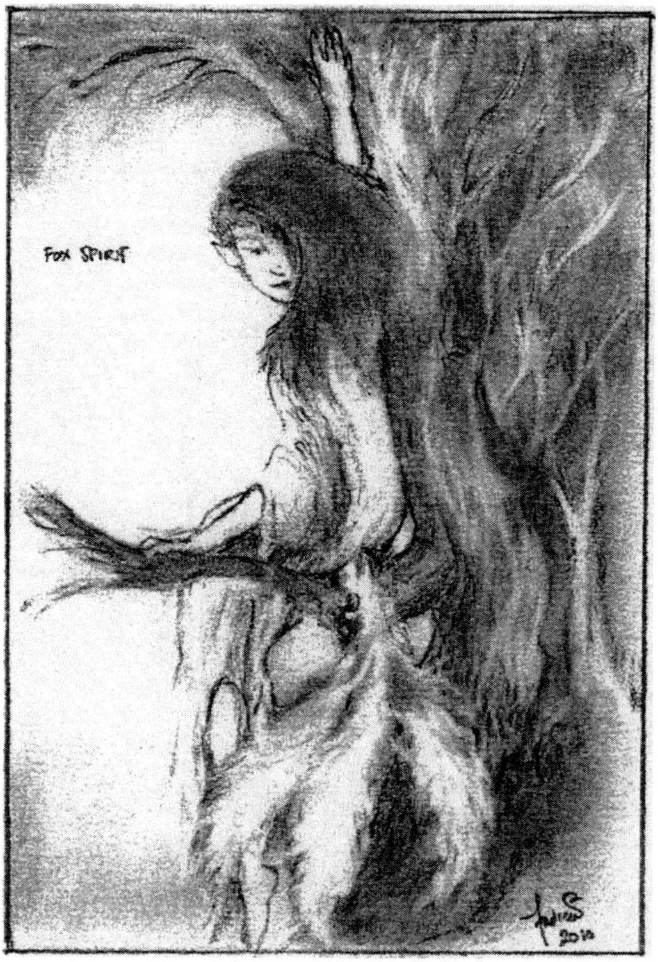

Figure 6.4 Pencil sketch of a mythological fox spirit. (Courtesy of Andrew Hock-Soon Ng.)

often powerful indictment of the state's failure to address its people's needs. They draw, however, on "popular" culture to disguise this criticism in order to appear "trifling" to avoid official censure. Figures like the fox spirit (see Figure 6.4) and the *raksha* have been part of China's literary tradition for centuries and are undoubtedly familiar to Chinese readership, but Pu's specific use of them in his stories has provided these monsters with added significance, thereby further reinforcing their propensity toward intimating surplus. In fact, some of his stories, such as "A Dream of Wolves," go so far as to implicate the narrative form with monstrosity itself.

As its title implies, "Dream" recounts the reverie of a man named Bai, whose son, Jia, is a magistrate. In the dream, Bai is visiting his son but discovers to his horror that the magistrate's house is littered with human bones and overrun by wolves, which are apparently Jia's attendants. Jia transforms into a ferocious tiger, but two warriors appear and disempower it by "knock[ing] out its teeth."[43] At this point, Bai awakens from his dream. Since dreams are portentous in Chinese belief (or, as Karl Kao puts it, dreams point to a "literalization of the metaphorical"[44]), it is unsurprising that Bai will soon after discover that his son has become deeply corrupted and is currently surrounded by a host of unsavory runners. Failing to persuade Jia to mend his ways, Bai falls ill and becomes bedridden. Not long after this, Jia is kidnapped and killed as punishment for his corruption by a band of self-proclaimed warriors. However, at this juncture, the story becomes slightly imprecise. Bai, we are told, has actually been misinformed, and in reality, his son is alive and well. But almost immediately after this revelation, the story again repeats Jia's kidnap and death (by decapitation), but for real this time. What is thus far a realistic tale becomes, from this point, increasingly surreal. Jia's head is reattached to his body by an official, after which Jia miraculously resurrects. However, because his head is affixed in the opposite direction, Jia is henceforth "more of a monster than a man."[45]

From this brief summary, it is already possible to see how Pu implicates the monster in the narrative form itself. Constructed in a series of narrative frames, "Dream" already implies excess; the fact that it blurs the distinction between dream and reality, and infuses what is otherwise an indignant look at state corruption with (black) comedy, further lends ambiguity to the text. We cannot even certify if Bai's misinformation is merely another dream, or if Jia's tragicomic end is actually his father's wishful thinking. That Bai becomes sick after learning of Jia's depravity (he recuperates only when he learns of Jia's death) may hint at the profundity of Bai's shame and helplessness that it is only through dreams that he can "rescue" his son. The repetition of a similar episode compels such an interpretive possibility. In a dream, Bai *would* know of Jia's fate even before it happens because foreknowledge of events is common in dreams. Also, only in dreams can the impossible be otherwise (such as returning from the dead). At the same time, so intense is Bai's disappointment of his son that he cannot allow Jia to become properly restored. Thus, Jia is turned into a monster in the narrative, which metaphorically suggests Bai's means of inverting moral and material monstrosities. In other words, to purify his son's soul, Bai must deform his body. Perhaps all this is nothing more than wish-fulfillment, but such a reading demonstrates Bai's success at simultaneously saving and punishing his son. More importantly, Jia's aberration can also possibly be read as reflective of the aberration that is the text, thus aligning form and content in a self-reflexive strategy prescient of postmodern literature. Pu's story, as such, is not just a monster narrative, *but a monstrosity itself.*

Though disparate in their historical and political settings, both the stories discussed earlier reveal the monster's incredible propensity to be paradoxical. As a literary trope, it camouflages attack against the status quo by pretending conformity. The fantastical qualities of Pu's story allow him to mock the government without attracting official retribution, while Sinbad's tale deflects, even as it exposes, his wickedness and contravention of Islamic principles. But for the monster's paradox to work, we must take into account the tale's immediate cultural moment. This does not mean that monster narratives cannot signify beyond their original contexts. But to read these narratives without considering their historical placements is reductive because it subtracts one crucial level of monster's paradoxical multiplicity. Moreover, such a reading also fails to capture the transformations in the monster's dialectics that often accompany sociopolitical shifts.

STASIS AND SILENCE: HISTORY AND THE ERASURE OF MONSTER NARRATIVES

Narratives like *The Ramayana, Journey,* and *Arabian Nights* have informed and defined the literary imagination of the Asian continent for centuries. In the case of the Indian epic, its influence in Southeast Asia is profound, spawning local versions of the tale throughout the region such as *Phra Lak Phra Lam* in Laos, *Reamker* in Cambodia, *Yama Zatdaw* in Myanmar, and *Ramakien* in Thailand. It has also defined several of the region's artistic expressions including dance (the *mak yong* in Malaysia and the *Khon* in Thailand) and theatre (the *kecak* in Indonesia). In fact, Wendy Doniger, a renowned scholar in Hindu mythology, has even suggested that the character of Hanuman, the monkey chieftain who aids Rama in his quest to rescue Sita, is possibly the inspiration behind Wu Cheng-en's Monkey.[46] *Journey*'s authority may not be as pervasive, but its fame throughout the Chinese *diaspora* even to this day is undeniable. Never out of circulation since its publication in the sixteenth century, *Journey* continues to play a significant role in China's cultural production hitherto, as evident in countless filmic and television adaptations (the first feature-length animated film produced in China, *Princess Iron Fan* [1941], is based on an episode from *Journey*), comic books, and even computer games. In the Middle East, *Arabian Nights* remains representative of the region's literary tradition, with many of its characters, such as Ali Baba, Sinbad, and Aladdin, having become integral to the Western cultural imagination as well.

Yet the power and endurance of these texts foreshadows a doleful consequence for subsequent monster narratives: in some cases, because foundational works like *The Ramayana* and *Jātaka* have established such potent, memorable creatures in the continent's literary traditions, and with such far-reaching influence, all subsequent monster narratives have become eclipsed by them. After such texts, significant monster stories that can attain the status of an epic and therefore define the region's literary tradition became more or less impossible. There are, of course, the folktales which have proved instrumental in transmitting, often via oral traditions, monster stories through the centuries, but these tales either pre-date the foundational texts (such as the fox fairy lore, which has a long history in East Asia and has possibly originated from Japan[47]) or may have been developed from these texts themselves, such as narratives featuring *rakshas* (the class of monsters under Ravana's command). *Journey*, to a large extent, could be said to combine both these features: it bases the character of Monkey on Hanuman while correspondingly incorporates many familiar creatures found in Oriental folktales. It seems, if my formulation is correct, that the appearance of a foundational text (which may accompany, or may be motivated by, an ideological shift) places stress on the possibility of cultivating further an assortment of narratives that showcase a multiplicity of innovative monsters.[48] So comprehensive and exhaustive are the representations of monsters in such works that it becomes subsequently impossible for later writers to come up with anything original, monster-type wise.

In other cases, the absence of significant monster narratives may be due to a radical shift in the region's ideological system, resulting in the elevation of certain texts and relegating others to inferiority or silence. The literary tradition of the Middle East is perhaps illustrative. Although *Arabian Nights* may be written at different historical periods by various hands, the fact that it is compiled during the Golden Age of Islam (Abbasid period, 750–1258 CE) and infused with the religion's perspectives has served to enshrine its importance. If Arabic folktales also survived, albeit increasingly Islamized, it is partly because the Arabs actually believe in the reality of creatures like the ghoul,[49] which are part of God's creation (13: 16).[50] Within this logic, then, new monsters are impossible for several interrelated reasons: first, the unreality of such creatures already disqualifies them from God's creation, and as such, they cannot take form even in art. Second, because art in Islam must complement what The Koran, considered the art *par excellence* in Islam because of its divine status,[51] has revealed, to use art to represent a nonexistent entity (reason one) would contravene Islamic teachings. Third, because Islamic art, as Edward Madden argues, "is the expression of a whole culture, intimately intertwined with religious, theological, and legal commitments," and as such, "is a way of expressing and celebrating the defining ideology of a community" rather than a means for individual expression, "the search for new artistic patterns is never great [while] repetition—or better, improvement and refinement—of classic forms is always prized, and skill in it constitutes the essence of art, whether it be literary, architectural, or decorative."[52] Accordingly, then, to institute new forms of monstrosity in literature could be construed as a "search for new artistic patterns" and therefore as self-promotion, and for these reasons, make such a pursuit suspicious and prohibited.

Such a restriction in depicting innovative monsters is not confined to just the literary traditions of the Middle East; in many areas where Islam has infiltrated and gained dominance, monster narratives must either be reconstituted to serve Islamic precepts or risk becoming silenced altogether.

If innovations in monster narratives have become impossible in the literary traditions of Asia beyond certain established texts for the reasons outlined above, the monsters in even such texts will experience considerable strains due to the impact of history in the last 500 years. Western Imperialism, which has infiltrated numerous aspects of Asian culture, has significantly manipulated several of the continent's principal literary works to demonize Asia's otherness in order to justify colonialism's mission to enlighten this part of the world (while safeguarding the West's boundaries and increasing its wealth and dominion). In the case of *The Ramayana,* its heroes are redrawn as monsters to potentially implicate Hinduism (and by extension its followers) as a religion of idolatry, superstition, and ignorance, and therefore unable to distinguish heroes/rightness from monsters/wrongness. Hanuman, for example, has been consistently portrayed as a monster in "popular journals, books and lectures of western Europe and American travelers to India over the past few centuries . . . through the deployment of a vocabulary of horror" characteristic of Gothic novels.[53] These travelers, deploring "religious otherness," in turn translate their experience "for readers back home as . . . dread horror in the face of monsters,"[54] thereby fueling the Western imagination with further proof of Asia's threat and the need to civilize and Christianize it. Similarly, the ghoul, more nuanced in its portrayal in Arabic stories, becomes transformed into a manifestation of pure evil when borrowed by Western writers for their enterprise in sensationalism.[55] If the Arabic ghoul is partial to human flesh (although the folktales rarely ever exploit this characteristic), under Western appropriation, its utter repulsiveness is confirmed by the fact that it dwells in cemeteries, feasting on corpses[56]—a trait alien to Arabic ghouls. Thus are Asian heritages pillaged and distorted (and the people disparaged) by Western colonialism in order to reinforce its agenda.

China's long literary acquaintance with monsters (and ghosts) more or less ceased in the twentieth century under Mao's overarching policies. If monster and ghost stories have always been an integral part of the country's literary tradition to suggest "how rare are times of peace and how rarely human beings and ghosts [and monsters] have been kept apart,"[57] after the May Fourth movement and the emergence of Communism, such creatures became associated with "the five ghosts"—"poverty, disease, ignorance, corruption, and chaos"—that had to be exorcised in accordance with Mao's "agenda of Chinese Enlightenment."[58] Aesthetics under this new regulating structure promoted forward looking (modernity), self-transcendence, and identification with communal unity. It became, as Ban Wang terms it, a "sublime" aesthetics "that furnishes a gigantic image of the People, the figure of the collective subject engaged in a world-transforming practice in order to carry out the telos of history."[59] As such, narratives that depict decadence, superstition, and the fantastic—all of which are important ingredients in monster and ghost stories—have no place: existing ones either had to be suppressed or reinterpreted for political assertion,[60] while innovations became a forbidden venture, punishable by death.

Somewhere along the Chinese civilization's etymological development, the term for monster, *taowu,* became cognate for "history" as well.[61] Curious as this may be, it is however profoundly accurate in more ways than one. Mao's century unequivocally captures this attribute of history, making History, in fact, the monster that will not only erase all others but *The Monster* that will come to tyrannize its people for nearly the rest of the century. Yet, this is not peculiar to Chinese history alone, as my discussion has thus far demonstrated. Because new sociopolitical systems require the mobilization of culture to reinforce their structures, art with its capacity to reach and influence the masses is a perfect vehicle to drive specific agendas. In the case of literature, narratives that can be used to forward a particular structure's cause are sometimes established as "foundational" texts, while those that question or potentially subvert the structure must be excised or carefully managed. Monster narratives, with their propensity for paradoxes, are an endangerment to the status quo, which is why it is unsurprising that they are also often a prime target for ideological repression. Banned, burned, and/or reinterpreted to suit shifting ideologies, monster narratives nevertheless reveal that rather than orchestrating terror; they actually reflect manifold anxieties in any given period of history. Whether expressed or repressed, such narratives tell us that what we have to fear are not stories, but *histories* and their predisposition toward oppression and destruction.

CONCLUSION: THE RETURN OF THE MONSTER

With the end of Maoism and the emergence of a global economy in which China desires participation, monster and ghost narratives have made a significant comeback since the 1980s. The literary movement known as New Wave Fiction (*Xinchia xiaoshuo*), whose practitioners include internationally acclaimed writers such as Can Xue, Mo Yan, and Su Tong, has resurrected tropes of the monsters and ghosts in narratives to profoundly probe and criticize the effects of Maoism on the Chinese people in often graphically disturbing and extreme ways. Directly repudiating the socio-realist genre that characterized Chinese literature for almost sixty years, New Wave Fiction instead celebrates what Ban Wang sees as three oppositional "aesthetic categories: the fantastic, the schizophrenic, and the grotesque."[62] However, such a positive turn does not suggest uncompromised artistic freedom. Contemporary authors in China may have a wider recourse to what they can write, but criticism against the government, even if done metaphorically, is still a punishable offence ranging from the banning of their works to imprisonment.

One writer who has suffered such a fate is Ma Jian. But if Ma's works are continuously banned in China, they are highly acclaimed in the West (Ma now lives in London) and reveal the aptness of the correlation between Chinese history and monstrosity. In his most recently translated novel *Beijing Coma* (2008), Ma pays homage to, and draws on, one of China's most ancient and beloved monster narratives, *The Classics of Mountains and Seas* (possibly first century, and perhaps the earliest monster text), an imaginary cartography of ancient China believed to be populated by all types of extraordinary beings such as "the piebald" that "looks like a horse; it has a white body with a black tail, a single horn and the fangs and claws of a tiger"[63]; the "ride-yellow creatures which look like a fox [*sic*], and have horns on their back"[64]; an animal-deity named "Awestruck," which "looks like an ox with [a] bright blue body, but has no horns and only one foot,"[65] and many more. In Ma's novel, the comatose protagonist Da Wei constantly resorts to this text in an attempt to imaginatively escape his lifeless body. It is perhaps unsurprising that he identifies with this outlandish Chinese geography and its panoply of monsters rather than with modern China, not only because he is as an embodiment of living-death, and is thus a kind of monster himself, but also because the history of modern China (specifically the Tiananmen Massacre of 1989) is what has both produced and marginalized a "creature" like him. By superimposing *Classics* onto his own body, Da Wei "discovered that all the wonders described in this book exist within me . . . . I know that to reach the soul, you must travel backwards."[66] In a way, Da Wei reclaims his body that has otherwise been manipulated, cheapened, and rendered useless by communism and modernity, and continues in his resistance against the status quo even in his paralyzed state. Da Wei is able to reject the overwhelming "Monster that is History" by working *through* a monster narrative that will fundamentally take him back to the core of his identity (his "soul"). The fact that Da Wei uses a monster narrative to reclaim a sense of a self against overwhelmingly debilitating circumstances suggests that monster texts may not just reflect cultural and personal anxieties but can function as a means for salvation as well. Monsters are a way back to a primal identity uncluttered by the impositions of ideology. *Beijing Coma,* in this sense, shows us that if monsters are products of ideologies, they are also a means by which ideologies may be transgressed and effect a kind of emancipation, however visionary or private.

If Ma uses a classical monster text to reflect upon, and subtly expose the lack in, history as a nationalist agenda, Salman Rushdie, in his novel *Shame,* constructs a monster using the conventions and vocabulary of the Gothic to criticize postcolonial nationalism. *Shame* is replete with the monstrous feminine, primary of which is the character Sufiya Zinobia, the eldest daughter (only a child) of one of the two patriarchs at war with each other over a South Asian government (allegedly Pakistan). Variously affiliated with avenging angels, werewolves, and vampires, she is a "latent monster,"[67] who takes pleasure in twisting the heads off turkeys[68] and murdering men.[69] Yet, despite the terror—"the Beast"—she obviously embodies, she cannot be discussed by her family, much less comprehended. This is not because she is "the unspeakable," but because "to comprehend Sufiya Zinobia would be to shatter, as if [she] were a crystal, these people's sense of themselves; and so of course they would not do it, they did not, not for many years. The more powerful the Beast became, the greater grew the efforts to deny its very being."[70] Sufiya, in the end, is a monster because she literally allegorizes her father's (Raza) shame; if Raza, in his pursuit of power and dominance, would resort to despicable and extreme acts for which he cannot be criticized or punished because of his wealth and status, his daughter, in becoming the Beast, signifies history's refusal to let Raza off the hook. Here, the monster that is history visits retribution onto Raza in the guise of his daughter.[71]

Rushdie will again turn to monsters for creative and critical purposes in his next novel, *The Satanic Verses* (1988), for which he will have a *fatwa* pronounced upon him by the then religious leader of Iran. Clearly, dabbling with monsters is a dangerous thing, not because monsters are distortions of truths, but because, as Sufiya Zinobia demonstrates, they question the dominant order or bring unwanted truths to light, which then necessitate their suppression. But there is no denying that monsters are again creeping, even if slowly, out of the closets of Asian literary traditions to do the kind of cultural work for which they are best known. The finesse with which they affect ambiguity and paradox in order to simultaneously criticize and conform makes them particularly potent and useful as reflections of contemporary anxieties. Take, for example, the *geongxi* (vampire) films popular in Hong Kong just before the island state's reclamation by China in 1997. That the vampires are identifiably Chinese could suggest the fear of being reabsorbed into a structure that would end the socioeconomic freedom enjoyed by the populace under British rule; at the same time, that the *geongxi*s are also imaged after the Western vampire (they have fangs and suck blood) could suggest the West's contamination of the Chinese culture, and, as such, are monsters that must be eliminated in order to restore the purity of the latter and to remove the last vestige of Imperial rule in the region. That the *geongxi* can play such a contradictory function is due to its hybrid nature of merging characteristics of Eastern and Western monsters. And perhaps this is the way innovation in the literary tradition of Asia can occur with regard to monster narratives. By hybridizing the familiar features of Eastern monsters with those of the West (a strategy that Rushdie also deploys), perhaps Asian (and Western) literatures can produce monster narratives which speak not only specifically to and of the issues faced by a nation/people struggling to come to terms with history but also to those pertinent to a postmodern, globalized world where the East–West dichotomy has increasingly collapsed, and where the idea of self has been stricken with the trauma of displacement, whether virtually or literally (as with the experience of diaspora).

NOTES

1. A preemptory and explanatory note before I begin: the term "monster" is very broad and can cover a range of meanings that are linked to forms of embodiment, ideology, morality, and so forth. This

chapter, however, is fundamentally interested in monstrous creatures—that is, mythological beings that have, for various reasons, attained the label of monster, and the significance they bear in the literary tradition from which they are derived.

2. Monster is derived from *monstrum,* from which the verbs *monstrare* ("to show" or "to reveal") and *monere* ("to portend") are formed.
3. Gilles Deleuze, *Difference and Repetition,* trans. Paul Patton (New York: Columbia University Press, 1994), 17.
4. Glennis Byron, " 'Where Meaning Collapses': Tunku Halim's *Dark Demon Rising* as Global Gothic," in *Asian Gothic: Essays on Literature, Film and Anime,* ed. Andrew Hock-Soon Ng (Jefferson, NC: McFarland Press, 2008), 32–45.
5. Quoted in Donald A. Mackenzie, *China and Japan: Myths and Legends* (London: Senate, 1923/1994), 54.
6. David William, *Deformed Discourses: The Function of the Monster in Mediaeval Thought and Literature* (Montreal-Kingston and London: McGill-Queen's University Press, 1996), 81.
7. F. J. Daniels, "Snake and Dragon Lore of Japan," *Folklore* 71, no. 3 (1960): 154.
8. Richard Kearney, *Strangers, Gods and Monsters* (London and New York: Routledge, 2003), 91.
9. Mackenzie, *China and Japan,* 61.
10. Mackenzie, *China and Japan,* 65.
11. Michel Foucault, *The Order of Things,* trans. unknown (London: Routledge, 1970/2002), 171.
12. Michel Foucault, *Abnormal: Lectures at the Collège de France 1974–1975,* trans. Graham Burchell (New York: Picador, 2004), 63.
13. Foucault, *Abnormal,* 63–64.
14. Kearney, *Strangers, Gods and Monsters,* 65.
15. Alain Grosrichard, "The Case of Polyphemus or, A Monster and Its Mother," trans. Marina Harss and Sina Nafaji, in *Cogito and the Unconscious,* ed. Slavoj Žižek (Durham, NC: Duke University Press, 1998), 118–119.
16. See volume three of Anthony Yu's four-volume translation.
17. Laurie Cozad, "Reeling in the Demon: An Exploration into the Category of the Demonized Other as Portrayed in 'The Journey to the West,' " *Journal of the American Academy of Religion* 66, no. 1 (1998): 128.
18. See volumes one and two respectively of Yu's translation.
19. Cozad, "Reeling in the Demon," 138.
20. Rob Campany, "Demons, Gods, and Pilgrims: The Demonology of His-yu Chi," *Chinese Literatures: Essays, Articles, Reviews (CLEAR)* 7, no. 1/2 (1989): 95.
21. Although there are scholars who argue that the religious element of *The Ramayana* is a later imposition, Sheldon Pollock provides a strong argument that suggests otherwise. See Sheldon Pollock, "The Divine King in the Indian Epic," *Journal of the American Oriental Society* 104, no. 3 (1984): 505–528.
22. P. Lal, ed. *The Bhagavadgita* (New Delhi: Roli Books, 1994), 49.
23. R. K. Narayan, *Gods, Demons and Others* (London: Heinemann, 1965), 100.
24. R. K. Narayan, *The Ramayana: A Shortened Modern Prose Version of the Indian Epic* (London: Penguin, 1972), 80.
25. Narayan, *The Ramayana,* 147.
26. More recently, modern Tamil literature has recuperated Ravana as hero, whose defeat in *The Ramayana* by a treacherous Rama is reflective of the Aryan infiltration into South India at the expense and elimination of Dravidian culture and tradition. For discussion, see K. V. Zvelebil, "Ravana the Great in Modern Tamil Fiction," *Journal of the Royal Asiatic Society of Great Britain and Ireland* 1 (1998): 126–134.
27. See the ancient text, *Jātaka: Or, Stories of the Buddha's Former Births,* ed. E. B. Cowell, et al. (Cambridge: Cambridge University Press, 1895–1913). Monkey may be a fictional figure reinscribed into the Buddhist structural order to demonstrate the encompassing and supreme nature of the latter, but in the case of the *naga,* or dragon, which, prior to the rise of Buddhism, was a local deity throughout various parts of India, it too must be redrawn as a potential threat to the "new religious force" in order for the latter to "[assume] the sacred place and region of an older deity," while allowing "the older

deity to continue in its original power [but] under new authority" (Lowell W. Bloss, "The Buddha and the Nāga: A Study in Buddhist Folk Religiosity," *History of Religions* 13, no. 1 (1973): 45).

28. Bernard Faure, *The Rhetoric of Immediacy: A Cultural Critique of Chan/Zen Buddhism* (Princeton: Princeton University Press, 1991), 131.
29. Ahmed K. Al-Rawi, "The Arabic Ghoul and Its Western Transformation," *Folklore* 120, no. 3 (2009): 292.
30. All these stories can be found in *Arab Folktales* (1986).
31. Jeffrey Jerome Cohen, "Monster Culture (Seven Theses)," in *Monster Theory: Reading Culture,* ed. Jeffrey J. Cohen (Minneapolis: University of Minnesota Press, 1996), 5.
32. Franco Moretti, *Signs Taken for Wonders: Essays in the Sociology of Literary Forms,* trans. Susan Fisher, David Miller, and David Forgacs (London: Verso, 1983).
33. Margrit Shildrick, *Embodying the Monster: Encounters with the Vulnerable Self* (London: Sage, 2002), 67.
34. Andrew Lang, trans., ed., *Tales from the Arabian Nights* (Hertfordshire: Wordsworth Classics, 1993), 167.
35. Lang, *Tales from the Arabian Nights,* 167.
36. Lang, *Tales from the Arabian Nights,* 168.
37. Lang, *Tales from the Arabian Nights,* 168.
38. Peter D. Molan, "Sinbad the Sailor: A Commentary on the Ethics of Violence," *Journal of the American Oriental Society* 98, no. 3 (1978): 237.
39. Molan, "Sinbad the Sailor," 246.
40. Lang, *Tales from the Arabian Nights,* 123, 124.
41. See *The Koran* (Dawood's translation, 1997, esp. 4:93, 6:151, and 17: 31).
42. Lang, *Tales from the Arabian Nights,* 160–161.
43. Songling Pu, *Selected Tales of Liaozhai,* trans. Yang Xianyi and Gladys Yang (Beijing: Panda Books, 1981), 106.
44. Karl S. Y. Kao, "Projection, Displacement, Introjection: The Strangeness of *Liaozhai zhiyi,*" in *Paradoxes of Traditional Chinese Literature,* ed. Eva Hung (Hong Kong: The Chinese University Press, 1994), 205.
45. Pu, *Selected Tales of Liaozhai,* 108.
46. Wendy Doniger, "Hanuman," in *Encyclopedia Britannica,* http://www.britannica.com/EBchecked/topic/254649/Hanuman.
47. T. W. Johnson, "Far-Eastern Fox Lore," *Asian Folklore Studies* 33, no. 1 (1974): 35.
48. Japan, for example, has an impressive array of folktale monsters, including the *tsuchigumo* (giant spider), the *oni* (ogre), the *kitsune* (fox spirit), the *kappa* and the *tengu* (human/animal hybrids), and the *obake* (shape-shifters).
49. Al-Rawi, "The Arabic Ghoul and Its Western Transformation," 294–295.
50. *The Koran,* trans. N. J. Dawood (Harmondsworth: Penguin, 1997), 176.
51. Ismail al-Fārūkī, "Islam and Art," *Studia Islamica* 37 (1973): 95–97.
52. Edward Madden, "Some Characteristics of Islamic Art," *The Journal of Aesthetics and Art Criticism* 33, no. 4 (1975): 423.
53. Timothy K. Beal, *Religion and Its Monsters* (London and New York: Routledge, 2002), 108.
54. Beal, *Religion and Its Monsters,* 110.
55. Ghouls feature, for example, in William Beckford's novel *Vathek* (1786), Thomas Moore's poem *Lalla Rookh* (1817), and more recently Neil Gaiman's *The Graveyard Book* (2008), and are alluded to in Emily and Charlotte Bronte's *Wuthering Heights* (1847) and *Jane Eyre* (1847), respectively.
56. Al-Rawi, "The Arabic Ghoul and Its Western Transformation," 299.
57. David Der-Wei Wang, *The Monster That Is History: History, Violence, and Fictional Writing in Twentieth-Century China* (Berkeley, CA: University of California Press, 2004), 263.
58. Wang, *The Monster That Is History,* 265.
59. Ban Wang, *The Sublime Figure of History: Aesthetics and Politics in Twentieth-Century China* (Palo Alto, CA: Stanford University Press, 1997), 8.

60. For example, in the preface to a 1961 collection of classical ghost stories, the translator unambiguously tells the reader that "There are no ghosts. Belief in ghosts is a backward idea, a superstition and a sign of cowardice" (Ho: 1), and argues instead that these stories must be read as political allegories in which ghosts represent the bourgeois, whom Marxism will eventually overcome.
61. Wang, *The Monster That Is History,* 8.
62. Wang, *The Sublime Figure of History,* 232.
63. Anne Birrell, trans., *The Classics of Mountains and Seas* (Harmondsworth: Penguin, 1999), 30.
64. Birrell, *The Classics of Mountains and Seas,* 117.
65. Birrell, *The Classics of Mountains and Seas,* 162.
66. Ma Jian, *Beijing Coma,* trans. Flora Dew (London: Chatto & Windus, 2008), 566.
67. Salman Rushdie, *Shame* (London: Picador, 1983).
68. Rushdie, *Shame,* 171.
69. Rushdie, *Shame,* 216.
70. Rushdie, *Shame,* 200.
71. For a more detailed discussion, see Andrew Hock Soon Ng, *Interrogating Interstices: Gothic Aesthetics in Postcolonial Asian and Asian American Literature* (New York and Bern: Peter Lang, 2007), 48–65.

CHAPTER 7

SLAYER AS MONSTER IN *BLOOD+* (2005–2006) AND *BUFFY THE VAMPIRE SLAYER* (1997–2003)

MARGARET L. CARTER

JAPANESE *ANIME* AND *MANGA* HAVE CROSS-FERTILIZED with American mass media for decades. As Susan Napier says, "By the late 1990s it was clear that anime both influenced and was influenced by a plethora of Western cultural products."[1] Particularly in regard to the vampire motif, Japanese horror has been heavily influenced by occidental vampire fiction and cinema, since nothing exactly like the European vampire exists in Japanese mythology. For instance, Hideyuki Kikuchi, author of the *Vampire Hunter D* novel series, acknowledges the Hammer *Dracula* films starring Christopher Lee as a primary source for his fiction. The title of the anime and manga series *Hellsing* alludes to Bram Stoker's vampire hunter Van Helsing, and the name of a major character in the series, Alucard, is, of course, "Dracula" reversed. Numerous other anime and manga use fangs, aversion to sunlight, capes, bats, crosses, and other images from Western vampire fiction. The increasing popularity of anime and manga with American mass audiences, rather than only a specialized fandom, entails an increase in reciprocal influence. In network television, *Buffy the Vampire Slayer* pioneered several tropes and narrative techniques relatively new to American television at the time this series premiered but were already common in anime. Notable among these are the teenage girl in a high school setting as a monster-slaying heroine with a hidden identity, continuity with complex plotlines and character arcs extended over multiple seasons, frequent deaths of major characters, and the mingling of disparate genres such as horror, romance, comedy, fantasy, and science fiction within a single series.

The vampire or half-vampire (*dhampir*) as hunter of vampires appears in several novel, anime, and manga series, for example, D in *Vampire Hunter D,* Alucard in *Hellsing,* and Miyu in *Vampire Princess Miyu.* Another such character, Saya in the movie *Blood: The Last Vampire* and the anime and manga *Blood+*, displays several striking analogies to *Buffy,* yet with subtle differences between the two series arguably attributable to cultural differences between their societies of origin. Although I have not encountered any explicit statement that Joss Whedon, creator of *Buffy the Vampire Slayer,* had acknowledged influence from anime, he was certainly aware of that medium. When adapting his theatrical film into a television series, he originally considered making "*Buffy* into a children's show, a girl-power version of *Power Rangers*,"[2] a program, of course, derived from Japanese television. Whedon definitely and deliberately "set out to create a truly cross-genre show" that "would integrate four distinct genres—horror, action, comedy, and drama."[3] *Buffy* was broadcast in Japan, as in many other international venues, and *The Anime Encyclopedia* suggests that *Blood: The Last Vampire* "is likely to be regarded in the U.S. as a Japanese rip-off of *Buffy the Vampire Slayer*" but with "demonic combat to put Buffy to shame."[4] The common element of a teenage girl slayer of vampires, however, is only the most obvious of parallels between the two works.

With the notable exception of *Vampire Princess Miyu,* most Japanese popular culture products featuring vampires derive their vampiric traits from Western sources. The *Vampire Hunter D* series and *Hellsing,* noted earlier, are only two among numerous examples of this phenomenon. As Wayne Stein notes in connection with vampire films, though, "the Judeo-Christian religious underpinnings of Westernized materials have not translated well with Asian audiences,"[5] as evidenced by the rather peculiar role (from a Western perspective) played by the Roman Catholic Church in anime such as *Hellsing*. Japanese writers and animators adapt the outward trappings of Western vampire lore to their own culture. In the original animated movie *Blood: The Last Vampire* (2000), the chiropterans—monstrous vampiric creatures, some of whom are capable of shape-shifting between human and bestial forms—are associated by analogy with invasion from the West. The story takes place in 1966, near the beginning of the Vietnam War, with much of the action set on a U.S. military base in Japan. The American authorities are secretly aware of the monsters' existence. Saya, posing as an ordinary high school student, has the mission of destroying the chiropterans that have emerged from hibernation. After their annihilation, the episode is covered up. The final scene shows an American bomber taking off for Vietnam. According to Christopher Bolton, "The ending leaves no doubt that vampirism is a metaphor for the U.S.-Japanese military relationship, though the vampire in this case could be either America or Japan."[6]

The later anime series *Blood+* (2005–2006) supplies the background on Saya missing from the short feature film. She herself is a chiropteran, as the movie reveals by referring to her as "the only remaining original."[7] In *Blood+* we learn that she and her twin sister (and deadly enemy) Diva are chiropteran queens, the mothers of the species, all other chiropterans being spawned from their blood by various means. An ordinary mortal fed with a queen's blood becomes a high-order chiropteran called a chevalier, utterly devoted to his queen. Later episodes reveal an artificially created group of chiropterans called the Schiff, who, while retaining more human traits than the bestial monsters Saya fights against, are physically somewhat fragile. Diva, having forcibly mated with Saya's foster brother and youngest chevalier, Riku, eventually becomes pregnant with the next generation of twin queens. *Blood+* has an international cast of characters. Many of Diva's followers as well as the personnel of Red Shield, the organization devoted to destroying her, come from Europe and the United States; in fact, one of Diva's chevaliers is an American naval officer. Since Diva and Saya were born and spent their childhood in France, in a sense *Blood+* presents vampirism as an invasion from the West. The series' action ranges widely over several continents, coming to a climax in New York.

In the early episodes of the anime, Saya suffers from amnesia, remembering nothing of her past before her adoption by a seemingly ordinary Okinawan family consisting of a widower and his two sons. When her first chevalier, Hagi, reenters her life and she must resume her crusade against the vampires, her memories gradually awaken. Actually well over a 100 years old, she had been in a state of hibernation before her foster father took her to his home. Over the course of the series, the conflict between Red Shield and Diva's followers builds to a final confrontation that destroys Diva but leaves her twin babies alive. Saya intends to die as well, but her surviving foster brother dissuades her, and she withdraws into hibernation once more. Her nieces, Diva's children, are adopted by her foster brother Kai.

According to Bolton, the film *Blood* is pervaded by "hope . . . tinged by such irony that it sometimes verges on nihilism."[8] The anime *Blood+*, on the other hand, concludes in a mood of reconciliation and peace. Bolton points out that Saya in *Blood* "sneers at the humans she protects and feels a kinship with the chiropterans she kills."[9] In the series, by contrast, she values her human family and yearns for a normal life. Both the movie and the anime foreground "the blurring of boundaries between the monsters and us" and portray Saya as a "hybrid . . . a creature somewhere between us and them."[10] Saya's own attitude, however, toward what Bolton calls "the ambiguity of [her] vampire identity"[11] appears more complex in the anime, as she resists the monstrous dimension of her nature and strives to hold onto her façade of humanity. Timothy Perper and Martha Cornog dwell on the point that "Saya is liminal: she can cross over between realms," not only between the supernatural and the scientific, high-technology realms but also between vampire and human. These authors note that a Western treatment of the story might build to a resolution of "a religious stereotype of heroic young women defying the vampires," a "vision of light conquering all" rather than the "liminal twilight realms" characteristic of the *Blood* universe (p. 296).[12]

At first glance, the early episodes of *Buffy the Vampire Slayer* (1997–2003) seem to present just such a heroic vision. The mantle of the Slayer, a female adolescent gifted with the power to destroy vampires and other demons, falls upon one girl in each generation (in theory, although in practice Buffy later loses that unique status). She has no choice about her role, even though she may not wish for it. Each Slayer has the guidance of a Watcher, who trains and advises her but usually does not engage in combat. Buffy's Watcher, Rupert Giles, and her two best friends, Xander and Willow, form an inner circle of people aware that supernatural evil exists below the seemingly normal surface of the town of Sunnydale. This circle later expands with the addition of other allies. Buffy's role as the chosen Slayer who defends humankind against supernatural threats appears to allow no ambiguity or liminality. As the series evolves, however, it problematizes this vision and the character of Buffy herself. Demons, first introduced as unequivocally evil and hostile to humanity, later prove to include a few neutral or benign species. One exception to the image of vampires as irredeemably evil appears in the first season—Angel, Buffy's protector and love interest. He is an exception, however, because he has been cursed with the restoration of his soul in order to make him suffer for his past cruelties. A later exception, Spike, presents a more intriguingly complex picture. Disabled by a microchip in his brain that prevents him from attacking human victims, he originally becomes Buffy's reluctant ally because he has little choice. In time, however, he falls in love with her, even though he still has no soul (whatever, precisely, "soul" means in the Buffyverse, an entity never clearly defined). He voluntarily seeks the restoration of his soul to become worthy of her. Ultimately, he sacrifices his life in the apocalyptic climax of the series, becoming instrumental in the destruction of a horde of vampires under the control of the First Evil.

The character of Buffy herself evolves in the opposite direction, from an apparently uncomplicated role as champion of good (despite how much her private life may be complicated by her secret identity as the Slayer) to a state of ambiguity that, during one phase of her life, so torments her that she plunges into a sexual affair with Spike simply in order to feel something (according to her friend Willow's assessment). Originally we witness Buffy engaged in an unambiguously righteous battle against vampires, demonic parodies of the dead whose bodies they inhabit, as symbolized by their instant dissolution into dust when staked. Later, though, Buffy's enemies include not only a variety of other supernatural monsters, but human villains who cannot be so cavalierly destroyed. She and her allies do not kill the mayor of Sunnydale, for example, until he completes the ritual of ascent to fully demonic status and becomes inhuman, a giant snake. Dark Slayer Faith's casual killing of one of the mayor's human henchmen, at a period when Buffy still maintains a relatively straightforward allegiance to the "good" side, offers a cautionary glimpse of what Buffy might become if she loses control of her power. Cryptically prophetic dreams in the Season Four episode "Restless" introduce Buffy to the First Slayer, the primal ancestress of the line, a savage figure whose entire being seems wrapped up in the drive to destroy. Later, in the Season Seven episode "Get It Done," we learn the true source of the Slayer's gift. In the prehistoric past, a group of male sorcerers, the Shadow Men, predecessors of the Watchers' Council, fused a young woman's soul with a demon. It is demonic energy that gives each Slayer the power to fight demons.

Just as Saya, the chosen warrior who uses her own blood to destroy chiropterans, is herself a chiropteran, Buffy draws her Slayer powers from the same source as the creatures her destiny demands that she destroy. As we learn in the Season Five episode "Buffy vs. Dracula," "her power is rooted in darkness."[13] Both Buffy and Saya are monsters fighting against monsters. Each has a double who uses the same kind of power in the service of evil rather than good. Saya's twin, Diva, originally an isolated, nameless girl whom Saya befriends after finding her locked in a tower, launches a campaign to annihilate humanity and overrun the world with chiropterans. Faith, another Slayer (created by a freakish sequence of events, although only one Slayer is supposed to exist at a time) at first accepted as Buffy's ally, turns against her and becomes the adopted daughter of the demonic mayor. She and Buffy ultimately clash in a confrontation that almost ends in Faith's death. According to Rhonda Wilcox, "Faith is a shadow and foil for Buffy."[14] Their status as doubles is emphasized in the Season Four episode "Who Are You," in which their personalities inhabit each other's bodies. Faith, with her mind in Buffy's body, heaps verbal and physical abuse upon "herself," her own body, currently possessed by Buffy's mind. The First Slayer may also be regarded as Buffy's double and shadow, the visible embodiment of what Buffy might become if she renounced her humanity to devote herself completely to destruction, even if in the service of good. As Wilcox notes, however, "Buffy refuses to be controlled by the First Slayer."[15] During the dream confrontation in the "Restless" episode, Buffy emphatically rejects the single-minded ruthlessness of the First Slayer: "I walk. I talk. I shop. I sneeze . . . . And I don't sleep on a bed of bones. Now give me back my friends!"[16]

This dialogue foregrounds Buffy's yearning to be normal, a desire expressed repeatedly from the beginning of the series. As Joss Whedon himself says, "The side of her that is Buffy is as important as the side of her that is the Slayer."[17] In the early Season One episode "Witch," she tries out for the cheerleading squad in an attempt to recapture something of the mundane popularity she enjoyed at her previous school before learning of her Slayer destiny. Later she runs against ultra-popular rival Cordelia for the Homecoming Queen position. At the end of the second season, her despair over the necessity to send her former lover Angel to Hell in order to save the town drives her to run away from home. In the Season Three episode "Anne," she takes a job as a waitress under an assumed name. This attempt at a normal life proves futile when she has to combat demons even in her new, low-profile role. The revealingly titled Season Six episode "Normal Again" finds her lapsing into an alternate reality in which her dead mother is alive, her divorced parents are still together, and her entire experience as the Slayer is only a psychotic delusion. Ironically, the "normal" life she reverts to in this fugue state makes her into a catatonic patient in a mental institution.

Saya, too, seeks normality through a mentally abnormal condition. Her amnesia at the beginning of *Blood+* may symbolize her drive to reject her chiropteran nature and her destiny as a killer of vampires. We first see her as a seemingly ordinary teenage girl, although suffering from amnesia and anemia, living with her adoptive father and two foster brothers, Kai and Riku. The advent of her chevalier, Hagi, stimulates her memories to begin returning in a gradual, fragmentary manner. She resists being torn from her contented, outwardly mundane life into the realm of supernatural violence for which her true nature destines her. The futile attempt to protect her family from that realm preoccupies her during the early episodes of the series. The death of her foster father from a chiropteran attack represents the first significant break, the point when she realizes she cannot escape her destiny. In the original *Blood* feature film, according to Wayne Stein, "Saya is very much in the tradition of the vengeful female ghost, a *yurei,* who seems possessed and intent on getting her revenge."[18] In the *Blood+* series, she does not display these personality traits until circumstances force her out of her family circle into her role as slayer of chiropterans under the guidance of Red Shield. In Season Three, after Diva rapes and kills Riku, Saya abandons Kai and her Red Shield mentors for a solitary identity as a slayer of chiropterans. Even when she rejoins her brother and friends a year later, she holds herself aloof like the "vengeful . . . ghost" mentioned by Stein. She rejects Kai's overtures, urging him to return home to Okinawa. Only when she becomes reconciled with him and her other allies and they begin to work together as a team again can they defeat Diva's forces.

Like Saya, Buffy surrounds herself with a family of choice rather than genetics. With her parents divorced and her mother first unaware of and then resistant to her Slayer identity, Buffy forms a surrogate family composed of her Watcher, Giles, and her closest friends, Willow and Xander. As Jean Lorrah points out, the "family" is later joined by Dawn (a disembodied energy entity transformed into a girl and accepted as Buffy's younger sister by alteration of everyone's memories), Spike, Tara (Willow's partner), Anya (a former vengeance demon in love with Xander), and others. A Japanese word often encountered in anime, *nakama,* embodies this concept of "family." Although literally signifying "crew, ally(/ies) comrade(s), or gang," according to the online *Urban Dictionary,* the word "has a deeper meaning, describing friends who are more like family."[19] The *Television Tropes* website (http://www.tvtropes.org) explicitly applies this term to *Buffy the Vampire Slayer,* citing the Season Five episode "Family," in which Tara's father arrives to take her home against her will. When he challenges Buffy's right to help Tara defy him, Buffy declares that she and her friends are Tara's true family. As Lorrah says, "The theme of a chosen rather than blood-related family develops throughout the first six seasons" and "family is what saves the world at the end of season six."[20]

Just as Saya in Season Three of *Blood+* abandons her family and allies to fight on her own, Buffy breaks away from her surrogate family at a point of crisis in Season Seven. In the episodes "Empty Places" and "Touched," she leaves home after a confrontation that transfers command of the group to a reluctant Faith. Only when Saya rejoins her people can the campaign against Diva's chiropterans move forward; while Saya is absent, David, her Red Shield mentor, succumbs to drunken inertia. Only when Buffy returns home and the group becomes cohesive again can the defeat of the First Evil be encompassed. In each case, disruption of the *nakama* threatens the heroes' hope of success, which the eventual restoration of the *nakama* ensures. In Buffy's world, the power of cooperation is illustrated by the spell performed by Willow in the Season Seven series finale, "Chosen." This magical rite transforms all potential Slayers into actual Slayers, distributing the power among them instead of leaving it concentrated in Buffy and Faith. With the burden of being the Chosen One lifted from her, Buffy at last has a chance at a "normal" life.

The shift from an uncomplicated division between "good" and "evil" characters to a more problematic paradigm, in which even the venerable Watchers' Council (whose mission is to supervise and mentor Slayers) becomes Buffy's enemy, is foregrounded by the embrace of former enemies such as Spike and Anya within the circle of "family." Characters such as Angel, Spike, Anya, and Oz (a werewolf, Willow's boyfriend for part of the series) suggest "that good and bad are not so far apart and that 'bad' is not simply the domain of the 'othered' bad guys but is, instead, the 'other' within."[21] Near the end of Season Six, Willow's shift to the dark side illustrates this principle. She uses her magic for destruction, and, as Lorrah's essay on "family" discusses, love saves Willow from herself and the world from her. In *Buffy,* according to Mary Alice Money, "Viewers are forced . . . to consider the possibility that . . . disposable or dangerous representatives of the Other just might be capable of humanity also."[22] The Schiff in *Blood+* at first appear both dangerous and disposable. Suspicious of both sides in the conflict, they seek the blood of a chiropteran queen to cure the Thorn, a fatal condition that dooms each of them sooner or later. Their attacks on Saya in search of a cure from her blood initially provoke violent reprisals from Red Shield. It later becomes apparent, though, that war need not exist between Saya's people and the Schiff. Through Kai's friendship with a Schiff girl, we learn along with Saya and her allies to view the Schiff as pitiable rather than evil. Saya and her "family" win them over by treating them as individuals worthy of respect and aid rather than the monsters Diva's followers created them to be.

In the final season of *Buffy the Vampire Slayer,* the diabolical entity known as the First Evil is evil by definition. Faith, although Buffy's nearly lethal enemy for part of the series, has the potential virtues and flaws of any human being. She commits evil because of life experiences that have warped her. The daughter, like Buffy, of a single mother, Faith grew up in a rough environment without the advantage of a loving parent–child relationship such as that between Buffy and her mother. Furthermore, Faith's Watcher died in horrific circumstances that left Faith tormented by guilt. She becomes an easy target for recruitment by the forces of evil acting through the mayor. Diva, similarly, is not inherently evil but becomes so through the trauma of her early life. Unlike Saya, she was not brought up in luxury with protective, affectionate companions but treated as a dangerous experiment or an exotic beast, kept in solitary confinement until discovered by Saya. Faith is eventually redeemed and joins Buffy's group. As Lorrah points out, "[I]f someone is a member of Buffy's family . . . it is always possible to be forgiven. Only people outside the family do not have that option."[23] For example, Spike, a formerly evil vampire, becomes redeemable as part of Buffy's *nakama.* Hostile beings, whether vampires, demons, or other creatures, who remain outside that circle must be annihilated. This worldview allows no room for reconciliation with the enemy, as appears to be offered to Diva in *Blood+*. Her death may be said to entail redemption in that her end makes possible the defeat of the chiropteran threat and therefore the peace and safety enjoyed by Kai and his family at the conclusion of the series. As Diva's last act, she bids farewell to her babies. Although she does not survive to become part of Saya's family, her children do.

The series finale of *Buffy* climaxes with the annihilation of the First Evil's vampire horde through Spike's sacrificial self-immolation, followed by the destruction of the entire town of Sunnydale. This apocalyptic imagery brings to mind the Christian trope of the destruction and resurrection of the universe in an ultimate battle between good and evil, reinforced by the frequent use of the word "apocalypse" in the dialogue of *Buffy*. This interpretation is strengthened by the epitaph on the heroine's gravestone at the end of the Season Five episode "The Gift": "She saved the world—a lot."[24] (She does not die permanently at that time, of course; like Saya in her cycles of dormancy and revival, Buffy "dies" to rise again more than once.) Despite the efficacy of crosses against vampires in the Buffyverse, the worldview of *Buffy the Vampire Slayer* remains secular. Buffy shows no evidence of being a practicing Christian. Demons prove to be, effectively, alien species, not fallen angels. Although Willow identifies herself as Jewish in the early seasons of the series, she also never draws upon religious faith to combat evil. Nevertheless, the "battle between good and evil" in traditional Judeo-Christian terms dominates the Buffyverse. The First Evil, Buffy's antagonist in Season Seven, constitutes a clear analogue to the Devil as conceived in Western mythology.

We do not witness this kind of apocalypse in *Blood+*, in keeping with that work's cultural milieu. According to Napier, "Neither traditional Buddhism nor Shinto envisions anything like the final battle between good and evil of Revelation."[25] At the end of *Blood+* Saya, too, saves the world, in her case not from a satanic figure like the First Evil in *Buffy,* but from Diva's plan to subjugate humanity under chiropteran domination. Saya also battles a horde of vampires, but without the transcendent overtones implicit in *Buffy*. It is worth noting that despite the secular worldview of the latter series, most of Buffy's opponents are framed as supernatural. She does sometimes confront misused technology and government conspiracies, but variants of traditional monsters pose the most prevalent threats. The threats battled by Saya arise from evolutionary mutations and warped science. Diva's minions, therefore, cannot be framed as an apocalyptic force on the level of Buffy's foes. In Diva's dying moment, as illustrated by the fact that her last thoughts are of her children, it is revealed that what she wanted most all along was a family, like Saya herself. Saya actually makes an attempt to save Diva from death, a gesture unimaginable from Buffy toward the First Evil. Western dualism appears to triumph in Buffy's victory. The source of evil is obliterated, or at least the current, local manifestation of it is, along with what is left of the town. Saya's victory, on the other hand, leaves her sister's twin babies alive. If Saya believes she deserves to die along with Diva in order to cleanse the world of chiropteran evil, logically the infant queens should die as well. In fact, that is Saya's initial plan. Instead, she decides to keep them alive and grant them the normal life with Kai that Saya had to renounce for the sake of her mission. The love of Kai and her devoted chevalier, Hagi, persuades her to let the babies live and refrain from seeking her own death. At the end of Buffy's saga, she has the freedom to seek her own path at last, no longer constrained by her Slayer destiny. Saya's story ends with a return to the family home in Okinawa, followed by her withdrawal to deathlike dormancy in a tomb, like a traditional vampire. The hope for her future rebirth, however, remains alive in the hearts of Kai, who brings her nieces to visit her sleeping place, and Hagi, who leaves a rose outside the crypt in tribute.

Stein suggests that in anime such as *Vampire Hunter D, Vampire Princess Miyu,* and *Blood: The Last Vampire,* "the Zen spirit of the samurai" combines with "the spirit of animism from Shintoism, and the code of honor from Confucianism," thereby "focusing on hunters looking for demons as a way to restore balance in nature."[26] The concluding images of *Blood+* convey a picture of just such "balance," in contrast to the final picture of Buffy and her allies poised in triumph over evil (although at the cost of terrible losses) against the background of the abyss that was once Sunnydale. The decision to let the infant queens live suggests a cycle of death and rebirth. The little girls will fulfill a happier destiny denied to Saya and Diva, the twin queens of the previous generation. In Buddhism, as Stein observes, "What really matters is returning reality to a state of harmony . . . . opposites can negotiate to restore harmony in the face of chaos." Saya's story, unlike Buffy's (at least as far as the television series is concerned, the Buffy "Season Eight" comic book series published since then lies outside the scope of this discussion), does not end immediately after the destruction of the opposing forces. The final image of *Blood+* suggests harmony, while the final image of *Buffy the Vampire Slayer* suggests victory.

It would not be accurate simply to place *Buffy* on one side of an occidental—oriental dichotomy, with an absolute opposition between good and evil derived from the Judeo-Christian tradition, and *Blood+* on the other side, with more fluid ethical and ontological divisions derived from Buddhist tradition. As we have seen, the similarities and differences in their approaches to evil and monstrosity are more complicated. Both Buffy and Saya gain their power to fight demons from demonic energies within themselves. Both of them draw strength from a *nakama,* a chosen "family" closer than genetic kin, which provides an ethical anchor in the midst of chaos. Like *Blood+*, *Buffy* allows for moral ambiguity in characterization and grants the possibility that seemingly evil characters may find redemption. At the same time, Saya fights to destroy predatory chiropterans just as Buffy fights to destroy predatory vampires, with each class of antagonists "othered" as monsters. Yet vampires in *Buffy* represent absolute evil on a different level from Saya's chiropteran foes, as demonstrated by the capacity for redemption shown by the Schiff, a few of Diva's chevaliers, and above all Diva's children. In *Buffy* only two vampires—Angel and Spike, because of their own unique circumstances—are exempt from the "othering" of vampires in general. When confronting Glory, a demonic deity in Season Five, and the First Evil in Season Seven, Buffy is clearly meant to be seen as engaged in crusades to save the world from apocalyptic disaster, a goal that requires complete destruction of the enemy. Although the consequences of Saya's potential defeat would be almost equally dire for humanity, her campaign against Diva's chiropterans does not share the transcendent quality of Buffy's battles. The closing scenes of *Blood+* frame Saya's ultimate goal as not merely the annihilation of the enemy, but reconciliation between opposites "to restore harmony in the face of chaos."

Acknowledgments

Other works consulted for this chapter include Christopher Golden and Nancy Holder, *The Watcher's Guide* (New York: Pocket Books, 1998); Nancy Holder, *The Watcher's Guide Volume 2* (New York: Pocket Books, 2000); Susan J. Napier, "Vampires, Psychic Girls, Flying Women and Sailor Scouts: Four Faces of the Young Female in Japanese Popular Culture," in *The Worlds of Japanese Popular Culture: Gender, Shifting Boundaries and Global Cultures,* ed. D. P. Martinez (Cambridge: Cambridge University Press, 1998), 91–109.

Notes

1. Susan J. Napier, *Anime from Akira to Howl's Moving Castle* (New York: Macmillan, 2005), 22.
2. Candace Havens, *Joss Whedon: The Genius Behind Buffy* (Dallas: BenBella Books, 2003), 32.
3. Havens, *Joss Whedon,* 39.
4. Jonathan Clements and Helen McCarthy, *The Anime Encyclopedia: Revised and Expanded Edition* (Berkeley: Stone Bridge Press, 2006), 63.
5. Wayne Stein, "Enter the Dracula: The Silent Screams and Cultural Crossroads of Japanese and Hong Kong Cinema," in *Draculas, Vampires, and Other Undead Forms: Essays on Gender, Race, and Culture,* ed. John Edgar Browning and Caroline Joan (Kay) Picart (Lanham, MD: Scarecrow Press, 2009), 236.
6. Christopher Bolton, "The Quick and the Undead: Visual and Political Dynamics in *Blood: The Last Vampire,*" in *Mechademia 2: Networks of Desire,* ed. Frenchy Lunning (Minneapolis, MN: University of Minnesota Press, 2007), 128.
7. Quoted in Bolton, "The Quick and the Undead," 127.
8. Bolton, "The Quick and the Undead," 133.
9. Bolton, "The Quick and the Undead," 129.
10. Bolton, "The Quick and the Undead," 129.
11. Bolton, "The Quick and the Undead," 129.
12. Timothy Perper and Martha Cornog, "Lurkers at the Threshold: Saya and the Nature of Evil," in *Mechademia 2: Networks of Desire,* ed. Frenchy Lunning (Minneapolis, MN: University of Minnesota Press, 2007), 296–297.
13. Quoted in Rhonda Wilcox, *Why Buffy Matters* (London: I. B. Tauris and Company, 2006), 83.
14. Wilcox, *Why Buffy Matters,* 49.
15. Wilcox, *Why Buffy Matters,* 165–166.
16. Quoted in Wilcox, *Why Buffy Matters,* 171.
17. Quoted in Wilcox, *Why Buffy Matters,* 171.
18. Stein, "Enter the Dracula," 246.
19. "Nakama," *Urban Dictionary,* accessed October 2, 2009, http://www.urbandictionary.com/define.php?term=nakama.
20. Jean Lorrah, "Love Saves the World," in *Seven Seasons of Buffy,* ed. Glenn Yeffeth (Dallas: BenBella Books, 2003), 167–168.

21. Tanya Krzywinska, "Hubble-Bubble, Herbs, and Grimoires: Magic, Manichaeanism, and Witchcraft in *Buffy*," in *Fighting the Forces: What's at Stake in Buffy the Vampire Slayer,* ed. Rhonda Wilcox and David Lavery (Lanham, MD: Rowman and Littlefield, 2002), 182.
22. Mary Alice Money, "The Undemonization of Supporting Characters in *Buffy*," in *Fighting the Forces: What's at Stake in Buffy the Vampire Slayer,* ed. Rhonda Wilcox and David Lavery (Lanham, MD: Rowman and Littlefield, 2002), 102.
23. Lorrah, "Love Saves the World," 168–169.
24. Quoted in Paul Ruditis, *The Watcher's Guide Volume 3* (New York: Simon and Schuster, 2004), 76.
25. Napier, *Anime from Akira to Howl's Moving Castle,* 250.
26. Stein, "Enter the Dracula," 242.

CHAPTER 8

"Shapeless Deformity": Monstrosity, Visibility, and Racial Masquerade in Thomas Grattan's *Cagot's Hut* (1823)

Daniel A. Novak

> Her stature was low, her complexion cadaverous, her eye sunken, and her countenance bore in every trait the imprint of disease and want. Her feet and legs were bare; a short petticoat just covered her knees; and over her head and coming half-way down her back, was a blanket or piece of coarse and filthy cloth. This she held folded round her waist, but as it lay open on her throat it exposed the hideous olive-coloured swelling called a *goître*, which protruded all around and joined the lower jaw and chin, giving to the whole face an air of shapeless deformity. I knew enough of the Pyrenees and their population to be certain that I gazed upon a *Cagot*.[1]

At first glance, the passage above from Thomas Grattan's 1823 novel *The Cagot's Hut* invokes assumptions familiar to the discourse of monstrosity—especially as it intersects with the kinds of biologically based colonial and racial discourse that Robert Young argues emerged in the mid-to-late nineteenth century.[2] The woman is described as primitive, diseased, lower class, immodest ("a short petticoat just covered her knees"), and visibly deformed. The narrator's status and ethnographic knowledge enable him to add up these signs as legible markers of her racial difference, declaring his certainty that she is "a *Cagot*."[3] Yet the passage above and Grattan's novel as a whole both anticipate the discourse of scientific racism and deviate from it. First, rather than being set apart by the darkness of her skin (as even "white" or passing figures like the Irish and Jews were imagined), the woman is visibly Other because of her "cadaverous" complexion. Nineteenth-century texts on the Cagot routinely cite their excessive whiteness, but the Cagot woman's body is both white and not white—excluded from the privileges of whiteness and doubly marked by a disease-like pallor and an "olive-coloured" goiter.[4] Second, while her bodily and racial difference is made visible in marks of disease, disability, and deformity (the *goître*), the effect of the whole is a kind of bodily incoherence—a "*shapeless* deformity" (emphasis added). This incoherence is produced by her body's excess—its swelling beyond its boundaries into illegibility.[5]

In addressing the curious case of the Cagots—an ethnic group of unknown origin, unclear history, and ambiguous race found in the Pyrenees on the west-coast of France and in the Basque region of Spain—Grattan's novel is in dialogue both with emergent racial theory and Romantic-era discourse on monstrosity, imagination, taste, the beautiful, and the sublime.[6] The monstrous body acted as a site for the intersection of discourses of taste and race.[7] As Paul Youngquist points out, this period "saw the installation of a norm of embodiment—call it the 'proper body'—that served . . . to regulate bodies in liberal society."[8] But what makes the representation of monstrosity different in Grattan's novel is that it theorizes monstrosity outside of visibility—a link that critics have traditionally associated with gendered and racial social norms. Whether acting as "over-determined" sites that bear the "marks of the constructions of femininity, race, and sexuality"[9] or as a vehicle for defining the "limits of the human" and the normal (Nussbaum 2003), monstrous bodies perform these functions most often through spectacle.[10] Instead, it is the Cagot's failure to inhabit a "normally" raced body—its incoherence—that marks them as monsters. If the monster is associated with the visibly "abnormal," the Cagot's body is "abnormal" in its failure to perform its abnormality properly.

In a way, the narrator's reaction to this abnormal abnormality is to attempt to figure the Cagot woman as the immediately recognizable object ("I gazed at a Cagot") of a gaze informed by ethnographic knowledge ("I knew enough of the Pyrenees and their population"). Yet, rather than try to render the Cagots as subjects of scientific knowledge—fixed and exposed—the rest of the novel labors both to hide their bodies and to mystify their racial and historical identity. When explicitly theorizing the nature of the Cagot's monstrosity and otherness, the narrator associates them with and defines them through tropes of disembodiment and invisibility. In the narrator's account, despite attempts throughout history to make visible the Cagot's monstrosity, the mark of the Cagot remains a sign of their unrepresentability. He notes their historical, "wild and impressive obscurity" and their status as "an anomaly in all the existing varieties of mankind, unaccountable and mysterious."[11] These tropes are reproduced in surprising ways throughout the novel. Even at close quarters with a Cagot girl, her racial monstrosity is explicitly associated with an imagined and invisible body.

Paradoxically, however, rather than working to critique assumptions about racial and bodily difference—that they are merely imaginary—it is this link to the imagined and imaginary that makes the Cagot and her monstrosity "real," accessible, and knowable to the narrator. Even when we find out that the woman we and the narrator thought was a deformed racial Other is a Spanish noblewoman in disguise, the narrator insists on imagining the Cagot girl as a separate and monstrous body. Instead of undermining the idea of Cagot-ness as performative and imaginary, her racial masquerade seems to render the monstrosity and racial difference of the Cagot more stable—less "wild and impressive" and more like the recognizably other, if "shapeless" Cagot woman in the quotation with which I began. The novel never returns to the question of the disguise and, in the end, this imaginative effort enables the narrator to maintain class and racial boundaries between lowly Cagots and beautiful Spanish nobles. But in the process of maintaining such boundaries, the novel ends up unsettling others, especially distinctions between the material and immaterial, visible and invisible, real and imagined. After all, the narrator can separate the "two" women only by imagining a virtual body and rendering the Cagot all the more indeterminate. It is this indeterminacy that itself represents a threat and comes to define the Cagot's monstrosity. Ultimately, the Cagots and the narrator's struggle to represent them challenge us as readers to rethink monstrosity not as something that must be seen but something that exceeds the visible—something that must be imagined.

"All That Can Excite the Vague and Shadowy Imaginings of Men"

Thomas Colley Grattan (1792–1864) was born in Dublin, and in 1818, he left for Bordeaux with the idea of joining the war of independence in South America. Meeting his future wife on the boat, however, he remained in Bordeaux and began as an author. It was Washington Irving who encouraged him to publish his collection of novellas and stories, and he met with success in England and America. He is perhaps best known for his friendship with the famous actor Edmund Kean, and Kean's disastrous, drunken performance in Grattan's play *Ben Nazir the Saracen.*[12] While Grattan's Irishness may play into this interest in the marginal figure of the Cagot, the opening of the novel immediately foregrounds the problem of nationality in its (somewhat complicated) historical and political setting. The narrator is an Englishman on holiday in the Pyrenees in 1822 and the novel is part of a series of novellas called *High-ways and By-ways; or, Tales of the Roadside, Picked up in the French Provinces by A Walking Gentleman.*[13] He finds himself ill and in need of shelter when he arrives at the "Hut" of the title, which serves as the pivot point of a Spanish political conflict that reaches its climax in 1823 when Louis XVIII sent his army into Spain to restore King Ferdinand.[14]

While the first part of the novel centers on the narrator's encounter with the political crisis and his time living with the Cagots, the second part is taken up with a domestic crisis entangled in a political crisis. To summarize, the lovers at the center of the story, Don Melchior and Malvide, are both children of Spaniards who came over with the French King Joseph after he was ejected from Spain, because of their dedication to reform and their resistance to King Ferdinand. Don Melchior entered upon a military career and eventually fought for constitutional forces in Spain. Malvide's parents came to France as reformers, but eventually became more allied with the monarchists. Knowing that her father won't approve of the match, Malvide keeps her secret love from her father while also refusing a secret marriage with Melchior. When her father attempts to marry her off to a French nobleman, she flees in disguise to the Cagot's hut where the two had met in secret before. While Spain's political history prevents an unambiguously happy ending, with "tyranny" winning in the end, the novel's romantic plot ends with parental tyranny defeated; the pair are finally accepted by her parents, legally married, and transplanted to a "regenerated Columbia."[15] Intractable "Old World" political conflicts are left behind for an uncertain but malleable future in Latin America.[16]

The Cagots and their "hut" are situated at the center of both the political and romantic plots. Not only is their hut the site for the lovers' illicit rendezvous, it is also located on the border between France and Spain. By placing them on a border that (until 1868) was still ambiguous, Grattan emphasizes and literalizes in geographic terms his image of the Cagots as metaphorically on the border, liminal in bodily, historical, national, and political terms—as a people without a nation and even without a history.[17] Moreover, in Grattan's account the Cagots emerge as a tangled mass of superstitions, historical speculations, and epistemological contradictions.[18]

The narrator tells us that because they were thought to contaminate the ground, they were "forbidden to walk with feet or legs uncovered."[19] The Cagot's white skin was thought to be a mark of leprosy. In the fourteenth century, they were "publicly sold as slaves . . . looked on as infamous and accursed."[20] They were limited to professions like carpentry or wood-cutting, while "every mean employment is confined to them; malady and misery are their only heritage."[21] Although linked to a range of religious and cultural others (Jews, Goths, and Saracens[22]), they were practicing Catholics who were discriminated against both outside and inside the church.[23] They were "admitted to the churches by a separate entrance, with seats apart, and even a distinct *benitier.*"[24] Grattan dramatizes these fears of "accursed" Cagot contagion when Spaniards encounter a Cagot woman. It quickly becomes clear that prejudice against the Cagots is not merely a matter of medieval superstition but very much alive in the nineteenth century: people make the sign of a charm against the "evil-eye,"[25] "exclamations of horror, invocations of saints, and threats of punishment were loudly uttered on all sides,"[26] and others fear her touch, receiving money from her with "contemptuous caution . . . as if its very touch carried infection."[27] In Grattan's account, then, the Cagots are seen as recognizably grotesque and diseased figures, whose contagion extended beyond the boundaries of their bodies and whose movement across spatial borders needed to be strictly policed.

The narrator, however, condemns these assumptions, arguing, for example, that the belief that they were afflicted with leprosy was generated by the combined forces of "conjecture and fiction."[28] Decrying the unjust treatment of this "rejected caste," he hopes that "by imagining the possibility of their amelioration, lead to plans for their relief."[29] He even asserts the Cagot's ethical strength, demonstrated in the face of oppression:

> There are to be found amongst these people—the most poor and wretched upon the face of the civilized earth—some of the finest primitive affections . . . we have at least the consolation of knowing that he possesses in himself the power of dissolving the shackles he has forged; and of burying the memories of his own injustice.[30]

The trope of shackles "dissolved" by the Cagots themselves offers a striking contrast with the image of the slave (in abolitionist publications) or the colonized subject—in need of others to help free them. It's unclear why the Cagots are figured as forging their own shackles (reminiscent of William Blake's "mind-forged manacles" in the poem "London") unless it is the "fear" born of generations of oppression "that persecution may attack."[31] Regardless, as an oppressed race, the Cagots seem rare if not unique in their ability to transcend social, political, and historical circumstance and free themselves by mobilizing a kind of Christian forgiveness.

However, even the narrator, who offers a generalized liberal sympathy, expresses his own involuntary "revulsion" at contact with the Cagots or anything they own: he "could not help shrinking from its acceptance; and had I not been so much indisposed, I should certainly have preferred trusting to a mountain walk, in search of other quarters, to coming into contact with any thing belonging to my revolting companions."[32] More important, in the same breath that he uses to combat the superstitious beliefs about the Cagots, he makes sweeping claims about their bodily monstrosity and their mental inferiority. Calling them "living libels on humanity," he asserts that "[t]hey are, without exception, deformed, infirm, imbecile; articulating imperfectly; afflicted with incurable and monstrous *goiters,* and uniting together the smallest possible portion of mental power, with the utmost excess of bodily degradation."[33]

The narrator's claim about the Cagot's legibility and visibility, as well as the link between the mental, moral, and physical, seems to echo both early nineteenth-century racial theory—George Combe's phrenological work in the 1820s, for example[34]—and how we most commonly understand monstrosity today—in terms of spectacle. Explaining this link between monstrosity and visibility, Chris Baldick writes, "[a]s Michel Foucault reminded us in his discussion of performances put on by the inmates of lunatic asylums until the early nineteenth century, a 'monster' is something or someone to be *shown* (cf. Latin, *monstrare;* French, *montrer;* English, *demonstrate*)."[35] Yet, if the Cagot's monstrosity and inferiority are immediately visible, it seems strange that "[t]he Dukes of Brittany fixed on them a *badge*—that last and worst mark of slavery and tyranny combined, for pointing out the victim to all the excesses of injustice."[36] The narrator cites the badge (which took the form of "the foot of a duck or goose"[37]) as a visible sign of their cultural degradation—"that last and worst mark of slavery and tyranny combined"—a degradation the Cagots shared with other outcasts, including Jews, Heretics,

Cagots, Lepers, and Prostitutes.[38] But the need for the badge also suggests the questionable legibility of the Cagot's "shapeless" monstrosity and the imaginative excess and projection that both surround the Cagots and constitute their racial and bodily difference. Paradoxically, however, it is the need to imagine and inscribe their visibility in the first place that marks them as monsters.

If the Cagot's body fails to embody its difference sufficiently, it also fails to record racial and cultural history. The narrator describes them as residing somewhere outside of history, "a race of beings whose very existence is an enigma that can never be solved."[39] While the Cagot badge speaks to the anxious need to make internal monstrosity visible, their historical obscurity makes them a site for imaginative and investment, as well as a subject for literary fiction. The narrator argues that he is "pleased" to have the origin of the Cagots remain "unexplained":

> To me it does not appear more extraordinary that they should have been as they now are from the first, than that they *are* as we now see them. And I am well inclined to let them rest in their present wild and impressive obscurity, an anomaly in all the existing varieties of mankind, unaccountable and mysterious, combining all that can excite the vague and shadowy imaginings of men, as beings "Who look not like the inhabitants of the earth,/And yet are on it."[40]

On the one hand, the narrator invokes a familiar racial trope of primitive stasis and a "natural" permanence of racial types. Yet, at the same time, he claims that there is nothing "familiar" about the Cagot, whether epistemologically, historically, or racially. They are an unrepresentable and unknowable "anomaly" whose obscurity is figured in positive terms—terms that echo the Romantic discourse of the sublime, "wild and impressive."[41]

In other words, their obscurity and mysteriousness, their irreducible and ahistorical otherness evokes less a scientific desire to uncover, expose, and define Cagot-ness, than animates a kind of literary and poetic imagination. The quotation at the end of the passage from *Macbeth* (Banquo's response to the three witches) is particularly telling in that the narrator turns the racial and cultural Other into the *otherworldly,* into a ghost, and a literary one at that.[42] If earlier the narrator had argued that the Cagots were immediately recognizable, here seeing the Cagot's bodily difference requires a different kind of vision—an ability to see what lies on the edges of the invisible. For the narrator, the fact that the monstrous racial body is a kind of ghost or specter makes it *more,* not less, "real" and recognizable. In other words, the narrator defines both monstrosity and race in terms of a liminal body, a body on the border between presence and absence, imagined and "real," visible and invisible.

"Seeing Is Not Believing"

But if in the abstract the Cagots are a kind of sublimely impressive mystery, in person they are *unsightly*—both deformed and unseen—and it is the lower-class female body that embodies this paradox for the narrator. When he turns to the husband of the Cagot woman, he argues that the men are less repulsive than the women: "Like most of the males of his unsightly race, he was diminutive, weakly, and dull, but not altogether so repulsive in appearance as those of the other sex."[43] Even before he meets her, the narrator finds the Cagot daughter of the Hut particularly disgusting and deformed. Yet, because he fears his own potential and uncontrolled desire for the Cagot girl, as well as the thought that others might see this desire, he avoids looking at her as much as possible. In other words, the body that is most "unsightly" is the one that one never bothers to look at very closely. As the mother mentions that she is alone with her daughter, he insists, "I was too ill to laugh outright, but I could not help smiling at this maternal alarm: the very notion of this daughter was so disgusting to me, that I for a moment felt utterly repugnant to enter the house."[44] The vehemence and frequency of these disavowals—later he assures the reader that while the girl "might have been about twenty" even if she were "a hundred, she had not been more secure from my inquiries or intrusion"[45]—betray his anxiety both about his own desire and the visibility of that desire.

When he does finally meet the daughter, he fears seeing her disfigured body yet finds that he is disgusted without needing to see her. Her throat is covered and "the *goitre* was not perceptible, and this lessened to some degree the rising nausea, which I found it so hard to suppress."[46] And, while her "other features appeared rather well formed," the narrator expresses a kind of paranoid terror at the unreliable control he exercises over his own gaze. He "was afraid to let [his glance] linger a moment longer, lest some movement might display the loathsome swelling, the very thought of which was sickening."[47] What is striking here is that the Cagot's unseen monstrosity and excessive body (the "loathsome swelling") evokes a kind of mimetic and involuntary sympathetic response in the narrator's body. His uncontrollable "rising nausea" mimics the (still unseen) swelling at the throat of the Cagot girl, as well as an involuntary sexual response. The body of the Cagot excites the imagination and the viewer's body, even and especially when one doesn't really see it. The imagined and imaginary nature of the Cagot's monstrosity also seems to render it strangely contagious and transferrable, echoing the tropes of infection and disease I discussed earlier. In the narrator's mind, it is almost as if even though one can't see the Cagot's deformity one can catch it.

The narrator returns again and again to this "involuntary" response, whether of revulsion or desire. Yet, he also consistently associates her body and its deformity with the workings of the imagination:

> [T]he damsel in question, but not in demand, was busily occupied . . . . I felt some qualms for the ingratitude that made me still look on her and think of her with an unaccountable feeling of loathing . . . . I could bear the presence of the old one better, for there was not any of those involuntary wanderings of thought with respect to her which one cannot suppress sometimes in relation to less antiquated females. Imagination could find no resting-place in her wrinkles, nor tread the mazes of her scanty grey hairs.[48]

Here, the Cagot girl emerges as at once monstrously embodied and imaginatively disembodied—present in space and time and a product of the "vague and shadowy imaginings" the narrator had associated with the ahistorical and otherworldly Cagots. The narrator seems conscious of the way in which the Cagot girl is a product of his imagination, but it is imagination and obscurity rather than literal "explanations" that he has already argued is the best way to understand the Cagots.

This logic gets applied to the Cagot's erotic appeal when the narrator upbraids his friend—a French sergeant—for flirting with a Cagot girl and for a kind of literalism and vulgarity that betrays a lack of aesthetic and erotic taste: "I was so provoked at this proof of gross want of taste—at the promiscuous gallantry which could make love to a *Cagot* . . . how can you look at, or think of this wretched Cagot girl, with her sallow cheeks and loathsome goiter?"[49] Note that the narrator does not seem to see the difference between the "cadaverous" Cagot woman from the scene I discussed earlier and the "sallow" girl—or at least he doesn't see it as a sign of racial difference. Instead, the description focuses on disease—the Cagot girl's "sallow, unhealthy color and swollen goiter." The sergeant, however, responds by eroticizing the Cagot's deformity not through the narrator's imaginative abstraction but through a form of bodily displacement: "beggars can't be choosers . . . . I worship the sex—and an idolater enough to admire a protuberance on the throat, just as much as though it were lower down."[50] Even the sergeant's metonymic logic is too literal and too visual for the narrator: "I shrunk involuntarily from her presence into the retirement of the bed-clothes. There was something nauseous to me in the notion of her sallow cheek, her lameness, and the hidden *goître,* which was exaggerated by imagination."[51] For the narrator, admitting that the repulsive, monstrous body is less seen than imagined paradoxically makes her body both more "real" and more "nauseous." As we saw before, the narrator suggests that imagination is the only way to see the Cagot properly. In this way, it is the hidden body of the Cagot that is more visible. That is, it is open to the projections and "exaggerations" of an imagination that can apprehend the "shadowy" racial identity better than direct sight.

Yet, as it turns out, both vision and imagination fail our narrator in reading the monstrous racial body. Despite his confidence in his ability to read the "index" of the Cagot woman's mind,[52] the woman that the narrator (and the reader) imagined to be the repulsive, "sallow" skinned Cagot daughter is actually a beautiful, olive-skinned Spanish-born noblewoman, Malvide in disguise. Fittingly, Malvide means "badly seen."[53] And he sees her badly indeed, mainly because he reads her through and *as* fiction. He proceeds to fantasize about the "concealed heroine, (for I was resolved that she *should* be one)" hidden in the house, reading scraps of letters, and watching with "a wistful glance . . . the door of the secret chamber, where I was convinced so interesting a subject of inquiry lay concealed."[54] Just as the narrator describes the influence of his active imagination in his account of the Cagot girl, here he not only admits that he is "resolved that she *should* be" a "heroine" but ties his own role to that of a reader rather than an actor in the narrative—a role highlighted by his reading "scraps of letters" as he imagines her story: "My one casual glimpse of her person, my ignorance of her name, her objects in concealment, and the causes which led to it, combined to throw an air over the whole situation, to which I cannot apply any other name than romantic, and tended to tinge my mind with a colouring that I must, I think, venture to call *chivalric.*"[55]

Moreover, while not enough to overcome his repulsion at seeing the Cagot girl, his literary interest in the hidden woman induces both a form of sympathy for the Cagot family and imbues them with an imaginative, poetic aura:

> It is in such times that the imagination fixes on some object, with an interest more than real—an exaggerated intensity, creating an atmosphere around, and giving to the meanest things with its influence, a character not properly their own . . . . And such was the state of feeling which procured for the Cagot family a degree of consideration on my part, that was due to my excited interest for the unknown female.[56]

Even better, his language in describing the workings of his imagination echoes romantic poetry—Wordsworth's "Ode: Intimations of Immortality in Early Childhood."[57] The Cagots are subject to a kind of double projection: their deformities are "exaggerated by imagination" and they are given a poetic "character not properly their own" by the halo of "exaggerated intensity" created by his narrative interest. This new "excited interest," however, allows him to distinguish between his earlier "unaccountable" feeling for the Cagot girl, as he draws unflattering comparisons between the two women: "I could not help from time to time drawing comparisons in my own mind, between her sluggard gesture and position, and the graceful figure I had seen in the same place the preceding night, its speaking attitude and eloquent contour."[58] If imagination paradoxically renders the (often unseen) Cagot girl *more* bodily and more monstrous, imagination turns the physical body of the (also often unseen) woman into the fluid and abstract shape of language: "its speaking attitude and eloquent contour."[59]

The true secret, of course, completely escapes the narrator—that Malvide and the Cagot girl are one in the same. After Malvide's lover Don Melchior is wounded by an assassin waiting in ambush near the hut, she rushes to his side in the costume of the Cagot girl:

> I had to suffer that wild but still incredulous conviction that made me certain of the fact discovered to me, but doubtful of my own intellect. The female before me was, I saw it, the *Cagot girl.* Her dress, her height, her whole appearance left no possibility of doubt, but her form of symmetry, her face of beauty, how could these be there? And . . . what was my amazement to see, instead of the gross deformity I had in fancy loathed, perfection that might invite a sculptor's hand, and make his heart thrill as he gazed. I hastily threw her cloak and hood over this rich field of beauty, which I felt to be already violated by the rude yet admiring stare of the astonished observers.[60]

While it seems as if the Cagot girl vanishes and the beauty appears, they converge again in the need for concealment, even if the reasons for concealment are widely different: "I hastily threw her cloak and hood over this rich field of beauty, which I felt to be already violated by the rude yet admiring stare of the astonished observers."[61] Whether badly seen because associated with a fictional body of an abstract "heroine" (Malvide) or because her monstrosity can only be imagined (the Cagot girl), for the narrator neither female body should be seen directly. The Cagot's otherness and the mysterious beauty of Malvide are best read not by sight but rather through imagination and fiction—the "vague and shadowy" poetic imagination. That both the monstrous and beautiful bodies are figured as hidden and invisible complicates the critical notion of the gendered scene of viewing, most famously described by Laura Mulvey. Rather than the eroticized object defined by her "*to-be-looked-at-ness,*" here and elsewhere in the novel, it is the unseen female body that carries an erotic charge.[62] In other words, both the monstrous racial body and ideal female beauty are seen to best advantage when not seen at all.

A few pages later, the narrator takes another look and describes his confusion in more concretely visual terms: "I could scarcely believe my eyes—those perjured evidences, which so lately told me that this heroine of mine was lame and loathsome and which now testified to her surpassing grace and beauty."[63] Yet, in explaining his theory of female beauty, he immediately figures this beautiful body in terms of its instability and vagueness:

> To my mind, *variety* in the face of a lovely woman . . . is the greatest possible charm . . . . But this is different far from that amazed delight with which we gaze upon the rare, yet to-be-met-with, specimens of beauty . . . by which we are every moment taken by surprise . . . Malvide was, to my taste, a sample of beauty's best variety. I cannot venture to describe the fluctuating charms of her countenance, which displayed an ever shifting sameness of loveliness, like the moving surface of the sea, each instant changing, but eternally the same.[64]

For our narrator, the beautiful female body is almost not a body at all, but rather "ever shifting" and "fluctuating." Strikingly, this definition of the beautiful female body overlaps both with the image of the "shapeless" Cagot body and the "enigma" or "obscurity" that comes to constitute Cagot-ness for the narrator. Or rather, the Cagot body's "shapelessness" compounds and makes monstrous the beauty of female disembodiment.

Here Grattan echoes Edmund Burke's definition of beauty in his *Philosophical Enquiry into the Origin of Our Ideas of the Sublime and the Beautiful* (1757). As Burke writes,

> But as perfectly beautiful bodies are not composed of angular parts, so their parts never continue long in the same right line. They vary their direction every moment, and they change

> under the eye by a deviation continually carrying on, but for whose beginning or end you will find it difficult to ascertain a point.... Observe that part of a beautiful woman where she is perhaps the most beautiful, about the neck and breasts... the variety of the surface, which is never for the smallest space the same; the deceitful maze, through which the unsteady eye slides giddily, without knowing where to fix, or whither it is carried. Is not this a demonstration of that change of surface, continual, and yet hardly perceptible at any point, which forms one of the great constituents of beauty?[65]

While the narrator doesn't mobilize the familiar tropes of the female body as "deceitful" or a snare or "maze," he shares in Burke's eroticization of a body and a "sex which is not one"—that is, neither a single body nor a body proper.[66] In Grattan's novel and in keeping with this association between the female body and vague fluidity, the narrator paradoxically sums up his sketch by defining her singularity in terms of her typicality: "I can go no further in this sketch.... I defy any or all to convert Malvide into aught but what she *was,* a beautiful—a *perfectly* beautiful girl."[67] What the body of Malvide and the Cagot girl have in common (besides the fact that they are the same person) is that even after breaking through the disguise, what you see is certainly not what you get. Looking at the Cagot, in our narrator's account, one only sees the "vague and shadowy" projections of the imagination. Looking at a beautiful woman, one sees something and somebody different at every glance.

Yet, while the novel aligns the monstrous female body and its opposite through a shared fluidity and "shapelessness," it never explicitly addresses and largely ignores the narrator's mistake. In a strange (even perverse) way, the narrator's misrecognition of deformity and race doesn't constitute a critique of the narrator's expectations for racial embodiment and deformity. Largely ignoring the discovery that the Cagot girl and Spanish noblewoman inhabited the same body, the narrator only refers to Malvide's Cagot disguise once more. Having asked Malvide to don her Cagot dress to satisfy his curiosity, he notes that "[m]ore than once did Malvide gratify my somewhat sceptical anxiety, by arranging her capulet as she was wont to do in her disguise, and sportively mimicking *her own* voice and gesture."[68] When she throws off the disguise, he "was again both satisfied and contented as to her identity."[69] Despite the fact that both monstrosity and idealized femininity are conceived of in the same terms and through the same figures—fluid, shapeless, and unstable—and despite the fact that the narrator witnesses her performing Cagot-ness, he goes out of his way to stress the distinction.[70] As the Cagot girl, she speaks in "*her own* voice" and makes the same "gesture[s]." When she "throws off the disguise" the narrator is convinced and "contented" that her "identity" as a Spanish noblewoman is secure. Instead of undermining a sense of the essential, if "unaccountable" monstrosity of the Cagots, the performative nature of "Cagot-ness" only serves to render it more stable and visible—the aspect of body proper with its "own" voice.

The narrator's association of the Cagot with the poetic imagination, then, ultimately threatens class and racial boundaries—boundaries that are awkwardly and tentatively restored in the end. The noblewoman remains idealized and disembodied while the "separate" Cagot girl comes to resemble the Cagot woman with whom we began—less a figure of the imagination than a literal body, recognizable even and especially in its shapelessness as lower class, primitive, and Other. At the same time, the ability to "see" the Cagot girl as a separate body rather than a disguise is perhaps the narrator's supreme act of literary and visual imagination. In this way, the Cagot body and its monstrosity remains fictional, imagined, and invisible. If we most commonly understand monstrosity etymologically, historically, and theoretically as something to be shown and seen, the novel challenges us to think through a kind of monstrous difference that exists outside of the sphere of the visible while also remapping the relationship between the particular and the typical, the material and the abstract, and seeing and imagining. Fittingly, the short story that follows this novel is entitled *Seeing Is Not Believing,* which might have served for the title of *The Cagot's Hut.*[71] Instead of challenging the logic of racial and bodily legibility (our "belief" in what we can "see"), the narrator redefines monstrosity *through* and *as* the immateriality and ambiguity of the deformed body—its constitutive obscurity and "shapelessness." Rather than "something or someone to be *shown*" in this novel, a monster is something or someone who must be imagined.

Notes

1. Thomas Grattan, *The Cagot's Hut,* in *Highways and By-Ways; or, Tales of the Roadside, Picked up in the French Provinces. By a Walking Gentleman,* third series, 1 (London: Henry Colburn, 1823/1827), 28.
2. As Robert Young argues, the late eighteenth and early nineteenth century was a moment when the kind of racial ideology and discourse associated with colonialism was in the process of being formed. While the 1820s had already seen efforts to link the physical, mental, and moral through phrenology, Young argues that scientific or "biological" racism and racial discourse was not really entrenched until the middle of the nineteenth century and maybe even the end of the century. Robert Young, *The Idea of English Ethnicity* (Oxford: Blackwell Publishing, 2008), 63.
3. On ethnography and the novel, see James Buzard's *Disorienting Fiction: The Autoethnographic Work of Nineteenth-Century British Novels* (Princeton, NJ: Princeton University Press, 2005). On the link between disability and race in nineteenth-century American discourse, see Doug Baynton, "Disability and the Justification of Inequality in American History," in *Race, Class, and Gender, in the United States: An Integrated Study,* seventh ed., ed. Paula S. Rothenberg (New York: Worth Publishers, 1998/2007), 92–101. Baynton explores the ways in which the "concept" of disability was widely used to argue for the disenfranchisement of women and African Americans. As he argues, more generally, "by the mid-nineteenth-century, non-white races were routinely connected to people with disabilities, both of whom were depicted as evolutionary laggards or throwbacks . . . . The issue of ethnicity and disability were so intertwined in the immigration debate as to be inseparable" (pp. 94, 99).
4. Francisque Michel's *Histoire des Races Maudites de la France et de L'Espange,* 2 vols (Paris, 1847)—a book on which many accounts of the Cagots are based—describes the Cagot's complexion as "complete whiteness almost like snow" (p. 7). This description runs through to the end of the nineteenth century, with the *Illustrated London News* noting that "unlike the pariahs of the East, they differ in no way, save in having whiter skin, from the rest of the inhabitants of the pyrenean borderland." See "The Cagots of the Pyrenees," *Illustrated London News* 96, no. 2662 (April 12, 1890): 535.
5. Ironically, the excessively swelling goiters are caused by the *lack* of iodine in the diet.
6. For a different reading of the relationship between monstrosity and the sublime, see Paul Youngquist, *Monstrosities: Bodies and British Romanticism* (Minneapolis, MN: University of Minnesota Press, 2003), 62; and Denise Gigante, "Facing the Ugly," *ELH* 67 (2000): 566. Gigante associates the creature with the Lacanian "real," "the unsymbolized: the repressed ugliness at the heart of an elaborate symbolic network that is threatened the moment he bursts on the scene, exposing to view his radically uninscribed existence" (p. 567).
7. *Frankenstein* (1818) immediately comes to mind, and the creature was also figured in racial terms, ranging from Irish to black and West Indian throughout the nineteenth century. See H. L. Malchow, "Frankenstein's Monster and Images of Race in Nineteenth-Century Britain," *Past & Present,* no. 139 (May 1993), 90–130. See also Elsie Michie, *Outside the Pale: Cultural Exclusion, Gender Difference, and the Victorian Woman Writer* (Ithaca, NY: Cornell University Press, 1993), L. Perry Curtis, *Apes and Angels: The Irishman in Victorian Caricature* (Washington, D.C.: Smithsonian Institution Press, 1997), and Chris Baldick, *Frankenstein's Shadow* (Oxford: Oxford University Press, 1990). However, a few years earlier (1810), the public exhibition of Sarah Bartmann (the "Hottentot Venus") in London associated her "monstrous" body with a form of "monstrous" sexuality. As Nussbaum argues, in the eighteenth and early nineteenth century, femininity itself was represented as deformity or disability—a "fair defect" (p. 17), while blackness of "complexion" (p. 18) was imagined as not just a sign of "visible difference" but also degeneracy (p. 18). On the Hottentot Venus, see Sander Gilman, *Difference and Pathology: Stereotypes of Sexuality, Race, and Madness* (Ithaca, NY: Cornell University Press, 1985).

8. Youngquist, *Monstrosities: Bodies and British Romanticism,* xiv. Youngquist notes "whiteness" as among the "rewards of proper embodiment" (p. xx).
9. Judith Halberstam, "Technologies of Monstrosity: Bram Stoker's 'Dracula,' " *Victorian Studies* 36, no. 3 (Spring 1993): 337.
10. See Halberstam, "Technologies of Monstrosity," and Felicity Nussbaum, *The Limits of the Human: Fictions of Anomaly, Race, and Gender in the Long Eighteenth Century* (Cambridge: Cambridge University Press, 2003).
11. Grattan, *The Cagot's Hut,* 47.
12. On Grattan and Kean, see Jeffrey Kahn's *The Cult of Kean* (Aldershot: Ashgate, 2006). Eventually, with the influence of King Leopold of Belgium, Grattan was appointed British consul to the state of Massachusetts, returning to England in 1846.
13. The novel was part of a set of stories that appeared over four years. *Cagot's Hut* was published in the first series, appearing in 1823. The second series appeared in 1825 and the third in 1827. It was republished by itself in 1847 and 1852.
14. In 1806, Napoleon exploited the tension in Spanish court between Charles IV (and his unpopular minister Manuel Godoy) and his son Ferdinand (and his supporters). In November 1806, Charles negotiated a treaty with France to conquer Portugal, but French troops continued to enter Spain. In the face of a popular uprising against his minister Godoy, Charles abdicated in favor of Ferdinand (called "the desired one"). At this point, Spain was occupied by French troops. Both Charles and Ferdinand realized that Napoleon's support would determine who kept the crown. Napoleon invited both to Bayonne in France and pressured Ferdinand to abdicate to Charles, who then gave the crown to Napoleon. Napoleon appointed his brother Joseph as king of Spain. Joseph posed as an "enlightened reformer" (p. 196), but there was resistance to Joseph in parts of Spain that were unoccupied. As we will see, the conflict is not merely between monarchists and constitutionalists, and in Grattan's novel, the supporters of Joseph are those in favor of constitutional reform. Moreover, those who rose up against Joseph used "revolutionary" words (p. 197), but their aim was conservative and monarchist "inciting the Spaniards to defend Religion, King, and Country against the godless French" (p. 197). Eventually, the Rebels formed a "Cortes" (p. 198)—a kind of parliament, including representatives from South American colonies. Members of the Cortes proposed instituting radical changes, and in 1812 they established a Constitutional Monarchy. With help from British and Portuguese forces, led by Wellington, they pushed the French out. By 1813, General Rafael de Riego proclaimed the Constitution of 1812 (p. 201), and Ferdinand finally agreed to lead by a Constitution. By 1822, however, there is resistance to the radicals and their perceived hostility to the clergy. "In 1822, the enemies of the constitution established a regency in northern Catalonia to rule for the King, who they said was no longer free" (p. 201). While the French army had stood by as neutral observers, in 1823 Louis XVIII sent his army into Spain to restore Ferdinand. Unlike the uprising against Joseph and French occupation, the Spanish people did not support the Cortes, which fled and surrendered. See Richard Herr, "Flow and Ebb 1700–1833," in *Spain: A History,* ed. Raymond Carr (Oxford: Oxford University Press, 2000), 191–204, and Henry Kamen, *A Concise History of Spain* (New York: Scribener's, 1973), 113–123.
15. Grattan, *The Cagot's Hut,* 128.
16. Columbia won independence from Spain in 1816 but by 1830 Venezuela and Ecuador seceded.
17. Peter Sahlins, *Boundaries: The Making of France and Spain in the Pyrenees* (Berkeley, CA: University of California Press, 1989), xv.
18. This is not to say that coherence is the norm for racial representation. As Robert Young argues in *The Idea of English Ethnicity* (2008), writers who focused on social factors over the biological were "no less prone to use the racialized language of the stereotype" (p. 69). More generally, he argues, racial knowledge has no "distinct source or centre" precisely because it draws its authority on a range of writings—writings themselves drawn from the "ubiquity" of claims about race (p. 45). At the same time, it is this general vagueness that renders the concept of race all the more tenacious.
19. Grattan, *The Cagot's Hut,* 45.
20. Grattan, *The Cagot's Hut,* 44.
21. Grattan, *The Cagot's Hut,* 45–46.

22. Grattan, *The Cagot's Hut,* 131–132.
23. For British readers, this renders them triply othered—simultaneously Muslim, Jew, and Catholic.
24. Grattan, *The Cagot's Hut,* 44. They were subject to almost every form of superstitious hatred and persecution from the middle-ages through the nineteenth century, even as late as the 1890s. An anonymously written essay in *All the Year Round* from 1878 claims that, both in the French Pyrenees and in Spain, Cagots are "shunned . . . to this day" ("The Cagots," 416–417). Other writers, like Elizabeth Gaskell for example, claimed they had monstrous goiters and were born with ears shaped like the ears of sheep with no tips ("An Accursed Race," 77) perhaps because they had nibbled one anothers' off ("The Cagots," 418). Gaskell mocks other myths about the Cagots including the idea that, as with the werewolves, the sight of the new and full moon induced a "violent delirium" called the "Cagoutelle" (p. 79), presumably after the tarantella. See "The Cagots," in *All the Year Round* 21, no. 518 (1878): 416–420; and Elizabeth Gaskell, "An Accursed Race," in *Household Words* 12, no. 83 (1855): 73–78.
25. Grattan, *The Cagot's Hut,* 80.
26. Grattan, *The Cagot's Hut,* 80–81.
27. Grattan, *The Cagot's Hut,* 85.
28. Grattan, *The Cagot's Hut,* 46.
29. Grattan, *The Cagot's Hut,* 48.
30. Grattan, *The Cagot's Hut,* 48–49.
31. Grattan, *The Cagot's Hut,* 48.
32. Grattan, *The Cagot's Hut,* 68–69.
33. Grattan, *The Cagot's Hut,* 42–43. The legal metaphor ("living libels") speaks to both the complicity of the law and state institutions in at least countenancing prejudice against them, and the irrelevance of the law to their social fate: "if law does not set its seal upon their brutalized condition, a proscription as powerful has stamped it with a fiat that seems as irrevocable as the wretchedness it perpetuates" (p. 46).
34. Robert Young argues that Combe "pioneered the linking of physical differences of the body with mental, moral, and cultural differences, both between individuals and between nations" (p. 63).
35. Baldick, *Frankenstein's Shadow,* 10.
36. Grattan, *The Cagot's Hut,* 43–44.
37. Grattan, *The Cagot's Hut,* 45.
38. Ulysse Robert, *Les Signes D'Infamie au Moyen Age: Juifs, Sarrasins, Hérétiques, Lépreux, Cagots et Filles Publiques* (Paris: Honoré Champion Librarie, 1891), 1.
39. Grattan, *The Cagot's Hut,* 42.
40. Grattan, *The Cagot's Hut,* 47. This quote is from *Macbeth,* as Banquo addresses the three Witches:

> How far is't call'd to Forres? What are these
> So wither'd and so wild in their attire,
> That look not like the inhabitants o' the earth,
> And yet are on't? Live you? or are you aught
> That man may question? You seem to understand me,
> By each at once her choppy finger laying
> Upon her skinny lips: you should be women,
> And yet your beards forbid me to interpret
> That you are so.
>
> (1:3; ll. 39–46)

41. In describing their historical obscurity, the narrator echoes language familiar from the discourse of the sublime. As Slavoj Žižek explains, "the paradox of the Sublime is as follows: in principle the gap separating phenomenal, empirical objects of experience from the Thing-in-itself is insurmountable . . . the Sublime is an object in which we can experience this very impossibility"; Slavoj Žižek, *The Sublime Object of Ideology* (New York: Verso, 1989), 203. While critics such as Denise Gigante

and Paul Youngquist have argued against conflating the monstrous body with the sublime object, the narrator of the *Cagot's Hut* tends to associate the Cagots with what one might call a sublime body. Youngquist, for example, argues that the Romantic embrace of the sublime acts to universalize and disembody a white norm, which "serves to culturally advance the cause of domination"—what he calls "white Romanticism"—while Gigante argues that the creature's problematic and excessive body in *Frankenstein* shouldn't be confused with the "Kantian sublime object" and is "not sufficiently accounted for by aesthetic discourse." See Youngquist, *Monstrosities,* 62; and Gigante, "Facing the Ugly," 566. Gigante associates the creature with the Lacanian "real," "the unsymbolized: the repressed ugliness at the heart of an elaborate symbolic network that is threatened the moment he bursts on the scene, exposing to view his radically uninscribed existence" (p. 567).

42. It is telling that this same passage is quoted in Sydney Owenson's *Wild Irish Girl* (1806) to describe the prince and princess of Inishmore. It is important to note, however, that while Grattan's narrator is describing the Cagots in general (as a type), Horatio (the narrator of Owenson's novel) is describing the *exceptional* household of Inishmore and especially Glorvina. In the passage, their otherworldliness is linked to their isolation as Horatio is surprised to find that they send and receive letters. He is "astonished that these beings . . . should hold any intercourse with the world"; *The Wild Irish Girl,* ed. Kathryn Kirkpatrick (Oxford: Oxford University Press, 1999), 66.
43. Grattan, *The Cagot's Hut,* 78.
44. Grattan, *The Cagot's Hut,* 61.
45. Grattan, *The Cagot's Hut,* 72.
46. Grattan, *The Cagot's Hut,* 64.
47. Grattan, *The Cagot's Hut,* 64.
48. Grattan, *The Cagot's Hut,* 71–72.
49. Grattan, *The Cagot's Hut,* 119, 124.
50. Grattan, *The Cagot's Hut,* 124.
51. Grattan, *The Cagot's Hut,* 97.
52. Grattan, *The Cagot's Hut,* 62.
53. Thanks to Sharon Weltman for this suggestion. A review of Grattan's volume uses this failure to see through Malvide's disguise as a prime example of the "improbabilities of character and situation" that haunt the novel, describing her disguise as "from the beginning . . . so transparent and so awkwardly managed, that no reader can for a moment be deceived by it." See "High-ways and By-ways," *Monthly Review* 6, no. 25 (September 1827): 105–116; quote at 106.
54. Grattan, *The Cagot's Hut,* 113, 116.
55. Grattan, *The Cagot's Hut,* 156.
56. Grattan, *The Cagot's Hut,* 157.
57. "To me the meanest flower that blows can give/Thoughts that do often lie too deep for tears" (ll. 205–206); William Wordsworth, *Selected Poems* (New York: Penguin, 2005), 163.
58. Grattan, *The Cagot's Hut,* 163.
59. Grattan, *The Cagot's Hut,* 163.
60. Grattan, *The Cagot's Hut,* 244.
61. Grattan, *The Cagot's Hut,* 244.
62. Laura Mulvey, "Visual Pleasure and Narrative Cinema," in *Feminism and Film Theory,* ed. Constance Penley (New York: Routledge, 1988), 62.
63. Grattan, *The Cagot's Hut,* 256.
64. Grattan, *The Cagot's Hut,* 257–259.
65. Edmund Burke, *A Philosophical Enquiry into the Origin of Our Ideas of the Sublime and the Beautiful,* ed. James Boulton (Notre Dame, IN: University of Notre Dame Press, 1968), 114–115.
66. I borrow Irigaray's phrase here in order to point out the way in which her theory of the female body, in some ways, recapitulates rather than disrupts the "phallocentric" tropes of femininity and female sexuality.
67. Grattan, *The Cagot's Hut,* 260.
68. Grattan, *The Cagot's Hut,* 260.

69. Grattan, *The Cagot's Hut,* 6.
70. For a different reading of the conjunction of race, gender, and class, see Anne McClintock, *Imperial Leather: Race, Gender, and Sexuality in the Colonial Contest* (New York: Routledge, 1995).
71. Of this story, the *Monthly Review* writes that "if possible . . . is still more fatiguing than the former one." See "Highways and Byways," 109.

Section III

In Between Fear and Desire

CHAPTER 9

APT PUPIL (1998): THE HOLLYWOOD NAZI-AS-MONSTER FLICK (EXTRACT)

CAROLINE JOAN (KAY) S. PICART AND DAVID A. FRANK

BRYAN SINGER'S *APT PUPIL* (1998) is certainly not the first film to tell the story of "Nazi as bogeyman" or of Nazism as evil incarnate corrupting the innocent . . . . [T]he narrative, visual coding, and marketing of the film as a horror film-psychological thriller rather than as a Holocaust "faction" (i.e., "fact" and "fiction") were so overt that numerous critics exploited the film's potential for quips and analogies. For example, J. Hoberman described *Apt Pupil* as a "naturalized *Nightmare on Elm Street*" and a "Faust story with a neat-o-Spielbergian resonance."[1] [. . .]

[. . .]

NOVELLA INTO FILM

Brandon Boyce's script for and Bryan Singer's film adaptation of *Apt Pupil* (Phoenix/TriStar Pictures, 1998) predominantly effaces the misogynistic threads in the novella. In particular, the most virulent and graphic misogyny toward Monica, Betty (Becky in the film), and the young Jewish woman are excised.[2] Instead, the film leaves the homophobia of the novella intact to signify monstrosity. The primary source of homoeroticism in the novella, the relationships Todd has with Dussander and the homosexual derelict, Archie (Elias Koreas), remain prominent in the film. In addition, the movie intensifies the connection between homophobia and the portrayal of male Holocaust victims. Lastly, a further instance of homoeroticism surfaces in the depiction of Ed French (David Schwimmer).

One factor that accentuates homoeroticism in the film adaptation is the proximity between male bodies within both the diegesis and spectatorship. Todd and Dussander are the only central characters in the novella, so it is not astonishing that they would remain prominent in the film adaptation. In fact, Singer saw this limitation to two main characters as a particular challenge with *Apt Pupil:* "The most difficult part of making this film is basically that unlike *Usual Suspects,* you're given only two characters.... So there aren't many places to go with the camera and storytelling."[3] Despite its wide-screen format, the film restricts most of the development of Todd and Dussander's relationship—framed mostly in close-ups[4]—within a crepuscular, dimly lit and claustrophobic bungalow, in which the hidden Nazi lives in obscurity, with the exception of the bus ride, dinner at the Bowdens', and the hospital scene.[5] This close proximity, framed in close-ups every time Dussander touches Todd,[6] intensifies a homoerotic intimacy, punctuated by dread of contact with the monstrous, which cannot be attained visually in the novella. Paul Emmons notes the intimidating effect of Dussander's proximity to Todd: "Kurt slowly approaches Todd as though to embrace him, only at the last second turning the gesture into a reach for an object behind the boy."[7]

Homoeroticism in the film is further created by the camera's gaze on Todd's body, a factor that is conveyed in the novella (e.g., the focus on the "moistness" of Todd's genitals and lower abdominal region[8]) but explored to a greater degree in the film. Jake Wilson draws attention to a memorable "pin-up shot," in which, "teenage hunk Brad Renfro [is] sprawled on his bed in his underwear, gazing up at the hovering camera."[9] Yet the knife cuts both ways: the "pin-up hunk" is thinly separated from the *eronemos* (beloved)—the "beautiful" boy-man who apprentices under the tutelage of the *erastes* (lover), whose mentorship includes the realm of sexual initiation. This relationship, within the contemporary characterization of male-male homoerotic relationships, is construed often as dangerously homosexual.

The film is quite different from the original script. In the script, Boyce describes a rumbling in Todd's room similar to an earthquake; Todd rises from his bed and begins to walk, suddenly finding himself in a much larger space. In the film, however, an arcing god's-eye-view long shot of Todd lying on his side in bed moves in slowly, in a manner just the opposite of Hitchcock's receding arcing shot of Marion's eye in *Psycho.*[10] [...]

The ever-encroaching camera and the lighting fetishize Todd's youthful body in a manner customarily applied to the female body, particularly in the shower or peeping-tom scenes in *Psycho, The Silence of the Lambs,* and *Schindler's List.* This insight may be applied to a broader number of scenes throughout the film, when Todd's white face, with its mild complexion and his white youthful body are fetishistically captured by the close-up and he is given to wandering about without a shirt on.[11] Wilson does not miss the implication of this structuring: "At times it's hard to say whether deviant sexuality is meant as a metaphor for evil or vice versa, given the film's fixation on Renfro's muscular body, pale fine skin, and rosebud lips (held vacuously open, like an actress playing a bimbo)."[12] Neither does Stuart Klawans of *The Nation* miss the significance of these scenes: "*Apt Pupil* devotes a lot of time to hinting that its clear-eyed hero, with his sensitive lips and lithe, hairless torso, might desire something other than the standard-issue girlfriend."[13]

We understand the homoerotic fetishism of Todd's body as one instance in a trend that is imposed on an assumed white masculine spectator and is complicit with a looming homophobia, which in turn is conflated with the evil of Nazism. Through this depiction, however, Todd enters the space of Mary Russo's "monstrous feminine."[14] [...]

[...]

Whereas the novella describes Dussander's transformation from a decrepit old man to a powerful SS officer, the film furnishes an image all too familiar from imposed-makeover scenes in such films as Hitchcock's *Vertigo* (1958) and Buñuel's *Viridiana* (1961).[15] Though the changes between the novella and the film are minimal, it is evident that in the film, Todd's demands are more dominant and voyeuristic. In the novella, Todd solicits Dussander to put on the uniform and when Dussander resists, Todd remarks that he has saved all summer to be able to afford it and shakes his head at Dussander's pleas. By contrast, in the film, Todd threatens to betray Dussander to the Israelis and declares, "I tried to do this the nice way, but you don't want it. So fine; we'll do this the hard way. You will put this on, because I want to see you in it. Now move!" [. . .]

[. . .]

However, between the novella and film there is a significant difference in what constitutes Todd's "abnormal" sexuality. In the novella, Todd begins to have misogynistic dreams, one of which includes the rape of a restrained and tortured Jewess . . . . The film replaces the rape scene with a homophobic shower scene, in which Todd witnesses the transformation of his peers into homoerotically coded Holocaust victims. One victim rubs his chest and gazes licentiously at Todd, while another victim, emaciated and octogenarian, stares ruefully through "night and fog."

This second shower-gas chamber scene, which is rife with references to both the gas chambers of the Holocaust and Marion's lethal shower in *Psycho* (staples in Holocaust and horror films), is described in the following way in Boyce's script:

> Todd gets under the nozzle and allows the warm water to blast the top of his head. He closes his *eyes*. Against the high tile walls the boys' *voices* echo loudly. A dozen running shower heads contribute to the din. Todd opens his eyes . . . .
>
> Writhing bodies, thin, malnourished. These are bodies he has seen before. The room is darker, concrete. The steam rises. Or is it steam? Smoke, thick smoke, surrounds him. The voices of the boys are more like screams.

One by one the boys file out of the shower. Through the heavy steam we see Todd virtually motionless under the raging steam of water. His eyes are clamped shut.

> Finally, Todd opens his eyes, realizing, suddenly, that he is alone. He turns the shower off. His skin is red and steaming from the prolonged exposure to the hot water . . . .[16]

No overtly naked old men are described in the passage cited above—only thin and malnourished ones.

Yet the film visualizes the grotesque geriatric body and lustful gaze prominently. [. . .]

[. . .]

NAZISM AND MONSTROUS SEXUALITY

In all of the above cases, one observes the recurring representation of sexual "abnormality," which is baffling to some critics[17] but which we read as a series of codes meant to signal Todd's descent into Nazism, as well as a recurring pattern of acting out the Holocaust. Indeed, not only does Todd spiral downward into the insanity of Nazism that Dussander represents, he also becomes sexually "abnormal." Throughout the novella, King establishes Dussander as a homoerotic surrogate and as a monster because he threatens heterosexual masculinity. However, we argue that this sexual abnormality is not by any means a result of Nazism, despite the insightful comments of some critics concerning the movement's suppressed homoeroticism.[18]

King and Singer employ landscapes of misogyny and homophobia, respectively, to increase the stakes of evil in their monsters. The ideological and social-structural implications of this formation are essentially problematic, for they apparently rely on the same heterocentric assumptions that give rise to fascist values, that is, the criminalization and extermination of individuals on the basis of sexuality. This equation of othered sexuality with evil is not surprising in the wake of a tradition of Holocaust historiography that has silenced the atrocities perpetrated against thousands of homosexual men, lesbians, and bisexuals in the process of the Final Solution. [. . .]

The spectatorial relation in *Apt Pupil,* in view of a LaCapran reminder that the victims' voices must not be silenced, seems markedly even less appropriate than *Schindler's List.* Yet unlike its famous docudrama predecessor, *Apt Pupil* makes little claim to authenticity or "historicality" in its commercial packaging. The only documentary footage is shown in the beginning, when credits roll, as we peep over Todd's shoulder and gaze through his eyes at the faded photographs of Nazis and camp inmates in which doctored images of McKellan are seamlessly inserted. Thus, unlike *Schindler's List,* which ends up being a false witness in its exacting pursuit of the look of "the real," *Apt Pupil* ends up honest in its unabashed display of its simulated ontology, steeped in the expectations and conventions of the horror-psychological thriller film. Like *Psycho* and *The Silence of the Lambs, Apt Pupil's* ending may be read as filtered through a conflicted lens, where evil (and vulnerability) are not simply out there but are part of us in our uncritical and voyeuristic consumption of these images.

The film's final scenes crosscut between Dussander's escape from his captors by suicide and Todd's escape from French by blackmail, in which he repeats some of the lines Dussander himself had used to counter-blackmail Todd into submission earlier: "[A scandal like] this will never go away not for you." The film ends with a dimly lit close-up of the dead Dussander's steely-eyed gaze. Yet it is clear that Dussander's spirit lives on through Todd. In other words, while the novella ends like a classic horror film, in which the monster has been successfully vanquished (the now deranged Todd being gunned down by a SWAT team), the film ends like a contemporary or "postmodern" Gothic narrative, in which the monster lives and is unveiled as part of ourselves rather than as an alien force out there.

[. . .]

Acknowledgments

Jason Grant McKahan helped us with an earlier version of this chapter. A more aesthetically oriented reading of *Apt Pupil,* with a critical analysis of the psychodynamics set up by films that focus on the ritualistic spectacle of sexualized torture, was co-written by Picart and McKahan and has been published with *Jump Cut.* See Caroline J. S. Picart and Jason G. McKahan, "Sadomasochism, Sexual Torture, and the Holocaust Film: From Misogyny to Homoeroticism and Homophobia in *Apt Pupil,*" *Jump Cut* 45 (September 2002): 23, http://www.ejumpcut.org/archive/jc45.2002/picart/index.html.

Notes

1. J. Hoberman, "Nazi Business," *Village Voice,* December 21, 1993.
2. There is a minor skirmish between Dick and Monica about her accumulation of bills, but Todd's hatred for his mother is no longer perceptible. In addition, Monica's mother and grandmother, Morris Heisel's wife, Lydia, Lydia's mother, Edward French's, Sondra, are not referenced.
3. Dan Scapperotti, "Stephen King's *Apt Pupil: Unusual Suspects* Auteur Bryan Singer on Adapting King's Timely Shocker," *Cinefantastique* 30, no. 9 (1998): 20–21.

4. Jake Wilson, "Apt Pupil," *Urban Cinefile,* November 9, 2001, http://www.urbancinefile.com.au/home/view.asp?a=2242&s=Reviews_Archives.
5. Had the earlier film adaptation been released, which was slated for 1988 but fell through after ten weeks of production, we would have seen Todd and Dussander congregate in exterior scenes such as a puppet show and a café! See Gary Wood, "Whatever Happened to *Apt Pupil?,*" *Cinefantastique* 21, no. 4 (February 1991): 36–37.
6. Richard Scheib, "Apt Pupil," *Science Fiction, Horror and Fantasy Film Review,* 1998, http://members.fortunecity.com/roogulator/horror/aptpupil.htm.
7. Paul Emmons, "Apt Pupil," *BigScreen Cinema Guide,* 1998, http://www.bigscreen.com/ReaderReview?movie=AptPupil.
8. Stephen King, *Apt Pupil,* in *Different Seasons* (New York: Signet, 1982), 189, 206.
9. Wilson, "Apt Pupil."
10. In *Psycho,* there is a match dissolve from the shower drain to Marion's eye (extreme close-up). The camera pulls away, arching slowly. The rotation stops as the camera continues to pull out, revealing Marion's face on the floor (close-up).
11. Fred McDonald, "Apt Pupil," Abingdon College and District Film Society Program Note, November 2, 1998, http://homepage.ntlworld.com/holtnet/abcdfs/prognote/apt_pupil.pdf.
12. Wilson, "Apt Pupil," from The Academy of Motion Picture Arts and Sciences.
13. Stuart Klawans, "*Scream* 4: The Holocaust?," *Nation* 267, no. 14 (November 2, 2002): 34.
14. Mary Russo, *The Female Grotesque* (New York: Routledge, 1995), 1–2, 6, 10, 12, 29, 37, 40, 53, 56, 63, 65, 93, 106, 120, 159, 164–165, 176.
15. In *Vertigo* (1958), John makes Judy dress up to resemble Madelein, while in *Viridiana* (1961), Viridiana's uncle makes her dress in his late wife's wedding gown. Compare a similar Pygmalion replication in Steve Cohen's *Devil in the Flesh* (1998), in which Debbie's grandmother makes her wear her mother's old cloths to school. Such scenarios are most common in pornographic films, such as *The Fever of Laure,* in which a client makes the prostitute Laure dress up as Alice in Wonderland.
16. Brandon Boyce, " 'Apt Pupil,' Based on the Novel by Stephen King," shooting script, February 3–March 14, 1997. From The Academy of Motion Picture Arts and Sciences script section.
17. See Scheib, "Apt Pupil": "What it all serves is a complete mystery." See also Klawans, "*Scream* 4": "And so I ask, Why does Bryan Singer do what he does? Why turn the Holocaust into a cross between Cujo and gay S&M?"
18. Christian Leopold Shea, "Apt Pupil," review of *Apt Pupil, Jaundiced Eye,* 1998, http://www.geocities.com/Hollywood/Hills/1670/aptpupil.html. Shea writes, "There was a strong element of homoeroticism in the Nazi cult of Aryan male body to begin with (see Leni Riefenstahl's *Olympia* for ample evidence of that!)."

Chapter 10

By Demons Driven: Religious Teratologies

Jason C. Bivins

Introduction

Perhaps no moment in the history of American religions captures enduring themes more than the overdetermined Salem Witch Trials. During these religio-moral spectacles of 1692–1693, a blend of exhortations concerning national destiny, scrupulous alterity, and high public drama combined to produce not simply corpses and social calamity but more significantly, a fascination with demonology and religious scapegoating that has over time become a recognizable part of American culture. Yet in these wild exchanges between piety, power, and demonology we find something not just American but perhaps something more generally Christian as well. This is not meant as a sophomoric denunciation of Christian imperial designs, as if nothing but the Crusades and the Witch Trials ever mattered anyway, but to suggest that the complicated textures of Christian identities and social engagements (especially in the United States) have depended on their monsters.

The fearful qualities of religions are well known. The study of religion has long reckoned with these features, focusing especially on religious *nomoi* as shields against fear and anxiety or on the ontological dread central to what phenomenologists call the religious experience of the "wholly Other." What is perhaps more pertinent, however, is the degree to which experiences of religious fright and terror facilitate the achievement of social order via the construction of perceptual, behavioral, and even emotional habits. Such experiences can either generate or legitimate prohibitions, imperatives, and epistemes in ways that are imbued with the particular urgency of fear.

Beyond this, specific attention to the discursive and iconographic construction of monsters reveals that religions make such embodiments of terror central to collective self-understanding, religio-political identity, and especially engagements with their others. In American religious history, these general observations have been powerfully and flamboyantly evident. While religious constructions of the monster have not been limited to Christianity alone, the intimate historic links between this complex tradition and sociopolitical discourse have often been fashioned in richly textured demonologies.

This chapter describes how specifically Christian expressions of fear-talk and teratologies have not simply shaped public perceptions about specific classes of humans (e.g., religious others from Catholics to Muslims) and behaviors (e.g., homosexuality) but also have generated complex religious identities simultaneously by rhetorics of embattlement and privilege, apocalypticism and amelioration, and attraction to and distance from the reviled. The specific shapes of these religious teratologies have transformed American culture in multiple ways, from the literary figurations of Indian and African American "monsters" in Puritan chapbooks and oratories to the lurid anti-Catholicism of the mid-nineteenth century; from the violence consistently directed against new religious movements to the hyperviolent imaginary of contemporary virtuosi of fear like Tim LaHaye and Glenn Beck.

Religions and Their Others

While "religion" as an interpretative category has been rendered quite malleable in recent decades (owing to genealogical investigation into its disciplinary emergence), it remains evident that complex relations between selves and others are vital to the construction and maintenance of religious identities.[1] Long a psychological truism, it is through our perception of and response to our others that identities are established, changed, and maintained. Especially intense moments of identity maintenance are occasioned by experiences of fear and vulnerability. Rooted in evolutionary biology, with collective development having been achieved at least in part through responses to the experience of predation, the cultural shapes of fear are clarified when interpreted through evaluative frameworks that rank and order perceptions and classifications according to taxonomies that can be aesthetic, moral, or political, for example. These cultural and learned dimensions of emotional life remain integral to understanding social interactions and agonisms particularly.[2] Human self-understandings, modes of interaction, emotions, and beliefs cannot be understood through their interiority but only as they are expressed in social performance, public comportment, or community interactivity. It is through what Arlie Russell Hochschild calls "feeling rules" that the religious self experiences revulsions, terror, and outrages, among other emotional states.[3]

Such experiences of "rules" and their social orders reveal, through their intersubjective blending of emotion, culture, and alterity, three important dimensions of religious teratologies: (1) their embodied resonance, or how the sensorium of religious experience is perceived and articulated through powerful experiences like fear; (2) their rootedness in specific practical and discursive traditions, which partly condition the dynamics of engagement with the sources of fear; and (3) their performative functions, or how at the heart of such experiences is an enactment (through ritual or other media) of strategies designed to name the inchoate and order the chaotic in ways shaped by specific social or cultural expectations.[4]

Through this lens we can see how specific narrations of evil and the monstrous—from canonical religious texts to popular entertainments—create an urgency or fright, which has regularly dovetailed with the socioethical imperatives of political religions. The perception of object-related fears is always context-dependent, shaped by cultural roles, expectations, and moralities that surround or link up to the emotional registers of human experience. Amid this confluence of factors, religions serve as one of the most powerful means by which moral and emotional agency are situated and constituted in cultural contexts that are intersubjective, historically patterned, and energized by those things which promise their doom.

These templates and patterns of interpretation help communities form ways of understanding our world and formulating convictions about it. In the context of teratologies, then, what is compelling about fear and its modes of interpretation are the responses it induces. The names and narrations given to these experiences, particularly as they are housed in religious traditions, invariably promise not just to name the fearful unknown but—by positioning this terror against pieties—to offer control and displacement as well. Looking closer into cultures of religious fear and teratologies later, what we see is not simply that these materials are energized and nurtured in context of sociopolitical urgency; they also reveal deep anxieties about identity and group boundaries.

Yet what is it specifically about religious monsters and fears that conveys such a sense of urgency or power? As John Corrigan and others have noted, religious cultures can generate or legitimate specific religious norms; they can, in ritual or performance, confirm membership in groups or one's own piety; they can, by association, mark off specific spaces or times as religious; and they can help culturally situated selves to generate cognitive and social judgments.[5] It is at the intersection of religious and "worldly" cultures, of individual and collective experience, of scripted and spontaneous emotions that the fearful narratives and representations of the monstrous go to work.

Such conjunctions become powerful when galvanized in response to perceived threats to identity. In specific instantiations of fear, narrative responses to those things named "monstrous" are couched in emotionally resonant language that affirms, and promises to protect, collective identity. Whether oriented to the cosmological or the mundane, the language of religious literatures and practitioners trades heavily in images of fear and trembling. See this in the foundational observation that "Fear of the Lord is the beginning of wisdom" (Prov. 1:7) and multiple subsequent biblical injunctions to remain obedient, lest wrathful judgments ensue. Many such images serve as reminders of bodily and epistemic limits, of the immensity of supernatural realities and our inability to name or fix them. In these moments, the sovereignty and boundedness of the flesh become not just inviolable but at risk. Those things and experiences designated as religious are often rendered distinctive through recourse to just these languages of powerful otherness.[6] Such experiences are recorded as especially powerful in monotheistic traditions, which knit together experiences of the *mysterium tremendum et fascinans* ("fearful and fascinating mystery") with moral obligation, piety, and safety. While such traditions cannot be reduced merely to command morality, pious fears are nonetheless commended to the faithful as registers of safety and of awareness: steadfast faith can serve as a strategy of avoiding dire consequences.

Indeed, it has frequently been observed—by canonical figures in the study of religion, as well as by contemporary researchers—that the experiences at the heart of religiosity are intimate with the fearful: for modern and early modern critics, the functional core of religious experience is to provide explanations of the fearful unknown and consolations in the face of uncertainty and death. The best-known formulations include Hume's notion that religious convictions are rooted in emotional "passions" and the "imposture" that seeks to account for gaps in knowledge; Freud's assertion that the experiences described as religious occur when the distinction between id and ego becomes unstable; and, less acerbically, Rudolf Otto's evocations of the holy's "bewildering strength" or overwhelming "awe or 'dread'."[7] Contemporary observers, less beholden to critical inveighing against religions or to vague postulations about the numinous, still locate religions in experiences of terror which can, via memory and repetition, underwrite the vigor of particular religio-social moralities.[8] These experiences of religious fear can be produced simply by inhabiting a specific religious *habitus,* which effectively communicates to believers practical and affective responses to circumstance, or they may facilitate in post hoc interpretations or rationalizations of experience.[9]

The appearance of monsters within a religious framework serves not only as a means of explaining or framing biological limits and inevitable mortality (by promising glimpses of possible fates to be avoided); the monsters teach and warn as limit-experiences of their own. Horrific and fearful figures—whether Satan or cultural monsters like heretics, the libidinous, or the foreign other—function to legitimate and justify through their ability to convey experientially what is elsewhere described in the language and symbolism of ultimacy. Their success—whether depicted in narrative or present through ritual enactment—turns often on the degree to which they are able to respond to social and political concern. As I note in *Religion of Fear,* however, they also emerge from and simultaneously address ambiguities of the self.[10] Particular constellations of fear-talk and religiosity have proven historically fertile in generating and sustaining religious monsters. Familiar examples stem largely from Abrahamic and, most commonly, Christian traditions: the potent demonologies of the high Middle Ages, the doomy mood of the Puritan commonwealths, or the nuclear tinge of mid-twentieth-century American apocalypticism.[11] This acknowledgment is not intended to suggest that in times of declension or deprivation the religious turn "naturally" to monstrous formulae; yet certain contextual and shaping factors are undeniably central to bringing the *monstrum* to life in the thick of religious convictions and perceptions.

Such emergences make sense given the narrative roots of monsters, as described by Timothy Beal[12] and Edward J. Ingebretsen.[13] The *monstrum* was originally understood as a divine messenger of sorts, as befits its derivation from the Latin *monstrare,* meaning to show or to warn.[14] According to Beal, "the monster often appears as an index of all that a particular culture projects as beyond its pale."[15] Monsters embody and constitute the racial, sexual, political, and religious other. Once established as threats, they justify often extreme social and political measures in the name of safety or purity. Indeed, the language and symbolism of risk—particularly, in the contemporary period, families and children at risk—is that without which teratologies cannot survive.[16]

In cultures historically obsessed with or driven by fear, the pedagogical function of monsters can be realized more effectively. American Christianities in particular have historically drawn from deep traditions—whose influence ranges from popular entertainments to national policy—which blend Gothic sensibilities, apocalypticism, and moral languages of retribution.[17] Americans not only have an insatiable appetite for disaster—from pandemics to mass killings to barbarians at the gates—but public cultures have regularly been defined by engagements with these real or perceived panics.[18] Such engagements serve a protective purpose, via negative transference, but more importantly they render the other fiendishly threatening.[19] Thus religions dramatize the need for identity maintenance, as the very fantastical nature of the discourse confirms, via its irregularity, the inevitable return to the normalcy at risk.

Religious habits of perception and practice contribute to these familiar social processes by investing the time and place with a specific ontological urgency. In ritual circumstances like exorcism, for example, sacred time overwhelms the profane, and the very religious engagement with the monstrously other confirms the sacrality of the cosmos.[20] They also reinscribe the context of the monstrous in such a way that it is larger than the social, directing attention away from the sources of its construction. The religious monster is understood as a material threat, an incarnation of evil; it is also a powerful part of a symbolic order.[21] When situated and articulated thus, representations of the monstrous can serve justificatory purposes (as in deliberations about launching war) and explanatory ones (invoking the need to redirect attention to a deity or to valorize a path already taken). Most commonly, those things that religions name as monsters or demons are, to cite Mary Douglas, "selected for special emphasis . . . either because they offend the basic moral principles of the society or because they enable criticism of disliked groups and institutions."[22] The religious monster is said to emerge from an order more real than the known, of an ontological depth and power that confers on their functions a gravity usually lacking in merely cultural monsters and their narrations.[23]

Religious monsters arrive or are announced framed by scriptural narrative, potent sacred imagery, and a religio-moral mood of preparedness to recognize their presence and meaning. Religious presuppositions facilitate such recognition, even as the emotional or social-critical response to monsters loops back to confirm the presuppositions themselves. Their admixture of emotional urgency, soteriological gravitas, and alterity lends to these creations an especially powerful pedagogical function. The most obvious level on which this occurs is through boundary-work, where the monstrous other teaches the self its ontological and behavioral limits. It is also cultural pedagogy, insofar as holy terrors remind us—through what Corey Robin calls "the clarifying knowledge that evil exists"—of the proper relation between purity and contagion, safety and risk, permitted and forbidden.[24] Perhaps most significantly, this is also pedagogy pitched at the level of reality itself, where the specific judgments linked with the monstrous—sexual, political, ritual—are housed in a broader cosmologic understanding of order and chaos, and the fate of the soul beyond the body.

The religious monster warns of God's order disrupted and promises its glorious restoration. Its success charts the degree of our fallenness. The capacity of the monstrous to dramatize and teach through awareness of our own misdeeds and temptations is central to their effectiveness. Their very threat to first principles and social stability reenergizes our commitment to these things, lends urgency to our efforts to distinguish ourselves from the monster. Sociologically, the monstrous other around which religions organize themselves—via prohibitions, ritual protections, and jeremiads—is frequently seen reflected in more mundane others like the apostate or the revolutionary, whose behaviors and judgments blur their identity with those of demons or damned. Where profane political fears turn on stereotypes that reinforce cultural presumptions about difference, religious monsters serve to write such engagements with others onto the universe itself, so that they perch outside conventional notions of time or place, presented to us as eternal and unchangeable.[25] The appearance of what religions literally and figuratively swear off is both crisis and opportunity, providing for the devout an occasion not simply to ban what is evil but—in naming it—to reassert foundational convictions and confessions.

In some senses, these templates that code the monstrous are housed in religious institutions and rituals such as casting out demons; for the most part, however, they are sustained in modes of perception and interpretation which flow from texts and iconography to become reproduced and legitimized through repetitive use, now clearly in the realms of politics and pop culture. The most potent and resonant religious teratologies have been Christian, perhaps nowhere more energized than in purportedly secular cultures that fuel the cultivation of distinctively religious identities. In the United States, these religiosities have also drawn energies from cultures of horror and the Gothic, which serve as an additional reservoir of symbols, metaphors, narratives, and sources of justification, moving fluidly within and alongside the religious. Marina Warner locates the beginning of societal law with the identification of monsters; yet in religious traditions the monster may also clarify laws and norms that supersede social values, thus marking the arrival of an order that frames and clarifies what the monster muddies or tears asunder.[26]

As Beal writes, "[b]y demonizing our monsters, we keep God on our side."[27] Such recognitions justify and rehabilitate God's purposes when these are called into question; serve as opportunities for conversion; address anomie and insecurity, experienced either socially or individually; and confirm that our cosmos is alive with sacred presence. In an endless process of warning and resolution wherein the fearful other's banishment purifies the fearful self, the monster actually cannot be banished completely since its very presence marks not the sacred's absence but its presence. Beal reminds that monsters are thus liminal, their arrival both conventionally threatening and a register of traditions wrestling with their ambiguities.[28] Religious teratologies, then—whether located in primal chaos monsters, Job's Leviathan, the dragon of the Johannine Apocalypse, or medieval imaginings of the Beast—move between the architecture of religious justifications and the dissolution of boundaries in the experience of terror.

Hell must be felt to be close by, its torments near, for us to require regeneration and new birth. American interpreters of religious monsters—from Cotton Mather to Tim LaHaye—have constructed sacred cartographies that require something horrible lurking in wait. These sensibilities have fed into a rich popular culture of horror and fright, and have drawn from it in turn. Literary and entertainment cultures have offered up an abundance of fearful narratives, whose mixture of revulsion and fascination with spectacles of doom (the sinning body brought low, the splattery crimes of the new city, the vengeance of unseen forces) owed equally to the influence of the Gothic and long-standing hellfire traditions.[29] Such imaginings of sacred terror range from Michael Wigglesworth's doom-fraught poetry to Hawthorne and Poe to Lovecraft and King, each of whose works appropriates primary religious tropes of terror that are integral to their wrestlings with identity.[30]

Contemporary religious teratologies are shaped not only by traditions of sacred reflection and literary darkness but also, beginning in the first decades of the twentieth century, by increasingly significant visual entertainments of popular horror. More than the Gothic or the chiliastic literature of Puritan New England, the religious tropologies of modern horror not only make central embodiments of the monstrous but dwell in a narrative space of retributive moralism that writes our mundane decisions into a cosmos of often grisly consequentialism. Thus, according to Ingebretsen, horror "tells a story, explains that story, and draws moral conclusions, simultaneously."[31] Modern American life is indebted and has in many ways taken shape through such horror formulae.

Religion's "Awful Disclosures"

The justificatory ends of religious monsters are achieved via the merging of social, cosmological, and political orders, the divine norms and judgments they embody both inflexible and endlessly applicable. The monster articulates religious discomfort with difference, and seeks to contain or eradicate it through the establishment of dread, prohibition, and God's fearful warnings. The monster's sheer abnormality in God's good order also, as both Beal and Ingebretsen show, embodies divine order in a kind of semiotic dualism, which demands of believers not simply attention but a kind of compliance. According to Ingrebretsen, monsters both metaphorical and real can be invoked to justify "a range of socially discounted but nevertheless tolerated behaviors—violences physical as well as rhetorical, social expressions of astonishment, scandal and insult, displays of sex as moral currency and economic exchanges."[32]

A full historical account of the sociopolitical uses of religious monsters is well beyond the scope of this chapter. Such a treatment would obviously range across the bestiary of chaos monsters in ancient Mesopotamian cultures, multiple mythological pantheons, Buddhist folk hells, fantastical colonialist responses to Hindu sacred beings, as well as the vast post-Johannine corpus of demonological literature.[33] Beyond malefic figures ensconced in myth or the enduring resonance of certain literary traditions (not just the Gothic, but also Dante, Blake, or the *Malleus Maleficarum*), religious monsters have been used consistently to undermine the "false gods" of competitor traditions, maintain behavioral boundaries (primarily sexual), and underscore sociopolitical distinctions as religious ones (particularly in the domain of race or ideology). How are actions like the castration of a Jehovah's Witness, the murder of a Sikh mistakenly taken as a Muslim, the burning of a convent, and other such outrages made possible?[34] Such acts of religious violence are always partly misrecognitions: monsters loom where only humans once stood. I explore these dimensions in a later section through the lens of American Christianities, because of these traditions' consistent uses of teratologies and because they have shaped political life in such powerful ways. Deprivation theory notwithstanding, religious monsters are energized in times of trial. Of late, American culture has been particularly conducive to nurturing such monsters.

One of the most powerful and enduring designations of the monstrous is achieved through rhetorical and symbolic constructions of "false gods." There are a few more effective ways of conveying to audiences that souls are at risk of damnation than to redescribe or reinterpret the object of their worship as illegitimate, monstrous, or demonic. The disciplines of the flesh and of the political have depended regularly on the dehumanization of those considered threats to social order, to orthodoxy, and to moral propriety. One key medium of constructing such threats has been the contention that the deepest commitments of one's others are shaped by something impure or malevolent. These strategies account for the fearful imaginings of the Puritan commonwealths, not only in obvious examples like the Salem Witch Trials of 1692–1693 (whose blessed rage for order depended on its demonologies) but also in, for example, Cotton Mather's boast following the war against the Pequot that several hundred souls were "brought down to hell," leaving the colonies safe from the savagery of Indian culture and religion.[35] We see them, too, in the virulent anti-Catholicism ranging from the mid-nineteenth century (where Nativist campaigns against arriving immigrants, including the burning of an Ursuline Convent outside Boston in 1934, found popular expression in *The Awful Disclosures of Maria Monk*) to the contemporary era (where fears of "popery" linger in popular evangelical works like Jack Chick's cartoon tracts).[36]

Many religious representations of monstrous others are aimed at policing or redrawing behavioral boundaries. The media through which these initiatives are pursued range from captivity narratives describing fearful Native American monsters to the recent explosion of Islamophobic blog content.[37] Much energy has focused on perceived sexual immoralities, as with the complex justification of certain "pro-life" Christian assaults on employees at abortion clinics (whom they regard as less than human, even monstrous for participating in such demonstrable evil) or Topeka's Reverend Fred Phelps invocation of divine hatred against the sexually "abominable," with his memorably toxic slogan "God hates fags."[38] Behind demon rum or fornication, in illicit entertainments or ritual out of bounds, there circulated rumors of monstrous practices ranging from cannibalism and child abduction to elaborate fifth column plots. In the fervid imagination of religious teratologists, the categories of heretic, outsider, and deviant collapse into each other. Once it is decided that before us stands not a fellow citizen or co-believer but a monster, great license is taken in actions against such threats. The mechanics of justification vary greatly, yet religious anxieties about demonology, devil worship, and the like are at work in a host of episodes of religious violence in the United States and elsewhere: in Nativist campaigns against racial others, the murder of Joseph Smith, the Nation of Islam's "white devils," the fantastical racial imaginings of the World Church of the Creator, the near extermination of Native American religions, or the heated demonological visions of contemporary conservatives like James Dobson, whose nationalist pieties depend on his lurid imaginings of sin, malevolence, and peril.[39]

Perhaps some of the most vivid of American Christian monsters are those that erupt directly into social and political life, drawing energy from the perceptual and representational strategies noted earlier. The category "monster" takes on abundant characteristics when invoked to make sense of, or stake out positions within, an unstable political structure. One of the most active cultural reservoirs of such imaginings has been in far right Christian cultures since the 1960s, blending extreme racism and anti-Semitism with Christian apocalypticism and paramilitary fetishes.[40] At the heart of these religio-political teratologies is the monster of government itself, made a hydra with financial, cultural, pedagogical, and administrative arms thought to undermine the authentic religiosity and sociality of "the common man." (Related to populist expressions circulating widely, the most extreme practitioners have found expression not simply in historic racist groups like the Ku Klux Klan or in demagogues like Gerald B. Winrod, Father Charles Coughlin, or Gerald L. K. Smith; we see them also in the complex exchanges between Christian Identity and religio-patriotic self-styled militias, particularly active just prior to the Oklahoma City bombings of 1995 and since President Barack Obama's inauguration [e.g., the

Hutaree].[41]) Indeed, the period since the September 11, 2001, bombings has proven extremely fecund for such imaginings in the United States. Energized by a vast culture of apocalypticism (which shares some elective affinities with earlier periods of fundamentalist anti-modernism), the (primarily Christian) discourse of the monstrous has woven into American engagements with the Gulf oil spill, the health care "debates" and their outrageous allegations of "death panels," the charged conversations surrounding immigrant and sexual others, the regular allegations that President Obama himself masks an infernal agenda, or with the Third Wave evangelical response to the Haitian earthquake.[42] Less obviously political are the representational grotesqueries that seek to portray specific religious constituencies—either entire traditions or specific expressions, as in the case of Islamophobia or Fundamentalist Latter-Day Saints respectively—as unfit for public life, as degraded, whose existence is a sign against some version of America's purported sacred history. Even conservative religion's complex engagements with pop culture have a deep politics, as I argue in *Religion of Fear*.[43]

Are religious monsters always political? Part of what is so resonant about religion's monsters after secularism is that they are, owing to the very technologies and discourses of the secular itself, eternally returning. Religious monsters not only thrive in a secular that suggests they have long since vanished but also depend on the secular as their own other, a context that perpetuates them and makes possible their lesser others, the gays, the pederasts, and the liberals. David J. Skal suggests that the experience of modernity, whose institutional and perceptual habitus removes humans from proximity to death, inevitably generates terrors and sideshows to rationality.[44] Indeed, in the context of purportedly secular public and political institutions it is via their lurid, vivid monsters that religions can announce and display their continued vitality.

Conclusion: Religion's Unstable Teratologies

This survey of religious monstrosities, primarily Christian American, reveals how centrally teratologies depend on religious rhetoric. In many cases, the articulation of this discourse rests on assumptions about what "religion" actually is. These practitioners are fascinated with the object of their terror and indignation, seeing in them nothing less than the other of "religion" itself, in "false" piety, abominable antireligion, or sociopolitical evils. What makes religious teratologies different from nonreligious instances is the broadening and deepening of the language of ultimacy in the face of these monsters, a consequentialism written across time and couched in a sacred cosmos. As David Frankfurter notes, teratologies emerge as "representations of local crisis and anxiety in totalized, cosmic terms."[45] This discourse is pitched in absolutist or cosmological terms because the monster convinces its audiences that ontological stakes are high. Establishing such urgency is precisely what lends to religious teratologies their justificatory edge, since actions undertaken in the defense of good order, divine law, or community piety—all of which we are told the monster makes vulnerable—can be legitimated, even if they seek to censure, expel, or even harm what is designated as monstrous.

Identifying the monstrous other—the secular humanist undermining education, the godless backslider, the cultist—explains distress in religious terms and works to reestablish religious identity at once. Against these figures, religious teratologies gain their energies from their warnings to the deviant or heretic that they risk God's wrath, made material in the monster. Religious teratologies both sharpen and muddy categories and identities: while they initially function to establish distance between the sacred and the material evil they identify, they also reveal—as authors from Kristeva[46] to Ingebretsen[47] demonstrate—the complex dependency of religions on their monsters. As symbols of crisis, religious monsters necessitate the work not just of the language of the sacred but the performance of identity itself, in what Kristeva calls "purification rites whose function is to separate this or that social, sexual, or age group from another one, by means of prohibiting a filthy defiling element."[48] The very materiality of evil demands such an engagement, even if it subsequently circulates at the level of the symbolic and the mediated. As Michael Rogin[49] and Corey Robin[50] have written with regard to political demonologies, the naming of the monster—as a figure that condenses and distils a range of inchoate fears and anxieties—help make firmer the foundations and first principles the monster is said to threaten. Religious agency thus turns on the degree to which it can contest the monstrous.

Yet it is at this very point that the mutual imbrication of sacred and monstrous is revealed once again. Beyond the sociopolitical aims and resonances of religious teratologies, they take shape on craggy boundaries that relate not just purity and defilement, salvation and damnation, but also the intimacy of these twinned others. This means more than simply the kind of mutual dependency so often remarked in studies of alterity (and which I elsewhere refer to as the Demonology Within[51]). It refers also to the animating, enlivening pleasures of these discourses, which I elsewhere call the Erotics of Fear.[52] Like the enemy one keeps close at hand, these grim narratives serve simultaneously as denials, projections, and fantasies that blur the boundary between material (and political) reality and the instability of the Gothic imaginary. The construction and projection of virtual, rhetorical, and narratological monsters is an enduring way by which certain American religious practitioners have posited the religio-ethical or the religio-political, and found their others wanting. The specifically religious shapes of American monsters have changed according to time period, medium, and the urgency of their articulation. Attending to their emergence illumines the darkness necessary to religious identity.

Notes

1. See, among other sources, Daniel Dubuisson, *The Western Construction of Religion: Myths, Knowledge, and Ideology* (Baltimore, MD: Johns Hopkins University Press, 2007); Tomoko Masuzawa, *The Invention of World Religions: Or, How European Universalism Was Preserved in the Language of Pluralism* (Chicago: University of Chicago Press, 2005); and Russell McCutcheon, *Manufacturing Religion: The Discourse on Sui Generis Religion and the Politics of Nostalgia* (New York: Oxford University Press, 1997).
2. The most visible popular example of such work is Pascal Boyer's *Religion Explained: The Evolutionary Origins of Religious Thought* (New York: Basic Books, 2001). Thomas A. Tweed's recent theoretical interventions, particularly in *Crossing and Dwelling: A Theory of Religion* (Cambridge: Harvard University Press, 2006), are animated by this literature.
3. See Hochschild's important *The Managed Heart: Commercialization of Human Feeling,* second ed. (Berkeley, CA: University of California Press, 2003).
4. In the vast literature on ritual, Catherine Bell's *Ritual Theory, Ritual Practice,* Revised Edition (New York: Oxford University Press, 2009), remains an excellent distillation of multiple approaches to performance and ritual life.
5. See John Corrigan, ed. *Religion and Emotion: Approaches and Interpretations* (New York: Oxford University Press, 2004).
6. See Timothy K. Beal, *Religion and Its Monsters* (New York: Routledge Press, 2002), 7.
7. See David Hume, *The Natural History of Religion* (New York: Oxford University Press, 1998), 27–29; Sigmund Freud, *Totem and Taboo* (New York: Norton, 1962) and *The Future of an Illusion* (New York: Norton, 1989); and Rudolf Otto, *The Idea of the Holy,* excerpted in *Theory and Method in the Study of Religion: A Selection of Critical Readings,* ed. Carl Olson (Belmont, CA: Wadsworth Publishing, 2002), 109.
8. See, for example, Harvey Whitehouse, "Rites of Terror: Emotion, Metaphor, and Memory in Melanese Initiation Cults," in *Religion and Emotion,* 133–148.
9. See Marcel Mauss's *The Gift: The Form and Reason for Exchange in Archaic Societies* (New York: Norton, 2000) and Pierre Bourdieu, *Outline of a Theory of Practice* (Cambridge: Cambridge University Press, 1977).

10. Jason Bivins, *Religion of Fear: The Politics of Horror in Conservative Evangelicalism* (New York: Oxford University Press, 2008).
11. See Paul Boyer, *When Time Shall Be No More: Prophecy Belief in Modern American Culture* (Cambridge, MA: Belknap Press of Harvard University Press, 1994) and Eugen Weber, *Apocalypses: Prophecies, Cults, and Millennial Beliefs Through the Ages* (Cambridge, MA: Harvard University Press, 1999).
12. Timothy K. Beal, *Religion and Its Monsters* (New York: Routledge Press, 2002).
13. Edward J. Ingebretsen, *At Stake: Monsters and the Rhetoric of Fear in Public Culture* (Chicago: University of Chicago Press, 2003).
14. See Beal, *Religion and Its Monsters;* and Ingebretsen, *At Stake.*
15. Beal, *Religion and Its Monsters,* 103.
16. René Girard's *The Scapegoat* (Baltimore, MD: Johns Hopkins University Press, 1989) remains a crucial source.
17. See, among many other sources, Sacvan Bercovitch's *The Puritan Origins of the American Self* (New Haven, CT: Yale University Press, 1975); John Putnam Demos's *Entertaining Satan: Witchcraft and the Culture of Early New England* (New York: Oxford University Press, 1982); Christine Leigh Heyrman's *Southern Cross: The Beginnings of the Bible Belt* (Chapel Hill, NC: University of North Carolina Press, 1997); George Marsden's *Fundamentalism in American Culture: The Shaping of Twentieth-Century Evangelicalism, 1870–1925* (New York: Oxford University Press, 1980); and R. Laurence Moore's *Selling God: American Religion in the Marketplace of Culture* (New York: Oxford University Press, 1994).
18. See Barry Glassner, *The Culture of Fear: Why Americans Are Afraid of the Wrong Things* (New York: Basic Books, 1999); Michael Rogin, *Ronald Reagan: The Movie, and Other Essays in Political Demonology* (Berkeley, CA: University of California Press, 1988); and Elaine Showalter's *Hystories: Hysterical Epidemics and Modern Media* (New York: Columbia University Press, 1998).
19. See James Aho's *This Thing of Darkness: A Sociology of the Enemy* (Seattle, WA: University of Washington Press, 1995).
20. See Andrew Cuneo's *American Exorcism: Expelling Demons in the Land of Plenty* (New York: Broadway Books, 2002).
21. David Frankfurter's *Evil Incarnate: Rumors of Demonic Conspiracy and Satanic Abuse in History* (Princeton, NJ: Princeton University Press, 2008) is a vivid comparative study of these symbolic logics.
22. Mary Douglas and Aaron Wildavsky, *Risk and Culture.* Quoted in Glassner, *The Culture of Fear,* xxvi.
23. Debbie Nathan and Michael Snedeker discuss similar processes at work in the construction of social panic surrounding "Satanic cults." They claim this panic functions in ways similar to what folklorists call a memorate, "the process by which an individual uses popular legends to explain an ambiguous or puzzling experience." See Debbie Nathan and Michael Snedeker's *Satan's Silence: Ritual Abuse and the Making of a Modern American Witch Hunt* (New York: Basic Books, 1995), 30.
24. Corey Robin, *Fear: The History of a Political Idea* (New York: Oxford University Press, 2004), 2.
25. See Leonie Huddy, "Fear and How It Works: Science and the Social Sciences," *Social Research* 71, no. 4 (Winter 2004): 802.
26. Marina Warner, *No Go the Bogeyman: Scaring, Lulling, and Making Mock* (New York: Farrar, Straus and Giroux, 1998), 3.
27. Beal, *Religion and Its Monsters,* 6.
28. Beal, *Religion and Its Monsters,* 146, 155.
29. See Mark Edmundson's *Nightmare on Main Street: Angels, Sadomasochism, and the Culture of the Gothic* (Cambridge, MA: Harvard University Press, 1999) and Walter Kendrick's *The Thrill of Fear: 250 Years of Scary Entertainment* (New York: Grove Weidenfield, 1991).
30. See Elisabeth Bronfen's *The Knotted Subject: Hysteria and Its Discontents* (Princeton, NJ: Princeton University Press, 1998).
31. Ingebretsen, *At Stake,* 43.
32. Ingebretsen, *At Stake,* 2.
33. It is well known, of course, that contemporary understandings and depictions of Satan far postdate early Christianity. See Weber's *Apocalypses* on this point.

34. Such strategies of religious alterity have a long and familiar history, it goes without saying. They are clearly evident, for example, in the demonization of Jews (in medieval blood libel and elsewhere). See Frederic Jaher, *A Scapegoat in the New Wilderness: The Origins and Rise of Anti-Semitism in America* (Cambridge, MA: Harvard University Press, 1996).
35. Quoted in Howard Zinn, *A People's History of the United States* (New York: Harper Perennial, 2001), 15.
36. See Jenny Franchot's *Roads to Rome: The Antebellum Protestant Encounter with Catholicism* (Berkeley, CA: University of California Press, 1994). On Chick tracts, see my *Religion of Fear: The Politics of Horror in Conservative Evangelicalism* (New York: Oxford University Press, 2008), 17–18.
37. Tracy Fessenden's *Culture and Redemption: Religion, the Secular, and American Literature* (Princeton: Princeton University Press, 2006) contains a brilliant account of captivity narratives. Rogin's study, *Ronald Reagan,* also remains definitive.
38. Panics emerging around embodiment and religious enthusiasms, too, have long turned on demonological claims and rendering monstrous what is considered religiously deviant. Ann Taves's *Fits, Trances, & Visions: Experiencing Religion and Explaining Experience from Wesley to James* (Princeton, NJ: Princeton University Press, 1999) vividly describes these panics during the First and Second Great Awakenings in the United States.
39. On white supremacist Christians, see Michael Barkun's *Religion and the Racist Right: The Origins of the Christian Identity Movement* (Chapel Hill, NC: University of North Carolina Press, 1997). Matthias Gardell's *In the Name of Elijah Muhammad: Louis Farrakhan and the Nation of Islam* (Durham, NC: Duke University Press, 1996) is an excellent introduction to the Nation of Islam.
40. See Michael Barkun's *A Culture of Conspiracy: Apocalyptic Visions in Contemporary America* (Berkeley, CA: University of California Press, 2003) and David Bennett's *The Party of Fear* (Chapel Hill, NC: University of North Carolina Press, 1988).
41. Mark Juergensmeyer's *Terror in the Mind of God: The Global Mind of Religious Violence,* third ed. (Berkeley, CA: University of California Press, 2003) remains an excellent resource for understanding these orientations. On Winrod, Coughlin, and Smith, see Barkun's *A Culture of Conspiracy* and Angela M. Lahr, *Millennial Dreams and Apocalyptic Nightmares: The Cold War Origins of Political Evangelicalism* (New York: Oxford University Press, 2007).
42. Elizabeth McAlister, an expert on Haitian religions, has assembled a comprehensive collection of writings on the Haitian earthquakes, notably featuring Pat Robertson's contention that these events represented God's judgment on vodou and other religions. The collection is available at http://emcalister.faculty.wesleyan.edu/writings-on-haiti-earthquake/.
43. Bivins, *Religion of Fear.*
44. David J. Skal, *The Monster Show: A Cultural History of Horror,* revised ed. (New York: Faber & Faber, 2001), 18.
45. Frankfurter, *Evil Incarnate,* 8.
46. Julia Kristeva, *Powers of Horror: An Essay on Abjection* (New York: Columbia University Press, 1982).
47. Ingebretsen, *At Stake.*
48. Kristeva, *Powers of Horror,* 65. Kristeva clearly has in mind Mary Douglas's important work here.
49. Rogin, *Ronald Reagan.*
50. Robin, *Fear.*
51. Bivins, *Religion of Fear,* 17–18.
52. Bivins, *Religion of Fear,* 17–18.

CHAPTER 11

AN AGE OF MECHANICAL DESTRUCTION: POWER TOOLS AND THE MONSTROUS IN *THE TEXAS CHAIN SAW MASSACRE* FILMS

IAN CONRICH

THE MODERN HORROR FILM IS MARKED BY ICONIC IMAGERY SUCH AS Freddy Krueger's razors-for-fingers glove in the *A Nightmare on Elm Street* series (1984–2010), Jason Voorhees's hockey mask in the *Friday the 13th* sequels and remakes (1980–2009), the distorted Ghostface mask of the killer in the *Scream* series (1996–2011), and Pinhead's multinailed facial and cranial features in the *Hellraiser* (1988–2011) films.[1] Central to these movies is a mixture of extreme imagination and familiar themes; a repetition and revisiting of effective images and situations, which at the same time are designed to exceed within a genre continually viewed as being close to a point of saturation.

William Friedkin's *The Exorcist* (1973) and Tobe Hooper's *The Texas Chain Saw Massacre* (1974) are frequently regarded as marking the start of the modern horror film, with its fascination for explicitly depicting unfamiliar physical forces toward the threatened body. The high cultural register of both films is apparent through their sequels, and the various parodies and imitations. In particular, *The Texas Chain Saw Massacre* spawned *The Texas Chainsaw Massacre 2* (1986), *Leatherface: Texas Chainsaw Massacre III* (1990), and *Return of the Texas Chainsaw Massacre* (1994), as well as a 2003 remake of the original, a 2006 prequel *The Texas Chainsaw Massacre: The Beginning,* and *The Texas Chainsaw Massacre 3D,* planned for release in late 2012. The films have created a chainsaw cult, which includes a variety of shorts, such as the *Texas Chainsaw Musical* (2007), and the feature films *Hollywood Chainsaw Hookers* (1988), *House of 1000 Corpses* (2003), *Chainsaw Sally* (2004), and *Chainsaw Cheerleaders* (2008). There is also the low-budget feature *Das deutsche Kettensägen Massaker* (*The German Chainsaw Massacre,* 1991), a locally made homage produced just after the collapse of the Berlin Wall. This film relocates the sociopolitical tensions of Hooper's original to a country in which former West Germans are shown slaughtering former East Germans as they cross the old border in their Trabants.[2]

The original *Texas Chain Saw Massacre* was partly inspired by the activities of the Wisconsin serial killer, Ed Gein. From there, the mask made of the skin of human victims—worn by the figure of Leatherface in the *Texas Chain Saw Massacre* films—was developed. Predominantly "faceless," as with other apparently indomitable modern monsters such as Voorhees and *Halloween*'s Michael Myers, and with a dehumanized epithet, Leatherface is another of the genre's simple yet original creations. Leatherface, as he was presented in the first film, is seemingly forever prepared for work wearing a slaughterhouse apron and/or a shirt and tie that suggest dedication and professionalism. But it is the chainsaw with which he is most associated, a mechanical weapon of choice, which he repeatedly parades in a frightening statement of brutal power. This chapter will focus on the monstrous, specifically the character of Leatherface, as articulated through a cycle of ideas and images presented within the *Texas Chain Saw Massacre* films. Incorporating a cinema and material culture of merchandise, props, and posters, this chapter will consider the ways in which a group of films have adapted and transferred key elements of the monstrous that are instantly recognizable within the modern horror genre—the mask made from human skin; the power saw popularized in the title of an infamous movie.

Mechanical Destruction as a Work of Art

In the late 1990s, New York's Museum of Modern Art (MOMA) added a copy of Hooper's *The Texas Chain Saw Massacre* to its permanent collection of films chosen for their significance and impact as modern artworks. For a film with a minimal narrative, *The Texas Chain Saw Massacre*'s design, appeal, its artistic ability to captivate, move, and register a striking visual and aural impression lies in its unrelenting terror and terrorizing, its incessant threat of unbelievable pain, and the almighty assault of the ever-whirring chainsaw. In fact, writing more than a decade before the film's induction into MOMA, Robin Wood had already argued that the film had "the force of authentic art," and that it was a transgressive text with a "spirit of negativity" and a "lust for destruction."[3]

Wood writes of an experience where he watched the film with an audience who "cheered and applauded every one of Leatherface's outrages."[4] As a modern work of notoriety and power, the film is clearly far from being contained within a Manhattan museum, with a cult of the chainsaw having now penetrated contemporary culture in a range of references from the stage performances of the pop artist Eminem to a series of comic books and artistic models and miniatures depicting Leatherface in fine detail.[5] It even inspired a computer game, made for the Atari console, and released in time for Christmas 1982 by Wizard Video Games. In the game, the player is encouraged to "[k]now the pleasures of total destruction," assuming the role of a chainsaw-wielding Leatherface, hunting down victims, including a character in a wheelchair. More recently, there was also a limited-edition pair of Air Force One Nike sneakers, designed by the company Sweatshop, with a stitched-skin effect around the shoe and a bloodied chainsaw replacing the Nike swoosh logo.

But can a film as populist as *The Texas Chain Saw Massacre* really be regarded as art? Walter Benjamin argued against the art status of film, due to mechanical reproduction being "inherent in the very technique of… [its] production,"[6] and as a necessary part of its consumption, thereby removing its aura as an original and authentic piece created within "the fabric of tradition."[7] Such arguments are persuasive, and are observable within a postclassical cinema that has become ever more "mechanized," increasingly reliant on technology for its look and effects, and synergistic, woven into a vast network of mass consumerism. Yet, contrary to Benjamin, there is no denying that elements of films have become highly valued and auctioned works of unique art. There are, for instance, art galleries selling coveted hand-drawn and painted animation cels (such as those for celebrated Disney films) and pre-production sketches and conceptual drawings (most noticeably for films in the *Star Wars* series [1977–2005]).[8] Crafted at a stage of production prior to the employment of a film camera, the cels and conceptual drawings are not alone in commanding high market prices as film originals. In recent years, movie collectables have also included original film props and costumes specifically crafted for and worn in films.[9]

Available props from *The Texas Chain Saw Massacre* films appear to have been largely restricted to the 2003 and 2006 productions. This is perhaps partly explained by the fact that the first four films were made before a true market for original movie collectables had emerged in the mid 1990s, and therefore items were only infrequently saved or reserved, and even then as mementoes by cast and crew. A visit to an online museum of movie props, yourprops.com, where collectors can display their treasures, reveals a few individuals with various items of chainsaw massacre clothing, a pillow from the Dodge van, a "dirty lantern," and a "SFX smoking chainsaw," from the 2003 remake, and Leatherface's carving knife and mask, from the 2006 prequel.[10]

Such cultural artifacts are transferred (and often exchanged) objects taken beyond the film screen and transformed into modern celebrations of screen creativity. Within the movie, they function in support of a larger experience and serve to enhance the manufacture of a fiction, which is then duplicated across numerous prints allowing for wide circulation and extensive recognition across different film markets. Yet, the "souvenir" film prop or original costume that is removed from the two-dimensional screen fiction is given a value as a three-dimensional object that neither needs the film camera or projector to continue its appreciation. The majority of these props are unique, though some are produced in multiples to function as reserve copies or for the creation of a particular effect. Many are made by skilled technicians and specialist craftsmen, and they carry an aura that comes from being an original and recognizable part of a singular screen production, a physical referent to an idolized moment or component of a film. Props by known special-effects artists, such as Carl Fullerton or Rick Baker, carry an extra value and are fêted as part of that filmmaker's oeuvre, and often placed on display at fan conventions. Moreover, there are the curated exhibitions, such as those displaying the costumes and props, the genuine craftsmanship and skill within the manufacturing of films such as *The Lord of the Rings* trilogy (2001–2003) and *Titanic* (1998). Significantly, such exhibitions have been presented in museum environments alongside other works of art and stunning craftsmanship. How these props are revered are, I would argue, part of a modern ritual located within their original use in the film, which is later part of a magical and perhaps religious process, with the "adored" objects functioning in support of a particular film cult and as an attraction pulling devotees toward conventions and exhibitions. Within this context, these visual and material objects display the aura identified by Benjamin as existing within the work of art.

A work of art can be popular and *The Texas Chain Saw Massacre* has been endured as both a critical and cult success. Around the film, and the versions that followed, there has emerged a chainsaw cult, with this extreme weapon of choice not only heralded in the films' titles but also foregrounded in an expectation of unspeakable horror in which the monstrous is partly defined by a threatened assault by power tool.

The Cult of the Chainsaw

At yourprops.com, one collector from Fort Worth, Texas, proudly displays a photograph of what is claimed to be an original chainsaw from the 1974 film. The photograph shows the power tool laid out on a platform surrounded by memorabilia from *The Texas Chain Saw Massacre.* This highly treasured item, which is the centerpiece of this fan's altar to the film, celebrates the chainsaw, above all else, as the most essential element of the production. Certainly, the chainsaw dominates the film's identity within a commercial marketplace. The emphasis within the titles of the films is not on the family, but on the power tool, and there is an exploitation factor to the word "chainsaw," which along with the word "massacre" suggests a relentless and unstoppable carnage.[11] The reportage style of promotion for the original film adds to the sensationalism, with the tagline "Who will survive and what will be left of them?," implying a situation of utter terror and near apocalypse. For this poster, the chainsaw extends out from the borders of the main image and acts both as an actual pointer to the title itself, which appears beneath, and as a challenge to the film's potential audience, with the chainsaw threatening to break out of the two-dimensional confines of the advert. This attempted effect was heightened in the American and French posters for *The Texas Chainsaw Massacre 2,* where a chainsaw is depicted ripping through the advert, which is designed as a door (in the former) and a wall (in the latter).

Indeed, the narrative images for the films continually foreground the chainsaw, where it appears prominent on almost every poster. For *The Texas Chainsaw Massacre 2,* the eagerly anticipated sequel to the first film, it was the return of the chainsaw that was announced as paramount. As the tagline declares, "After a decade of silence . . . the buzz is back." Positioned below this, on the most widely circulated design of poster, are five members of the Sawyer family of cannibals, in a posed group shot similar to an organized family portrait, with the chainsaw included in the image as an essential addition to the family unit. This is underlined in the poster for *Leatherface: Texas Chainsaw Massacre III,* in which a chainsaw positioned diagonally across the advert and in front of a shadowy presentation of Leatherface dominates the image, with "The Saw is Family"—a line spoken by Drayton Sawyer in the previous film (Part 2)—clearly engraved on to the steel length of the tool.

Subsequent posters for the series isolate either Leatherface as the sole family member of note or the chainsaw, or both. Two later posters for *Return of the Texas Chainsaw Massacre* both centralize an image of the chainsaw, with one presenting the power tool as a lipstick-chainsaw hybrid "applied" against a woman's large pouting red lips. In the poster for *The Texas Chainsaw Massacre: The Beginning,* a back shot outline of a potent figure that is deduced to be Leatherface walks toward the distance carrying a chainsaw. The man, whose face we cannot see, is presumed to be Leatherface because of the chainsaw; crucially, without the weapon this figure would be anonymous. Here, in this poster, the centrality of the chainsaw to the films is apparent, for it defines Leatherface and is the index to his monstrosity. The chainsaw, though, in these films is a force of its own and I would argue that any notions of the monstrous must see beyond Leatherface and recognize the horrendous power of this tool as well.

The immense threat of mutilation and bloody death that a chainsaw presents, and the ease with which it can wreak destruction, means it is a preeminent horror weapon. *The Texas Chain Saw Massacre* led to copycat titles such as *The California Axe Massacre* (1977) and *The Hatchet Murders* (1975), which foregrounded in their names the extensive use of a particular lethal weapon.[12] But only *Driller Killer* (1979) came close to delivering a similar height of notoriety, with a marketing campaign that promoted terror from a serial killer's relentless use of another power tool. Furthermore, of the horror films of the modern era, which have been dominated by serial killers and slashers, few movie monsters across a series have been so associated with such an iconic weapon. While Leatherface, at times, turns to other weapons and devices, such as hammers and meat hooks, for immobilizing his victims, it is the chainsaw that is most trusted by this monster, and it is never too far away. The chainsaw "dance" performed by Leatherface (see Figure 11.1), as he wiggles, jerks, and gyrates his body while wildly waving the chainsaw above his head, reveals a deep and unnatural pleasure that he holds in this power tool. In fact, Leatherface is so attached to this weapon, his "little buddy" as it is called in the 2006 film, that even after his chainsaw-wielding arm is completely hacked-off in the 2003 remake, he bends down with his undamaged left hand to collect the power tool before continuing with his assault. Only Freddy Krueger, and his razors-for-fingers glove, is as synonymous with a singular weapon and, even then, Freddy's methods of dispatching his victims regularly incorporate a range of other weapons and a richness of devices that benefit from the dreamscape in which he operates.

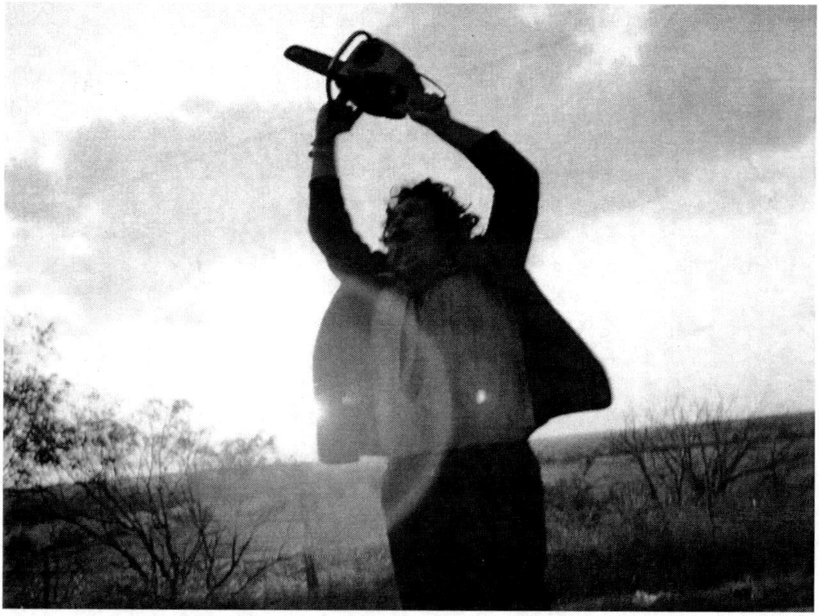

Figure 11.1 Power from the preeminent horror weapon in the chainsaw "dance" in *The Texas Chain Saw Massacre* (1974). (Courtesy of Vortex.)

Like Freddy's razors-for-fingers glove, Leatherface's chainsaw can be heard but not seen. In an environment of darkness or spatial uncertainty, the screech of Freddy's razors-for-fingers along surfaces, or the buzz of Leatherface's chainsaw motor from an off-screen position, creates an aural warning to the impending horror of a terrifying weapon that could suddenly appear. Leatherface tends to work in isolation and in rooms that are separated from the rest of the home. At the end of a corridor, which has been established with several long shots, and behind the metal slaughterhouse–style sliding door that firmly slams shut in *The Texas Chain Saw Massacre,* the buzz of Leatherface's chainsaw as he sets to work on his next helpless victim establishes a terminality from which there is little chance of survival. In these spaces, he can work largely undisturbed, with no need to disguise the noise of his saw. Significantly, unlike many other horror-film slashers, stalkers, and killers, there is a lack of stealth within Leatherface's approach, which adds to the raw horror of the situation.

The idea for the chainsaw assault came to Hooper in a moment of consumer suffocation, when he was trapped in the hardware department of a large store. Surrounded by chainsaws, he fantasized as to how they could be used to escape past the holiday season crowds.[13] Like many titular monsters whose appearance is restrained, or withdrawn, until a particular point in the film when the full horror can be unleashed, the chainsaw in the first film does not emerge until almost a third of a way into the movie. Leatherface is initially introduced wielding a slaughterhouse hammer, but it is his extended chase of Sally (Marilyn Burns) through the surrounding woods, while wielding a revved up chainsaw, combined with the final sequence which culminates in his chainsaw "dance," that became a key part of the film's signature. As if to authenticate the other films in the series, the signature chainsaw chase of a screaming teenager through the woods is replayed in all but the second film, while the chainsaw "dance" is reenacted several times and even transferred to the female victim-survivor Vanita "Stretch" Brock (Caroline Williams) in *The Texas Chainsaw Massacre 2.* She survives by becoming empowered by the saw, taking on the role of the chainsaw-killer and slaying Chop Top. Similarly, the film's other hero, Lieutenant "Lefty" Enright (Dennis Hopper), returns the terror of the chainsaw to the family of cannibals, arriving at their lair armed with three chainsaws and engaging in a swashbuckling duel of power tools with Leatherface, and ultimately defeating him with the blade cutting straight through the monster's belly. The chainsaw is a highly efficient tool that is commonly employed in agriculture, forestry, or the slaughtering industry, and it is associated with a slicing through matter with greater ease. It tends to be used as part of an extended job, in which there is an expected repetition, which is reflected in the fast-turning circularity of the blade. It is a circularity that is carried within the films, in which the myth of the monstrous Leatherface is revisited, replayed, and reimagined.

Reimagining Leatherface

As the series moves from *The Texas Chain Saw Massacre* (1974) through to *The Texas Chainsaw Massacre: The Beginning* (2006), it attempts a narrative circle, with the latter production starting at the birth of Leatherface in 1939 and ending a few years prior to the 1973 film. In many such extended film series, the narrative structure does not hold up to scrutiny with plot inconsistencies, discontinuities, and changes, and *The Texas Chain Saw Massacre* films are no exception. What is most striking in the Leatherface series is the fluidity in kinfolk, with the Sawyers, later renamed the Hewitts, consisting of at least 18 family members (not counting others introduced in the comic books), some of whom are explained through references to deviant sexuality, such as incest, inbreeding, and being the offspring of rape.

Actually, one of the few constants throughout the series is the chainsaw itself, with the figure of Leatherface, who is prominent in all six films, forever being adjusted to the point where it is best to refer to a series of Leatherfaces. Compared to horror's classical or golden age, modern horror films have a greater tendency for developing and rebooting the most successful screen monsters. Jason Voorhees was suddenly given the power of parody and irony with a clear vein of humor introduced to the *Friday the 13th* series, starting with *Friday the 13th Part V: A New Beginning* (1985). Rob Zombie's reboot of *Halloween,* meanwhile, saw a Michael Myers leviathan bulked-out and given significant extra height in *Halloween* (2007) and *Halloween II* (2009), where he was now played by former professional wrestler 6ft 8in Tyler Mane. By contrast, the changes to Leatherface through the six films to date are numerous, with the productions attempting an exploration of the psychology and nature of the man behind the mask while also extending the legend.

Leatherface is the modern horror film's original monstrous-sized human fiend, with 6ft 4in actor Gunnar Hansen playing the character in the first film. Hansen says that his size was a factor that helped him get the role: "[t]hey loved the fact that I filled the doorway."[14] His powerful presence is most emphasized in the film in the way that he pulls the screaming and flailing Pamela (Teri McMinn) back into the dreadful house and then lifts her up onto a raised meat hook. Against Leatherface, she appears petite and helpless, his thick arms smothering her body and his brute strength managing to effortlessly lift her off the ground as if she was a rag doll.

However, this butcher also has a bit of a paunch—Carol J. Clover sees it as "baby fat"—difficulties speaking, and a low level of intelligence, with subsequent interpretations focusing more on his weaknesses, reimagining him as an impotent and obese retard.[15] Hooper describes Leatherface as a "big baby" and, in Part 3, he is totally confused by an electronic speak and spell machine, with his repeated attempts at typing the word "food," under the image of a man, rejected as incorrect.[16] In the same film, he is referred to as "Junior" and is depicted as a backward child who remains attached to the wheelchair-bound maternal Mama Sawyer. Among other names, he is called a "dumb ass" in Part 2, and he is shown being chastised by his brother for his oafishness and for making mistakes. The belittling and taunting that he receives from his brothers includes prodding and pushing that only emphasize his corpulence.

Originally, it was intended that Leatherface had spoken lines, but these were replaced by having him make noises, such as pig squeals and gibberish sounds. Apparently, Hooper removed Leatherface's speech as it would have meant there was "too much intelligence in the character."[17] Hansen, who played the original Leatherface, has said that the character "knows what he wants to say, but he can't get his mouth to make the right sounds. He has the idea of speech, but he can't express it—he just makes sounds randomly."[18] This becomes worse over the first four films and Leatherface is often reduced to just grunts, yelps, screams, and primitive noises.

Moreover, there is in the first four films an effeminate side to Leatherface, which Clover views as "gender distress."[19] In the first film, he is the family member most associated with the home and the kitchen, the cook who prepares the food, and who, according to Hansen, dons his "pretty woman [mask] . . . because we had company and he was getting all dressed up for dinner."[20] Hansen argues that Leatherface is "not effeminate, just androgynous," but acknowledges that in Part 4 "he's played very effeminately."[21] Interestingly, Leatherface had appeared more feminine in the first film, with a scene showing him powdering himself and, as a "woman," preparing for the special dinner. The footage, though, was cut and it has only reemerged as a bonus scene on the DVD release for *The Texas Chain Saw Massacre*. By contrast, in Part 4, Leatherface is shown wearing a wig of female hair and adding lipstick to his female skin-mask while admiring his appearance in a mirror. The opening shot to this scene is ambiguous, with an extreme close-up of the lipstick being applied, thereby obscuring the rest of Leatherface and leading the viewer to briefly assume that the character they are watching is a woman. In preparation for this dinner, he also paints his fingernails, and puts on a dress with a plunging neckline. The dress reveals a female bodysuit complete with breasts, which is also made of human skin, and on to which Leatherface dabs a bit of perfume around his neckline and into his cleavage.

Clover also views killers such as Leatherface as the male "propelled by psychosexual fury."[22] Judith Halberstam takes this further into an argument for "monstrous gender, a gender that splatters, rips at the seams, and then is sutured together again as something much messier than male or female."[23] She is particularly drawn to *The Texas Chainsaw Massacre 2,* for its sexualization of Leatherface and the way in which he is romantically drawn to Stretch, the female DJ to whom the key parts of the Leatherface identity—the chainsaw and mask—are transferred. Chop Top childishly mocks Leatherface as having "got a girlfriend," after seeing him refuse to harm Stretch, a woman whom he is also seen to kiss. Earlier, Leatherface had discovered the terrified Stretch hiding, and gifted her a freshly cut mask, from the skin of her still-alive colleague. Forced to wear the mask to survive she agrees to also dance with her new partner, as Leatherface twirls her around. In this film, it is the infamous radio station scene that explicitly demonstrates Leatherface's psychosexuality, as he presses his extended tool—his dormant chainsaw—against Stretch's inner thigh and then up against her crotch. Stretch realizes the power of the chainsaw for Leatherface's ability to function, and tells him he is "really good" and "the best." Stimulated, he frustratingly finds that his saw will not start, its lack of power making him appear impotent. When the saw does start, he waves and thrusts it in front of Stretch but he does not kill her and leaves in a hurry. As Clover puts it, "immediately after ejaculation Leatherface becomes palpably less interested in his saw."[24]

The 2003 and 2006 films lose much of the comic eccentricity of the previous productions, such as the near-pantomime of Part 2, and curious moments like when Leatherface, in a moment of satisfaction, slaps palms with his brother Chop Top. In rebooting the series, Leatherface's character is streamlined and refocused by removing almost all of the black humor associated with his cumbersomeness and idiocy. A noted exception was the need in the 2006 prequel for Leatherface to chainsaw the good left leg of his uncle Monty, after a moment in which he had botched a bit of impromptu "surgery" on the damaged right leg.

It is not until the series is rebooted, with the 2003 Michael Bay-produced glossy remake, that Leatherface is hypermasculinized, with 6ft 5in bodybuilder Andrew Bryniarski playing the remodeled and new hulk. With the physique now of a bodybuilder, Leatherface has lost his paunch and femininity, and while still displaying learning difficulties, he is now suffering mental deterioration—a result of his extreme affliction—as well as appearing more a force of hatred and vengeance.[25] In the prequel, he is reminded by his brother of the bullying that he endured at school, as a way of inciting him to use his chainsaw for the first time as a killing tool. Earlier, the murder of his first victim within the film, the intimidating boss of the meat works who is bashed to death with a slaughter-hammer, is presented as especially justified. Years earlier, the bullying boss had oppressed Leatherface's birth mother and showed no concern as she suddenly went into labor, with the newborn child later disposed in a dumpster for waste meat. Like Freddy Krueger, Leatherface is a bastard child, and his adopted brother describes him as "the ugliest thing I ever saw." The montage of images in the opening credit sequence establishes, predominantly through childhood photos, a young boy who grows to realize that a disability has marked him as monstrous. It is Leatherface's disfigurement from birth, his degenerative facial disease, which is the reason for his wearing of masks.

Behind the Mask

From the very first film (1974), there were multiple Leatherfaces, with this monster owning then three quite different masks: the killing mask, the old woman, and the pretty woman.[26] Scriptwriter Kim Henkel said that "Leatherface is one of those characters who is what he wears—his character changes according to the face he puts on."[27] Elsewhere, I have written about *Friday the 13th*'s Jason Voorhees and the importance of the mask for modern horror film monsters: "[l]ike *Halloween*'s Michael Myers, and *The Texas Chain Saw Massacre*'s Leatherface, [for whom the] executioner's mask establishes a cold, mechanical and faceless killer devoid of personality."[28] On reflection, it was wrong to see Leatherface's mask as being so vacant and lifeless, with his range of facial disguises (in combination with clothes and mannerisms) providing a degree of information as to the monster behind the mask. Hansen, the first actor to play Leatherface, has talked at length about the way in which he approached this challenging character:

> What I took to be the great disadvantage for me—that I had neither voice nor face for the character and all I had was my body to play the character with—was actually a great advantage in fact: it forced me to spend the time trying to figure out the character physically. So I had a very strong idea of his personality . . . I had really worked on figuring out how I was going to represent the character physically . . . The whole idea [of Leatherface] was that the mask reflected who he was now—my feeling was that under the mask was nothing—if you take the mask away there's no face there—that's how I tried to play him . . . So the mask defines who he was.[29]

Furthermore, in the commentary for the DVD of *The Texas Chain Saw Massacre,* Hansen says to Hooper,

> you told me that the whole idea is that the mask is because he has nothing inside. I mean that the mask is the personality. So he changes faces depending on what he's trying to do. Now he's being domestic. He's been making dinner and so he's got the old lady mask on, an apron, and a giant wooden spoon. He moves different [*sic*] too.[30]

On one level, Leatherface's mask establishes an exterior personality, an outer identity, albeit stolen, flayed from a victim. In Part 6, for instance, Leatherface removes the face of Eric

(Matthew Bomer), which he takes as his first mask, while being secretly watched by Eric's girlfriend Chrissie (Jordana Brewster). Before Eric's facial skin is removed, it is inspected by Leatherface, who appears to assess the quality, appropriateness, fashion, and fit of his soon-to-be new attire. Having then acquired the features of a handsome and virile young man, and having just moments earlier discovered the power of the chainsaw for carving through human flesh, he emerges from his basement workshop, committed and confident as the monstrous Leatherface, his new identity completed with the mask and power tool. Such a mask has an aesthetic appeal for Leatherface, who is drawn to certain skins for their physical effect and the way in which they present for him an ideal that he believes improves his appearance.

Beyond the exterior, there is contrary to the statements from Hansen and Hooper, a viewed inner personality. This is spied through little holes in the mask for his eyes, and most visibly around the oral region, with Leatherface often licking his lips and teeth with a craving and desire. In Part 5, after Leatherface has been emasculated, with his chainsaw-wielding arm hacked off, and his attacker has escaped, a close-up of his mask establishes that he is now extremely angry, with the face beneath the mask able to reveal an unusual amount of information about this monster's heightened emotions. The mask in this reboot is more fearsome than those previously in the series, with Leatherface given large stitches worthy of Frankenstein's monster, and thicker and stronger features, as opposed to the slackness of his facial outline in the first film: now he exhibits a greater defined forehead, chin, mouth, and nose, a protruding brow, and deeper and darker recesses for his eyes. The result is a disguise that conveys more about the man beneath who, through a better-fitting acquired skin, is able to now fill out the mask.

A range of Leatherface masks appear throughout the six films and the acquired faces of assorted victims allow Leatherface to express himself differently, inhabiting alternative identities. They also allow the viewer to gain a degree of understanding as to Leatherface's personality. The mask may also be seen to guide or assist a gender performance, with the facial skin of a matriarchal woman worn to accompany a particular domestic activity, or the face of a younger woman applied for a special occasion and when there are guests for dinner. The effeminate Leatherface, with bodysuit, breasts, and a chiffon dress revealing cleavage, who loses at the end of Part 4, holds the palm of his hand to his face in distress, while drooping the chainsaw in his limp right hand. Such a conclusion could not be more different to the one presented at the end of the hypermasculine Part 5. Significantly, the mask is a crucial, though not solitary, part of a larger performance of the monstrous, with clothes, mannerisms, and tools—whether it be a kitchen spoon or buzzing chainsaw—revealing Leatherface's personality.

With the mask the membrane between outer and inner personalities, both taken and hidden, and which alternate across different genders and ages, Tamao Nakahara is correct to argue that Leatherface's identity is "always unstable and fragmented."[31] Indeed, for Part 3 in the series, Leatherface was, for the first time, given a mask of parts: as production designer Mick Strawn said, "it was supposed to be a bunch of skins sewn together, twisted and torn."[32] Like the stitched together or repaired flayed face, Leatherface is a patchwork of parts that cannot achieve completeness. He is a composite character and that has become part of his appeal, against which the simplicity of the saw is juxtaposed.

In an attempt to give added depth to the character, the series has explored his workshop or den, the spaces in which he tortures and slaughters, or in which he makes-up and reflects on his appearance. The design of these rooms is important, from the water-drenched basement in which Leatherface operates in Part 6 to the dressing room with the old gramophone, playing slow music, as Leatherface applies makeup in Part 4. Within these private spaces, Leatherface is shown—in Parts 3 and 5—manufacturing his mask. In Part 3, the cutting and stitching together of parts of facial skin presented within the opening credit sequence defines this monster's centrality, alongside the centrality of his mask to the film. The cutting is done with care and precision, and contrasts with the mask that is ripped off in Part 2 and presented to Stretch. In Part 5, the film extends the establishment of a space that defines Leatherface's identity and work, with him seated at a sewing machine table crafting a new mask in a workshop surrounded by tools and body parts in jars and on trays that suggest within this "laboratory" there is a professionalism and organization to this evolving monster.

The 2003 and 2006 films, Parts 5 and 6, in which the series was rebooted, are particularly drawn to developing the legend of Leatherface and the Hewitts (previously the Sawyers), filling in the narrative gaps as to who Leatherface is, where he was born, what is his relationship to his family, how he came to employ a chainsaw as a killing tool, and why he wears a mask. As Kim Newman argues, though, such mythmaking is not required and the point of the films is, in this context, lost by the reboots: "the whole point of the chain-saw family is that they just are, and we don't need (or want) to know where they came from and how they came to be that way."[33]

Part 5 in the series goes where no film in the series had gone before and lifts off the mask to reveal the true face of Thomas Hewitt. His appearance recalls Erik, the Phantom of the Opera, whose mask is a permanent cover for a severe facial disfigurement. In those films, though, and most memorably in the original 1925 Lon Chaney silent version, the mask is dramatically stripped off Erik's face by Christine who sees to her horror and to the audience's horror the extent of Erik's deformity. After four *Texas Chain Saw Massacre* films, the filmmakers of Part 5 evidently believed that a similar dramatic and horrific revelation would be achieved by lifting off Leatherface's mask. But the impact is strangely muted, and the revelation is easily forgotten. In my article on the *Friday the 13th* films, I argued that "more frightening than the mask is the concealed face . . . the 'face shot' that the audiences expect."[34] Leatherface appears different and, for such a monstrous masked figure, audiences and fans have not expected or demanded a facial exposure. His identity has been built around a series of masks that have helped establish a character that goes beyond the more mono-dimensional masked killers like Jason Voorhees and Michael Myers.

As with those successful series, characters have been altered and extended, and as with *The Texas Chain Saw Massacre* films, the monsters have been highly popularized and developed into modern bogeymen, recognizable on a global level. Leatherface is not the only monstrous character in *The Texas Chain Saw Massacre* films but he has become the series' most recognized and most easily transferred figure. Much of the power to adapt and reimagine this character comes from the monstrous form that he is given through his mask of human skin and his chainsaw. For these are what significantly define Leatherface, and as observed in the marketing of the series, they are key factors in the promotion of a promise of the monstrous.

Acknowledgments

I would like to thank Rick Simon and Roy Smith for their helpful comments and suggestions.

Notes

1. Note Jason did not acquire his trademark hockey mask until *Friday the 13th* Part 3 (1982).
2. The Trabant is a car associated with a manufacturing industry in the former East Germany. Made of poor materials, with few accessories, and distinctly lacking in design values, it has become an icon of car production ineptitude.
3. Robin Wood, 'Introduction,' to *Planks of Reason: Essays on the Horror Film,* ed. Barry Keith Grant (Metuchen, NJ: Scarecrow Press, 1984), 191.
4. Wood, 'Introduction,' 191.

5. Posters and figurines have been produced capturing Eminem's infamous stage performance, in which he not only wielded a chainsaw but referenced Jason Voorhees and the *Friday the 13th* films through the simultaneous wearing of a hockey mask.
6. Walter Benjamin, "The Work of Art in the Age of Mechanical Reproduction," in *Illuminations,* ed. Hannah Arendt (New York: Schocken Book, 1988), 244.
7. Benjamin, "The Work of Art in the Age of Mechanical Reproduction," 223.
8. See, for instance, the film artwork sites on the Internet at http://www.animationartgallery.com/ and http://www.cartoon-factory.com/.
9. See, for instance, Prop Store at http://www.propstore.com, where Jason's machete used in *Friday the 13th* (2009) sells for £2929 (http://www.propstore.com/product-Jason-Voorhees—Derek-Mears—Machete.htm), an original Creeper latex mask from *Jeepers Creepers* (2001) sells for £1019 (http://www.propstore.com/product-The-Creepers—Jonathan-Breck—Finale-Prosthetic-Mask.htm), and a complete Pumpkinhead monster suit from *Pumpkinhead: Ashes to Ashes* (2006) sells for in excess of £5000 (http://www.propstore.com/product-Pumpkinhead-Complete-Costume.htm).
10. See http://www.yourprops.com/view_items.php?movie=texas+chainsaw&keywords=&do=search&index_from=100.
11. The sensationalism of the word "chainsaw" is realized in the title of Carol J. Clover's study of the horror genre, *Men, Women, and Chain Saws: Gender in the Modern Horror Film* (London: British Film Institute, 1992).
12. The *California Axe Massacre* was originally released as *Axe,* and *The Hatchet Murders,* or *Dario Argento's Profondo rosso,* was originally released as *Deep Red.*
13. Stefan Jaworzyn, *The Texas Chain Saw Massacre Companion* (London: Titan Books, 2003), 28.
14. Jaworzyn, *The Texas Chain Saw Massacre Companion,* 37.
15. Clover, *Men, Women, and Chain Saws,* 27–28.
16. See Tobe Hooper in the documentary *Texas Chainsaw Massacre: The Shocking Truth* (1974/2000).
17. Jaworzyn, *The Texas Chain Saw Massacre Companion,* 43.
18. Jaworzyn, *The Texas Chain Saw Massacre Companion,* 43.
19. Clover, *Men, Women, and Chain Saws,* 27.
20. Jaworzyn, *The Texas Chain Saw Massacre Companion,* 45.
21. Jaworzyn, *The Texas Chain Saw Massacre Companion,* 45.
22. Clover, *Men, Women, and Chain Saws,* 27.
23. Judith Halberstam, *Skin Shows: Gothic Horror and the Technology of Monsters* (Durham, NC: Duke University Press, 1995), 143.
24. Clover, *Men, Women, and Chain Saws,* 28.
25. Leatherface's obesity is replaced by the obesity of his birth mother in Part 6, and the morbid obesity of the bizarre Tea Lady (Kathy Lamkin) in Parts 5 and 6, whose size recalls the physical difference of circus sideshows.
26. These three mask descriptions were given by Gunnar Hansen; see Jaworzyn, *The Texas Chain Saw Massacre Companion,* 45. In the commentary for the DVD of *The Texas Chain Saw Massacre,* Hansen refers to the old lady mask as part of his "grandma" "get-up." See also Tamao Nakahara, "Making Up Monsters: Set and Costume Design in Horror Films," in *Horror Zone: The Cultural Experience of Contemporary Horror Cinema,* ed. Ian Conrich (London: I.B. Tauris, 2009), 149.
27. Jaworzyn, *The Texas Chain Saw Massacre Companion,* 43.
28. Ian Conrich, "The Friday the 13th Films and the Cultural Function of a Modern Guignol," in *Horror Zone: The Cultural Experience of Contemporary Horror Cinema,* ed. Ian Conrich (London: I.B. Tauris, 2009), 179.
29. Jaworzyn, *The Texas Chain Saw Massacre Companion,* 43.
30. Nakahara, "Making Up Monsters," 149.
31. Nakahara, "Making Up Monsters," 149.
32. Jaworzyn, *The Texas Chain Saw Massacre Companion,* 184.
33. Kim Newman, "Review of The Texas Chainsaw Massacre: The Beginning," *Sight and Sound* 16, no. 2 (December 2006): 81.
34. Conrich, "The Friday the 13th Films and the Cultural Function of a Modern Guignol," 180.

Section IV

Queer Theory and Boundary Crossings

CHAPTER 12

"WAY TOO GAY TO BE IGNORED": THE PRODUCTION AND RECEPTION OF QUEER HORROR CINEMA IN THE TWENTY-FIRST CENTURY

HARRY M. BENSHOFF

THIS CHAPTER IS AN UPDATE TO MY BOOK *MONSTERS IN THE CLOSET*: *Homosexuality and the Horror Film,* which argued—drawing upon Robin Wood's famous formulation of the movie monster as white patriarchal capitalism's repressed Other—that monstrous figures in American cinema were and are informed by their given era's social understanding of homosexuality, or more broadly queerness.[1] As the twenty-first century begins, various aspects of contemporary and historical queer cultures continue to be brought into the mainstream, including those surrounding the figuration of the "monster queer." *The Rocky Horror Picture Show* (1975)—a film that forthrightly exposes the queerness inherent in the horror genre—is an excellent barometer of such social changes. Produced by a major Hollywood studio (20th Century-Fox), it bombed upon its initial release. Then, finding a smaller, appreciative, and queer audience, it became the most celebrated cult film/midnight movie in history. Today, it is arguably more popular and well known than ever, repeatedly airing on basic cable and available via most DVD outlets. Most recently, it served as the basis for the FOX-TV hit *Glee*'s Halloween episode, albeit in truncated form. What was too queer then now seems almost quaint. This chapter examines how the monster queer continues to come out of the closet, and how recent horror films and fan bases have frequently been forced to acknowledge his or her presence. While queer audiences may variously celebrate or decry these developments, for straight fans of the genre, these more overtly queer horror films sometimes bring discomfiture, being in the words of one such fan, "way too gay to be ignored."[2]

Probably the most important factor to contribute to the increased visibility of queer horror has been the proliferation of LGBTQ media itself, in both traditional and new media forms. As this niche market has expanded, queer horror has become one aspect of its diverse economic base. Gay and lesbian DVD retailers such as Wolfe and TLA have devoted entire sections of their catalogs to queer horror. Gay and lesbian film festivals from London to Los Angeles have programmed queer horror events, including talks, features, and short film parodies like *Traditional Family Vampires* (2000) and *Out of the Coffin* (2006). Queer Canadian filmmaker Bruce LaBruce has taken up the undead as subject matter, releasing *Otto; or Up with Dead People* (2008) and *L.A. Zombie* (2010). Automat Pictures, a production company in Los Angeles, is producing *Queer for Fear,* a documentary that will bring together clips, scholars, and filmmakers in a discussion of queer horror. In the avant-garde world, Charles Lum's *Indelible* (2004) intercuts splatter scenes from 1970s horror classics with cum shots from gay porno videos, suggesting the repressed connections between sex and violence that arguably define the horror genre in the first place. The website deadguyscinema.com features similar fare in exploitation form, selling homemade videos that commingle gay sex with torture and murder fantasies. More generally, websites such as unspeakablehorror.com, queerhorror.com, and campblood.org feature reviews, chat rooms, and blogs all devoted to queer horror.

Slightly more above ground, there are an increasing number of independent (and in most cases straight-to-DVD) slasher films that feature openly gay and lesbian characters (as opposed to more broadly queer ones), such as *Make a Wish* (2002), *Hell Bent* (2004), *Fraternity Massacre at Hell Island* (2007), and *The Gay Bed & Breakfast of Terror* (2007). *Creatures from the Pink Lagoon* (2006) is a campy gay black-and-white pastiche of 1950s/1960s horror films, and *Cthulhu* (2007) updates H. P. Lovecraft by centering on a gay protagonist. The bargain-basement production *Skull & Bones* (2007)—made by gay men obviously fascinated with horror films and serial killers—is about two working-class homicidal homosexuals who slice, dice, sodomize, and "zombie-fy" privileged Yale undergrads as well as the politics they represent.

In more mainstream developments, one of the first shows to be produced for the gay subscription television service Here-TV! was *Dante's Cove* (2005), a supernatural soap opera. It was followed by *The Lair* (2007–2009), with a theme about a gay vampire nightclub. The even more mainstream *True Blood* (HBO, 2008-) features gay and queer characters both monstrous and human, while the whole show works as an allegory about vampires and other denizens of the night "coming out of the coffin" and assimilating into the mainstream (or not). In 2005, the national gay weekly *The Advocate* commented on this trend, helpfully listing "horror and thriller [film] essentials" for the LGBTQ community while plugging twelve new books of queer horror fiction from eight different publishers, for reading "once you've exhausted your Anne Rice and Clive Barker collections."[3] In Hollywood and elsewhere, there is an increasing coterie of openly gay horror writers and directors, including Clive Barker, Don Mancini, Kevin Williamson, Sam Irvin, Alejandro Amenabar, Paul Etheredge, David DeCoteau, and Victor Salva.

This atmosphere now allows someone like Don Mancini, the writer of the popular *Child's Play* films (1988, 1990, 1991), to give freer reign to his camp sensibilities. The franchise's latest entries, *Bride of Chucky* (1998) and *Seed of Chucky* (2004), are wicked satires of all things heterosexual. In *Seed,* for example, murderous living dolls Chucky (Brad Dourif) and Tiffany (Jennifer Tilly) give "birth" to a doll-child named Glen/Glenda (voiced by former *Lord of the Rings* hobbit Billy Boyd) who—as its name implies—has a sexual identity crisis. Deciding that they want to have human bodies once again, the three dolls capture the *actress* Jennifer Tilly (playing herself), impregnate her with Chucky's sperm, and watch as her "voodoo pregnancy" yields human twins. By the end of the film, Chucky has been dispatched, Tiffany the doll has taken over Jennifer Tilly's life and career, while the spirit of Glen/Glenda uneasily inhabits the human (?) twins. Also starring in the film as a sleazy paparazzo is John Waters, the grandfather of cinematic sleaze and deliberate queer camp. Although its producers were concerned that the film was turning out "too gay" (as reported on the DVD's bonus materials), it was nonetheless marketed at gay pride parades with special *Seed of Chucky* condoms that exhorted recipients to "Get a Load of Chucky!"

Lagging somewhat behind the commercialization of queer horror is a discussion of its politics. As the aforementioned *Advocate* essay queried, "in an era of 'positive images' for gays and lesbians, can queer characters still get chopped up in horror movies?"—or, as it later asks, wear the killer's "hockey mask?"[4] Do horror films still play on homophobic fears, as Robin Wood originally asserted? Perhaps those concerns are becoming less important as the number and range of LGBTQ images in popular culture continues to expand, although some films still ignite that sort of controversy. Israel Luna's *Ticked-Off Trannies with Knives* (2010) recently witnessed angry protests from the transgender community when it played at the Tribeca Film Festival. *2001 Maniacs* (2005) features a gay male victim who is skewered through the anus with a long sharp pole that then comes out his mouth, arguably "fit punishment" for his homosexuality. The French slasher film *High Tension* (2003) revealed its killer to be a psychotic lesbian, a fact that did not please some queer watchdog groups. On the other hand, a few openly gay filmmakers have been able to insert relatively "normal" (or at least nonmonstrous or "deservedly" victimized) gay characters into their films. Kevin Williamson, who wrote the *Scream* trilogy (1996, 1997, 2000), characterized a gay teenager in his recent werewolf saga *Cursed* (2005)—and the young man even got to survive the film's bloody climax.

Despite the rise of overtly LGBTQ horror—some of which challenges or complicates the genre's usual queerphobic formulas—the use of queer connotation to "monsterize" violence and villainy continues apace in many mainstream horror films, such as Eli Roth's "torture porn" *Hostel* films (2005, 2007). In the first film, one sadistic murderer/torturer is coded as a gay man, while the second features an extended lesbian bloodbath—literally. The cocky Roth apparently enjoys flaunting his status as a big cinematic prick, and has circulated a sultry publicity shot of himself wearing a huge prosthetic penis. The fact that the good-looking Roth has a gay male fan base—despite his films' arguable homophobia—suggests the complexities of queer horror's production and reception in the twenty-first century. Straight white male filmmakers who make films with heterosexist agendas (acknowledged or not) are still more readily financed by Hollywood backers and accepted by genre fans, gay and straight alike. Horror films that break with the genre's usual "us-them" binaries (or attempt to tweak the hetero/sexist formulas of the genre) often fail to find financing or else do poorly at the box office. For example, Joss Whedon's *Alien: Resurrection* (1997) screenplay attempted to blur queerly all sorts of generic binaries, producing sympathetic human–alien and human–machine hybrids opposed by the evil forces of white patriarchal capitalism, but the film failed to earn back domestically its production costs.[5] Similarly, Jennie Livingston, the lesbian director of the New Queer Cinema documentary hit *Paris Is Burning* (1990), has reported Hollywood's reluctance to finance her idea for a horror film about a queer psycho-killer who only attacks straight white men.[6]

The two case studies that comprise the remainder of this chapter explore these and other issues in the production and distribution of twenty-first-century queer horror. Director David DeCoteau produces slick-but-shallow homoerotic horror films that are popular in the straight-to-DVD market (and on gay subscription television), even as they cause a form of homosexual panic for some straight male genre fans who unsuspectingly encounter them. On the other hand, writer-director Victor Salva struggles to maintain a career in more mainstream Hollywood filmmaking, despite his past history of being convicted and serving time for having had sex with an underaged male.

DAVID DECOTEAU: STRAIGHT-TO-VIDEO BEEFCAKE HORROR

The undisputed king of contemporary homoerotic horror is Canadian-based producer-director David DeCoteau. As one of his fans succinctly sums up the DeCoteau formula, all of his films feature "Hot stupid guys with great asses running around in their underwear."[7] A sampling of DeCoteau films that follow this formula includes *Voodoo Academy* (2000), *The Frightening* (2002), *Wolves of Wall Street* (2002), *Leeches!* (2003), *Speed Demon* (2003), as well as the six films that comprise *The Brotherhood* franchise (2000, 2001, 2002, 2005, 2009, 2009). There are also a few DeCoteau films that exploit a female version of the same formula, such as *The Sisterhood* (2004) and *Witches of the Caribbean* (2005). While making most of these films, DeCoteau initially denied their homosexual content—ostensibly because they never featured overtly gay or lesbian characters—featuring only sexy young men or women in various comprising same-sex positions motivated by some sort of supernatural plot point.[8] More recently, after gay fans complained about such a disingenuous stance (and straight male viewers began to complain about the homoeroticism of his films), DeCoetau has made more overtly gay horror films. His recent Edgar Allan Poe adaptations—*The Raven* (2007), *House of Usher* (2008), and *The Pit and the Pendulum* (2009), all made in collaboration with the gay production/distribution outlet Regent Entertainment—feature openly gay characters in extended same-sex makeout scenes. As of 2010, instead of making "straight" horror films with gay appeal, DeCoteau now makes gay horror films that he and his producers hope might still be accessible to straight audiences—thus the gay sex scenes always end or fade to black before coitus can occur.[9]

The incredibly prolific DeCoteau has directed over 80 films since the mid-1980s. Early in his career, he worked as a production assistant for Roger Corman's New World Pictures, and in the mid-1980s he began directing both gay and straight video porn tapes. He then became involved in Charles Band's low-budget production/distribution company Full Moon Entertainment, for whom he started directing horror films; DeCoteau still occasionally directs entries in their popular *Puppet Master* franchise (1991, 1998, 1999, 2010). DeCoteau has also directed a slew of standard (i.e., female objectifying) soft-core sexploitation films such as *Beach Babes from Beyond* (1993), *Test Tube Teens from the Year 2000* (1994), and *Bikini Goddesses* (1996), often under pseudonyms like Ellen Cabot, Julian Breen, and Victoria Sloan. One of his earlier claims to fame was the Full Moon-distributed *Sorority Babes in the Slimeball Bowl-O-Rama* (1988), a *Gremlins*-style knockoff that has earned a place in cult film history mostly because of its memorable title. As he was coming out of the closet professionally in the late 1990s, DeCoteau made one "serious" independent movie, *Leather Jacket Love Story* (1997), a gay romance which played mostly at queer film festivals. In 1999, apparently opting for commercial genre success over the independent art film, DeCoteau created Rapid Heart Pictures, his own boutique production company specializing in the production of beefcake horror films.[10]

DeCoteau's films are part of the ongoing hegemonic negotiation of exactly what the phrase "queer horror film" might actually signify. What chiefly distinguishes them from most other low-budget horror films—both contemporary and historical—is the way that DeCoteau fills his screen with sexy young men rather than nubile young women. Like many other queer horror films, DeCoteau's are often perched precariously on the edge of the homosexual–homosocial divide. This is, in fact, the very formula of *The Brotherhood* films and many of DeCoteau's stand-alone titles. Each of these films is about a young man being drawn into a monstrous homosocial space: a fraternity of vampires, a coven of warlocks, or a Wall Street law firm made up of werewolves. In each film, the monstrous homosocial group, dominated by a powerful alpha male, seeks out a young male novitiate in explicitly homoerotic ways. In *The Brotherhood,* for example, a slow-motion shot-reverse-shot exchange between a head vampire and his desired fresh meat exploits but inverts the usual dynamics of the male gaze, objectifying and fetishizing a male body rather than a female one. Then, as the hunky young protagonist of each film is drawn further into the monstrous group's homosocial circle, a ritual soft-core "orgy" scene—conceived of by DeCoteau as a showstopping erotic production number—occurs. In these scenes, the members of the monstrous homosocial group (now all wearing designer underwear) exchange bodily fluids or some other intimate token in order to fully integrate the newbie into the clan.

Perhaps in order to diffuse the explicit homoeroticism of these scenes (a move usually too little and too late by this point in the films), a woman or two is often tossed into the mix as the alleged target of the males' sexuality.[11] However, women are used in these homosocial exchanges as Eve Sedgwick has famously suggested: as objects through which the men triangulate their own needs and desires.[12]

Perhaps unsurprisingly given his prolific output, DeCoteau's films are often quite formulaic. The quality of the scripts seems to be the most variable thing about them: while his young actors are uniformly beautiful, and his direction and cinematography often quite stylish, his scripts range from clever (the zombie boy-band plot of *Ring of Darkness* [2004]) to almost nonexistent (the slasher/revenge "motif" of *Beastly Boyz* [2006]). Most of the films are shot in approximately one week wherever cheap (but good-looking) locations can be found: empty high school locker rooms, stately mansions, prep school campuses, and so on. Mostly the films copy the look and feel (and marketing strategies) of theatrical teenage horror films from the late 1990s, such as *I Know What You Did Last Summer* (1997) and *The Faculty* (1998). Indeed, like those films, DeCoteau's can easily be identified by their repetitive cover designs—usually four or five of the nubile cast seductively posed below or around some signifier of horror such as a monstrous face, a scary mask, or a Satanic symbol.

It is partly because of the copy-cat marketing strategy that DeCoteau's films often find themselves in the DVD players of unsuspecting straight male horror movie fans, where they frequently cause a form of "homosexual panic."[13] As such, straight male fans of B horror have repeatedly used the Internet to denounce or condemn DeCoteau, and to warn other straight men to avoid his films. For example, *Leeches!* was called by one such fan "a heterosexual male's nightmare," precisely because it contained "scene after scene of guys in showers, gays in speedos [*sic*], guys in tight boxers . . . ."[14] Comments on BadMovies.Org about *Leeches!* attest to some men's defensive feelings of aversion and hostility toward anything perceived as gay: "I have been following your website for years and in all my time I have never been visibly bothered by any of the movies except for now . . . . I want to hurt this movie. But I can never hurt it the way its hurt me."[15] Instead of being "Laughable-Horror-Flick[s]-With-Bikini-Clad-Babes"[16] as such fans expect, DeCoteau's films use sexy young male characters to overtly "homosexualize" the horror film's more metaphorically queer tropes, such as the erotic exchange of bodily fluids, mysterious supernatural rituals, or beastly transformations and attacks. As one such fan put it, "when I rent a horror movie I want to watch a horror movie, not homo-erotic porn hidden under a very thin layer of 'horror'."[17] Once again demonstrating the dynamics of defensive homophobia, straight reviewer Andrew Borntreger wrote that "all of [DeCoteau's] recent films seem to share a common theme, and that theme causes me great anguish . . . . Insidiously, this movie causes me distress by replicating the style of countless titillations, but by using a male subject."[18]

Once recognized by viewers, the specter of homosexuality in any given DeCoteau film can then be spotted across the text. Other gay-panicked reviewers of *Leeches!* (2003) read its monstrous leeches in explicitly sexual and phallic terms, noting that the film's DVD menu—depicting a screaming open-mouthed pretty boy confronted by a blood-swollen leech—suggests queer monster fellatio. At another point in the film, a young man comes home, strips to his underwear, and falls asleep on his bed. Straight reviewer Andrew Borntreger describes the scene in feverish detail: "The leech slowly crawls up the napping, nearly-naked young man. This was accomplished with a latex leech hand puppet passing up the soon-to-be victim's thighs and back (of course he is sleeping on his stomach; of course). I just know that the director would slip on that special effect glove and say something like, 'Oh no, it's time for Mr. Leechy to come visit!' " Borntreger continues, "DeCoteau gleefully donning the leech glove sprang to mind every time an attack happened, and I always envisioned him grinning like a madman and wearing red devil horns as he waved the latex hand puppets in the air. The man has become my personal Satan. Damn him."[19] (Speaking of the same special effect, Posiedon-3 on the *IMDb* quipped that "they could have left off the gloves and called this 'Letches!' just as easily."[20]) On the same message board, poster Nik "screamed" out in capital letters that "LEECHES ARE KILLER PENISES! THIS MOVIE IS ABOUT AIDS OR SOMETHING!" Again illustrating the curious dynamics of queer horror (and defensive homophobia) Nik continued, "it's easy to imagine straight boys seeing this film, feeling creepy and grossed out, without ever realizing it's because of the hidden gay agenda."[21]

That said, other female and queer horror fans have used the same forums to critique such homophobic perspectives, in the process addressing and exposing the (hetero)sexist conventions of both fannish discourse and the horror film itself. For example, Midnight writes that

> As a gay horror movie fan, I think the little boys on here complaining about seeing scantily-dressed males is hysterical. The prior poster said he wanted horror, not "thinly-disguised gay porn" or words to that effect. Funny, he doesn't seem to mind the hundreds upon thousands of horror films that are basically excuses to show teen sex and bare lady-boobs. I've sat through a lot of such movies and never saw a reason to whine about it. I defy this poster—or any other poster—to tell me why a very small number of horror films that show men as sex objects for a change make them *that* uncomfortable.[22]

Although the posters on this particular site did not then engage in a discussion of homophobia as a defense mechanism against repressed same-sex desires, they did begin to realize the ubiquity of female objectification in the horror genre. Reviewer Borntreger admitted that "Now I know how my wife feels when I watch movies like *Hard Bodies* or *Hollywood Chainsaw Hookers*."[23] ShifterCat suggested a utopic solution to the whole problematic dynamic of the male gaze: "I look forward to the day when a camera lingering on an attractive male happens just as often as a camera lingering on an attractive female, so that even if someone isn't interested in that sort of body they won't freak out about the 'inversion'."[24]

David DeCoteau's beefcake horror films have caused some interesting anomalies in the usual patterns of horror film reception, and in some ways suggest a "coming out of the closet" for both horror movies and horror movie fans. The films' overt homosexualization of the genre's usual queer dynamics makes the old "reading too much into things" argument obsolete and untenable, and challenges straight male fans to confront the genre's frequently heterosexist and queerphobic formulas. On the other hand, some gay horror movie fans feel that far from de-repressing the homosexuality in the genre, DeCoteau's films don't go far enough. Still, whether "way too gay" or not gay enough, David DeCoteau films appeal to "horror fans who enjoy the opportunity to make politically/socially/subversive readings of film texts—because your work is pretty much done for you."[25] While they are unlikely to queer the horror genre overnight, David DeCoteau's beefcake horror films nonetheless contribute to the ongoing hegemonic negotiation of homosexuality, the horror film, and the multifarious interconnections between the two.

Victor Salva: Outing the Monster Queer at the Multiplex

Contemporary horror film auteur Victor Salva has a sexual history that—once known—impacts upon the production and reception of his work. In the late 1980s, Salva (then about 30) was arrested for having had sexual contact with Nathan Winters, the 12-year-old star of *Clownhouse* (1989), Salva's feature horror film debut. Salva claimed that the sex was consensual, but pled guilty to lewd and lascivious conduct, oral copulation with a person under 14, and procuring a child for pornography (Salva had recorded the act). Salva served 15 months of his three-year sentence and completed parole in 1992. Since then Salva has gone on to write and/or direct several other horror/thriller/fantasy films, including *Nature of the Beast* (1995), *Powder* (1995), *Rites of Passage* (1999), *Jeepers Creepers* (2001), *Jeepers Creepers 2* (2003), and *Peaceful Warrior* (2006). Most of his films focus—in either manifest or metaphoric terms—on issues related to intergenerational abuse and/or intimacy between men. The *Jeepers Creepers* films, Salva's most well-known films to date, center on a predatory, male-coded monster who specifically tracks and kills teenage boys for their desirable body parts.

All of which is to say that Salva's films do seem to reprocess issues related to his own sexual history. Salva, who now self-identifies as gay, explores within his films the various types of relationships that can exist between men of different generations. Even more so than DeCoteau's, Salva's films blur the borders between male homosociality and homosexuality, and tend to focus on queer outsider figures who are feared and/or hated by "normal" people, whether they be sympathetic (as in *Powder*) or monstrous (as in *Jeepers Creepers*). This formula allows the films to expose and explore the brutality and homophobia inherent in much contemporary masculinity, even as it also can literally "monsterize" other forms of male–male intimacy. Yet, what makes Salva's films different from most other queer horror films is the fact that they cannot escape the public's knowledge of Salva's criminal conviction. Internet chat rooms are awash with denunciations of Salva and his films. To reference Foucault's concept of the author-function, one might say that knowledge of Salva's sexual history affords audiences the chance to label and categorize his work as that of a "child molester" (as opposed to a great artistic genius).[26] This naming "authorizes" viewers to acknowledge the queer horrors that lurk in Salva's films—queer horrors that they might just as easily have overlooked in similar films by unknown filmmakers.

For example, Salva's debut feature *Clownhouse*—made before Salva went to prison—was not denounced upon its premiere, even though it is just as homoerotic as his later films. The film centers on three adolescent brothers, who are terrorized by three escaped lunatics disguised as circus clowns, a fictional gloss on the real-life case of the homosexual serial killer (and clown) John Wayne Gacy. (Casey, the youngest brother, is played by Nathan Winters, the 12-year-old with whom Salva had sexual contact.) The film begins as a shirtless Casey has a nightmare about a menacing clown, and in his fear Casey wets the bed. The next morning, as oldest brother Randy masturbates off-screen, middle brother Geoffrey—in his underwear—helps Casey change the sheets, and Salva includes a shot that reveals Casey's bare bottom. Later in the film the three boys share a bathroom scene, in which Casey is naked in the tub while the two older boys discuss whiskers and pubic hair. Why the lunatic-clowns decide to attack the boys is never fully explained; however, "Cheezo's" almost lewd and lascivious "come on" to Casey at the local circus—coyly beckoning to him with pursed lips and leering grins—does suggest a homosexual element, as does a bit of gender-bending dialogue that describes him as "just a man with paint on his face." In fact, the clowns' white face paint becomes a motif representing their (homo)sexual menace: when the boys find and examine it with their fingers, the framing of the shots makes the white stuff highly suggestive of semen. These fairly blatant homoerotic motifs went unremarked upon in most of the film's original reviews. *Variety* simply deemed the film a "serviceable but formulaic old-dark-house opus that could flush out a little theatrical business with kids before finding its appropriate resting place in home-vid stores."[27]

Indeed, *Clownhouse* may well have died a dusty death in "home-vid stores" had not Salva continued to make films after being convicted and serving time in the early 1990s. His little-seen second feature, *Nature of the Beast* (a.k.a. *Bad Company,* 1995), takes its inspiration from the old campfire story "The Hatchet-Man," and borrows considerably from the homoerotic road movie *The Hitcher* (1986). True to generic form, sex and violence are conflated throughout the film, as its criminal characters share the road as well as a homoerotic and increasingly violent pas de deux. Initially, the film suggests that frumpy salesman Jack (Lance Henriksen) has stolen a million dollars from a casino, and that sexy drifter Adrian (Eric Roberts) is an axe-wielding murderer, among whose first victims was a 19-year-old boy named Danny. When Jack first spots Adrian on the side of the highway, an old-fashioned song about a "Lover Boy" is heard on the car radio. Adrian has already hitched a ride with a trucker who made a pass at him, and he directly asks Jack if he's a "fag." Adrian constantly taunts Jack, tossing a Gila monster into his lap and making suggestive comments such as, "I'll show you mine if you show me yours" and "You wanna get bloody with me?" Gerald and Dahlia, two hippies in a "love van," wonder aloud if Jack and Adrian are lovers, and when Adrian does drugs and has three-way sex with Gerald and Dahlia, Jack acts like a spurned lover. The rocking of the "love van" as Adrian engages in his ménage á trois echoes the first murder in the film, during which the rocking of the car was caused by a violent murder, not sex. Ultimately, a not-rather-convincing twist at the end of the film reveals that Adrian is in fact the thief and that Jack is the Hatchet-Man. Jack kills Adrian and returns to his "normal" life as a husband in a generic suburb, suggesting that his psychotic male violence and confused sexuality is an endemic, if hidden, element of the middle-American landscape.

Salva's next film *Powder* was released widely by Disney and exhibits many of Salva's signature themes: troubled father–son relationships, the brutality of male homosocial groups, a sympathetic young male protagonist who is shunned by "normal" people for being different, and significant amounts of beefcake. "Powder" is the nickname of Jeremy Reed (Sean Patrick Flanery), a bald albino teenager who can read others' thoughts and seems to be charged with an electrical force, a phenomenon partly explained in a flashback in which his mother was struck by lightning while pregnant with him. When his mother dies giving birth, Powder is abandoned by his father and raised by his grandparents. The body of the film begins when Powder's last grandparent dies and he is transported to a state school for boys. Powder is also befriended by a high school science teacher (Jeff Goldblum), who figures out that Powder's lack of body hair is due to the fact that "he *is* electrolysis." Throughout the film, Powder transforms several lives via his magical powers, and at the end he is struck by lightning and apparently subsumed into the heavens. Before that moment, however, there is a final homoerotic confrontation with the state school boys that begins with Powder gazing longingly at a shirtless boy in the locker room. The scene is depicted via a slow-motion subjective shot that is marked as Powder's gaze. When the other boys see Powder looking at their buddy in this way, they taunt him as a "Peeping Tom" and a "faggot." They drag him outside, strip him naked, and dump him into a puddle. As Powder calls upon his powers, the boys' medallions, earrings, and (most audaciously) buttons and rivets on their jeans begin to unsnap, drawn toward the electromagnetic Powder. Then a blast of energy throws them all backward and Powder lands again in the puddle with an orgasmic, slow-motion splash.

As this brief description attests to, Powder is a metaphoric fantasy figure meant to stand in for any number of "real life" social issues (much as do comic book movie characters like the *X-Men* [2000]). As one critic put it, "*Powder* is an archetypal story that gets into everyone's blood."[28] While Powder's sexual difference is made fairly explicit, racial difference is also hinted at by Powder's pale skin color. Further nominating the possible Others Powder might represent, the boys call him a "vampire from outer space" and suggest he might have cancer or "some kind of disease," perhaps AIDS. The Sheriff's dying wife thinks Powder is an angel, while other townspeople think he is a demon. Powder is also quite clearly a Christ figure, having been created out of the union of an earthly mother and heavenly forces. He lays hands on the sick and dying, and espouses the connectedness and beauty of all living things. In other words, Powder is a queerly liminal figure, a hybrid perched between god and man, man and boy, straight and gay.

It was during the wide release of *Powder* that Salva's public relations crisis began. Nathan Winters and five of his friends picketed screenings of the film in Los Angeles. They were determined to call attention to Salva's sexual history and shame the Disney corporation for having hired him in the first place.[29] Winters's protest ignited a firestorm of controversy and outed Salva to the media.[30] Disney/Hollywood made no official comment, although they did remove Salva's credit from some of the film's newspaper advertisements.[31] Perhaps surprisingly given the film's homoerotic themes, *Powder* became a small hit. It opened in second place behind *Get Shorty* (1995), and racked up 21 million dollars in its first two weeks. Intriguingly, according to *Variety, Powder* scored best with young males 12–17.[32]

That said, the publicity about Salva's sexual history colored many filmgoers' and critics' responses to *Powder* in very specific ways. Manohla Dargis in the *LA Weekly* called the film "weird, weird, weird, a truth that would hold even if the director weren't also a convicted child molester."[33] *Variety* took to the street to interview "average" filmgoers for their responses to the film. Lan Ngyuen, a 22-year-old female from Los Angeles was quoted as saying, "During the movie, I kept on thinking 'child molester,' especially during scenes when (Powder) is naked and another where a guy is changing and Powder is staring at him. But I wouldn't have thought that had I not known."[34] These comments are worth unpacking. Had this particular viewer not been aware of Salva's sexual history, she would have found nothing remarkable about the film's objectification of young male bodies, and would have overlooked the (fairly obvious) sexual desire with which Powder gazes at another teenage boy. Furthermore, the scene in question is *not* a scene of intergenerational desire—the characters are supposed to be age-equivalent peers—thus these comments invoke and reinscribe the old "homosexuality and pedophilia are the same thing" canard. Similarly, *Variety*'s review of the film noted the scene "that has Powder innocently viewing another boy taking a shower may disturb audiences who have read the news stories about Salva."[35] Use of the word "innocently" is very interesting here—it seeks to deny the fact that Powder might sexually desire the other young man (as such as gaze would not be "innocent") while also suggesting that Powder's "innocent" gaze is actually Salva's criminal, pedophilic one.

Because of the publicity, *Powder* was not received as a film with mildly homoerotic elements that could be (and routinely would have been) overlooked. Instead, the film's homoeroticism was now "evidence" of Salva's pedophilic inclinations, and vice versa.

Once aware of Salva's background, *The Northeastern News* could write that "Powder's delicate features, blood red lips, pale skin, and complete lack of body hair conveys a very sensual idea of a prepubescent child. As well, Goldblum runs his hands over Powder's smooth head and soft hands in an eerie picture of pedophilism."[36] (In fact, Sean Patrick Flanery was 30 years old when he played the teenage Powder.) In one of the more thoughtful reviews of the whole situation, Joe Morgenstern in *The Wall Street Journal* noted that he had seen the film and liked it before he became aware of Salva's past. Then, considering the film again in light of that, he realized that

> it's quite impossible to separate the substance of [Salva's] vision from what we've learned about his troubled life. In the young and innocent Powder, Mr. Salva has created a magical child, an idealized child whom he treats with tenderness, even reverence. Is this a conscious attempt at expiation, an unconscious effort of overcompensation, or, yet again, an artist reprocessing his obsessive past? No way to know, no way not to wonder.[37]

Salva followed *Powder* with a smaller, more realistic father-and-sons thriller entitled *Rites of Passage* (1999). Although it premiered at several film festivals, the film received little-to-no theatrical distribution in the United States, perhaps because of its frank exploration of how contemporary masculinities are colored by homosexuality, homosociality, and homophobia. Tellingly, it was Salva's next two films—the *Jeepers Creepers* films—that became his most financially successful, perhaps because they more readily fit the mold of the horror genre's classical binary structure: queerly coded monster attacks "normal" heterosexual characters.[38] Both films center on a male monster of indeterminate origin, who awakens from a death-like sleep every 23 years in order to feed on humans for 23 days. However, the Creeper is discerning in his appetites—he only wants "certain things from certain people"—most often the organs or limbs of frightened young men that he has chosen via their scent. (The Creeper has three nostrils that pulsate and quiver when he is aroused.) Although the Creeper has apparently killed and eaten women in the past, it is made quite clear in both films that he prefers young men, pointedly ignoring or deliberately turning away from available female prey. In the first film, the Creeper is apparently after the eyes of young Darius Jenner (thus explaining the film's title), while in the second film the Creeper has designs on a group of teenage athletes he has trapped inside a school bus. Like a classical Hollywood movie monster, the Creeper's desire is a queer jumble of violence, appetite, and sexuality.

As might be apparent from that brief description, both *Jeepers Creepers* films are steeped in queer male sensibilities. They are ripe with beefcake as teenage boys take off their shirts (or have them ripped off), exposing their bare chests. Darius (Justin Long) has a rose tattoo (a reference to Tennessee Williams?) around his navel which both films fetishize—in the second film the Creeper has reworked the young man's belly skin into a throwing star—like weapon. Both films feature scenes in which teenage male protagonists empty their bladders by the side of the road, and the homosocial–homophobic banter between the characters—"dick licker, ball sniffer, ass kisser, butt picker"—constantly evokes denigrated queer sexualities. The name of the athletic team in *Jeepers Creepers 2* is the Bannon Bantams, and the boys are proud to be the "Fighting Cocks." The films also make male homosexuality manifest in several ways, even as they center on a more metaphorically queer monster. For example, in *Jeepers Creepers 2,* the character Izzy is directly accused of being gay ("Izzy or Izn't he?"), an assertion the character neither denies nor admits. In the first film, Darius and sister Trish play a guessing game with vanity license plates, and Darius reads the plate "6A 4EVR" as "Gay Fever" or "Gay Forever," while sister Trish suggests the correct interpretation in "Sexy Forever." Furthermore, Darius is not overtly heterosexualized by the films—no mention is made of his romantic or erotic life even though his sister's is discussed—thus leaving open the possibility that he might be gay. And a running motif about his "rosy pink jockey shorts" (allegedly created by a washing machine mishap) hints at that idea, as does the Creeper's attraction to the same article of clothing. As one witness describes the Creeper sniffing Darius's dirty laundry, he was obviously "likin' it too!"

The Creeper's attacks themselves are often figured as incorporating same-sex fears. When he beheads a policeman in the first film, the Creeper appears to make love to it—a la Salome kissing the severed head of John the Baptist—before biting out the dead cop's tongue. Most audaciously, in *Jeepers Creepers 2,* the Creeper sniffs out his objects of affection from behind a window at the rear of the school bus. In a series of shot-reverse-shots, the Creeper leers at the boys and then winks at one, smiles at another, and wiggles his index finger at a third. After ignoring the females and motioning aside one male student who apparently is not to his liking, the Creeper makes his desire felt for a fourth boy by slowing licking the glass in front of him, a move the others will later refer to as the Creeper's "tongue action." This particular sequence occurs not long after Izzy—the possibly gay student—has had a confrontation with the homophobic Scott. Izzy asks Scott if the very idea of a homosexual makes him "nervous," and the proximity of this exchange to the Creeper's sexualized attack draws a firm link between real-life fears of male homosexuality and the more metaphoric menace of the Creeper. The same note is sounded when a teammate refers to the nerdy team manager as having been "sniffin' jock straps"—again making a connection between the athletes' homophobic idea of gay male sexuality and the actual practices of the Creeper.

Most intriguingly from an auteur standpoint, the queer Creeper is an artist as well as a monster. His lair beneath the abandoned church is filled with bodies he has preserved over the centuries and stitched together in a sort of ghoulish "Sistine Chapel" mosaic. His weapons are handcrafted tools made from his victims' remains. The Creeper is also rather campy as he toys with his victims, sometimes posing as a scarecrow, or in one case whistling the title tune on his way to a kill. He also seems to enjoy listening to nostalgic records as he goes about his business. Complicating the Creeper's nasty persona is a small strain of religious symbolism—the initials *JC* do suggest Jesus Christ, and in the set piece that opens the second film, the Creeper-as-scarecrow is filmed in a Christ-like fashion, flanked by two other scarecrows in a triptych that seems to suggest the crucifixions at Golgotha. Similar imagery also occurs at the end of the film, as the dormant creature is nailed to a wall and put on display as a sort of fallen angel, literally a "Bat Out of Hell."

As with *Powder,* Salva's past history authorized a queer reading of the films. The *LA Weekly* noted that *Jeepers Creepers 2* contained "an odd strain of juvenile homoeroticism that feels particularly unsavory in a movie made by a convicted pedophile."[39] On the less-decorous Internet, posters continue to construct Salva as a pedophile auteur, some seeing his films as fairly explicit commentaries on what they perceive to be Salva's ongoing "sickness." For example, one entire thread on the *IMDb*'s *Jeepers Creepers* message boards is simply entitled "the creeper is GAY." In fact, one rather remarkable post explains in exquisite detail how the first film is really

> a very warped revenge on Nathan Winters. . . . Y'see, the Creeper is Victor Salva, or at least a fantasy version of Victor Salva who can totally dominate his intended victims and never be caught. . . . Naturally in Victor Salva's fantasy version, the police are powerless against the Creeper (this [is] an expression of his resentment toward his former jailers. He did serve time), and the monster heroically escapes with his sexual conquest. The fact that Darry [the young male victim] is revealed to be naked at the Creeper's and that we're not shown *everything* that the Creeper has inflicted on him, in my mind, is a pretty good indication that the Creeper either raped Darry or has necrophilic tendencies as well as cannibalistic ones.[40]

Of course, monsters throughout the history of the genre have been cannibalistic, necrophilic, rapists, but that fact does not perhaps become obvious (or at least worth commenting upon) until the victim is male and the monster/director is known to be queer.

Speaking on the social construction of pedophilia, Harris Mirken, associate professor of political science, has noted how pedophilia is usually framed in terms of

> absolute good and evil. Real discussions of pedophilia, as opposed to ritualistic condemnations, are almost non-existent. There are no commonly used neutral labels [and] definitions are characteristically vague, so that statistics from the mildest activities can be blended with images from the most atrocious. Six- and thirteen-year olds are grouped in the same category ("Child") and images of intergenerational sex acts that take place with pubescents and post-puberty teens are routinely projected back onto very young children. In the same way as adolescents are merged with little children, all sexual activity is equated with violent or coerced sexual activity.[41]

Indeed, many of Mirken's observations can be readily demonstrated in the Internet chat room response to Victor Salva. For example, chat room participants often "inflate" the level of Salva's crime: rather than refer to it as sexual fondling and oral contact with one 12-year-old boy (as the criminal charges reflect), Salva and his films are denounced "because he *rapes* 12 year old *children* [emphasis added]."[42] Similarly, hyperbolic language is used to describe the vast and therefore disturbing gulf between Salva and his alleged victims: as one Internet writer wrote about the making of *Jeepers Creepers II* documentary, "Watching this 500-pound guy drool over some 98 pound kid who looks 14 is creepier than anything in the movie."[43] And despite decades worth of education to the contrary, homosexual identity is still directly associated with pedophilia in many peoples' minds, as another Internet writer concludes about Salva: "he did rape a 12 year old boy. *that* makes him gay."[44]

Of course, homosexual intergenerational intimacy is also accorded more drastic and negative social meanings than is heterosexual sex between men and women of different ages, as can readily be attested to the fact that many states have higher age of consent laws for homosexual acts than they do for heterosexual acts. This issue also plays out on Victor Salva message boards. One writer, daring to defend Salva and his films, compares him to Roman Polanski:

> roman [Polanski]
> 13 year old girl
> gave her coke
> fled the country to avoid incarceration
> people on his forum talking about how great his movies are
>
> victor [Salva]
> don't know how old boy.
> videotaped it.
> did his sanctioned time
> people on his forum talking about how evil he is.

As this writer concludes, "i guess it makes a difference that roman did it with a girl."[45]

The production and reception of Victor Salva's horror films reveals several significant things about contemporary sexuality and the horror film. One is the continued conflation of pedophilia with homosexuality, and the presumption that intergenerational sex is far worse when it is homosexual rather than heterosexual. The films also suggest the reluctance of many viewers to acknowledge the repressed queer core of the horror genre itself: terrible sexualized things happen to both men and women in the horror film, with women being the usual victims. It is perhaps a function of the genre to displace "real life" rape or abuse onto fictional monsters, but such a displacement is also an invitation to take pleasure in such images. Salva's homoerotic horror films underscore our patriarchal culture's relative comfort with that process when those abused bodies are female, that is, "acceptable" objects of the straight male gaze. Those dynamics are rarely commented upon by the genre's fans—unless the sexualized spectacle is of abused male bodies, as in the films of David DeCoteau or Victor Salva. Their horror films make the homoerotic manifestly homosexual, opening up a space for a critique of the genre's usual hetero/sexist dynamics.

To their credit, both DeCoteau's and Salva's films often explore this eroticization in relation to a broadly queer continuum of masculinities and sexualities—identities and subject positions that cannot be simply reduced to that of gay male or pedophile or even homosocial buddy. The fact that the discourse surrounding the reception of their films attempts to do precisely that—denounce them as overtly homosexual and/or pedophilic—is itself exemplary of the processes by which our culture maintains a comforting distance between its everyday, unremarked-upon eroticization of (female) youth and the ever-popular narrative of the monstrous (queer) child molester.

NOTES

1. Harry M. Benshoff, *Monsters in the Closet: Homosexuality and the Horror Film* (Manchester: Manchester University Press, 1997). See also Robin Wood, *Hollywood: From Vietnam to Reagan* (New York: Columbia University Press, 1986).
2. H. A. Huffman, "WOW, Giant Leeches . . . Attacking Pretty Boys?," December 14, 2003, *Amazon.com* Customer Reviews of *Leeches!,* accessed October 26, 2004, http://www.amazon.com/review/R1RNOGGT0WG2UU.

3. Sean Abley, "Arts and Entertainment: Scary!" *The Advocate,* November 8, 2005, 58–60.
4. Abley, "Arts and Entertainment," 58.
5. According to the *IMDb,* the film cost approximately $70 million to make and grossed slightly under $48 million domestically. See "Box office/business for *Alien Resurrection* (1997)," *IMDb,* accessed July 20, 2010, http://www.imdb.com/title/tt0118583/business.
6. Livingston shared that anecdote with me during a personal discussion at the University of Santa Cruz in the late 1990s. She has yet to make another feature film.
7. ApolloBoy109, "I Just Never Stopped Laughing. I Loved it," December 1, 2004, *IMDb* User Comments for *Leeches!,* accessed July 20, 2010, http://www.imdb.com/title/tt0339288/usercomments?start=20.
8. For example, on the audio commentary track for *The Brotherhood,* DeCoteau states, "I don't think there's any gay anything in this movie."
9. A discussion about this occurs on the DVD commentary track for *The Raven.*
10. For more on Rapid Heart, see http://www.rapidheart.com. DeCoteau's films are frequently made via financing and distribution deals with companies known for LGBTQ niche marketing, including Regent Entertainment and its subsidiaries Here-TV!, LOGO, and OutTV Canada. These films have also appeared on the SyFy Channel and are widely available at video stores and through most rental services.
11. *The Brotherhood II* does without the female "beard." Instead, four nearly naked men in the campus swimming pool get drunk and drink each others' tears—one boy even licking it directly off the face of another.
12. Eve Kosofsky Sedgwick, *Between Men: English Literature and Male Homosocial Desire* (New York: Columbia University Press, 1985).
13. I use the controversial term "homosexual panic" here to refer to the ways that some men become angry, violent, or fearful when confronted with homosexuals—or in this case homosexual or homoerotic imagery. Such a reaction is often theorized to be the result of such men's own repressed same-sex desires. For an overview of what some theorists call "defensive homophobia," see John P. DeCecco, ed., *Bashers, Baiters, and Bigots: Homophobia in American Society* (New York: Harrington Park Press, 1999). These dynamics have also been proven in the laboratory. See Henry E. Adams et al., "Is Homophobia Associated with Homosexual Arousal?" *Journal of Abnormal Psychology* 105, no. 3 (1996): 440–445.
14. C. Seggelin, "Plastereddragon," "Ack!! The Badness!!! The Aching Badness!!," online posting for *Leeches!,* November 12, 2003, Amazon.com Customer Reviews of *Leeches!,* accessed October 26, 2004, http://www.amazon.com/Leeches-Julie-Briggs-II/product reviews/B0001IXU6W/ref=cm_cr_pr_link_next_3?ie=UTF8&showViewpoints=0&pageNumber=3&sortBy=bySubmissionDate Descending.
15. El Rico, "Reply #5," June 9, 2009, *BadMovies.org* Comments for *Leeches!,* accessed July 20, 2010, http://www.badmovies.org/movies/leeches/index.html?start=0.
16. Seggelin, "Plastereddragon."
17. Rembrandt36, "Reply #9," June 10, 2009, *BadMovies.org* Comments for *Leeches!,* accessed July 20, 2010, http://www.badmovies.org/movies/leeches/index.html?start=8.
18. Andrew Borntreger, "Review of Leeches!" June 8, 2009, *BadMovies.org* Comments for *Leeches!,* July 20, 2010, http://www.badmovies.org/movies/leeches/index.html?start=0.
19. Borntreger, "Review of Leeches!"
20. Posiedon-3, "The Leeches Aren't the Only Things That Suck!," October 17, 2007, *IMDb* User Comments for *Leeches!,* accessed 20 July 2010, http://www.imdb.com/title/tt0339288/usercomments?start=10.
21. Nik, "Reply #7," June 9, 2009, *BadMovies.org* Comments for *Leeches!,* accessed July 20, 2010, http://www.badmovies.org/movies/leeches/index.html?start=0.
22. Midnight, "Reply #10," June 11, 2009, *BadMovies.org* Comments for *Leeches!,* accessed July 20, 2010, http://www.badmovies.org/movies/leeches/index.html?start=8.
23. Bornterger, "Review of Leeches!"
24. ShifterCat, "Reply #19," June 25, 2009, *BadMovies.org* Comments for *Leeches!,* accessed July 20, 2010, http://www.badmovies.org/movies/leeches/index.html?start=16?

25. Traveshamockery, "Campy/Homoerotic Classic," August 27, 2007, *IMDb* User Comments for *Leeches!,* accessed July 20, 2010, http://www.imdb.com/title/tt0339288/usercomments?start=10.
26. Michel Foucault, "What Is an Author?," in *The Foucault Reader,* ed. Paul Rabinow (Harmondsworth: Penguin, 1977/1984), 101–120.
27. Cart., "[Review of] *Clownhouse,*" *Variety,* February 1, 1989, no pagination.
28. Quoted in the *Powder* Pressbook, accessed at the Margaret Herrick Library, Los Angeles.
29. Disney was at that point in time already the subject of right-wing condemnation and boycotts over alleged subliminal sexual material in *The Little Mermaid* (1989) and *Aladdin* (1992), as well as its release, via recently acquired Miramax, of *Priest* (1994) and *Kids* (1995).
30. Literary scholar James R. Kincaid suggests that such media frenzies allow America to be both titillated by and distanced from the implication of childhood sexuality. In a telling turn of phrase, Kincaid argues that we "wouldn't be telling this tale of the exploitation of the child's body if we didn't wish to have it told . . . . what these stories do for us is keep the subject hot so we can disown it while welcoming it in the backdoor." James R. Kincaid, *Erotic Innocence: The Culture of Child Molesting* (Durham, NC: Duke University Press, 1998), 6.
31. James Bates, "No Credits Where Credit Due," *The Los Angeles Times,* October 30, 1995, no pagination.
32. Ted Johnson, "Salva Salvos Continue," *Variety,* October 26, 1995, no pagination.
33. Manohla Dargis, "[Review of] *Powder,*" *LA Weekly,* November 3, 1995, no pagination.
34. Ted Johnson, "*Powder* Rolls $7 Mil Amid Flap," *Variety,* October 30, 1995, no pagination.
35. Joe Leydon, "[Review of] *Powder,*" *Variety,* October 30, 1995, 72.
36. Anni Clark, "Lightning Strikes *Powder* with Pedophilia Theme," *The Northeastern News,* November 1, 1995, 20.
37. Joe Morgenstern, "[Review of] *Powder,*" *The Wall Street Journal,* October 27, 1995, no pagination.
38. In order to shoot the first film in Florida, the local film commission had to debate whether or not Salva's production represented a menace to their community. "After seriously considering the various factors—the time since the crime, the three years of prison Salva served and verifying that the script contained no children or sex—the commission approved the project." However, Commissioner Jude Hagen registered Salva as a sex offender in Florida and kept police informed of his whereabouts, and the Marion County School Board refused to allow teenagers from Dunnellon High School to visit the set. "On Location," *The Hollywood Reporter,* July 18, 2001, no pagination.
39. Scott Foundas, "[Review of] *Powder,*" *LA Weekly,* August 29, 2003, no pagination.
40. Raiderofthelastfries, "Re: Some New (?) Thoughts on the Meaning of the Movie," April 3, 2004, *IMDb* User Comments for *Jeepers Creepers* (2001), accessed October 26, 2004, http://www.imdb.com/title/tt0263488/board/nest/3334638.
41. Harris Mirken, "The Pattern of Sexual Politics: Feminism, Homosexuality and Pedophilia," *Journal of Homosexuality* 37, no. 2 (1999): 12.
42. Theo Robertson, "Re: Ok SHUT UP," April 28, 2004, *IMDb* Message Board for Victor Salva, accessed October 26, 2004, http://www.imdb.com/name/nm0759207/board/nest/7987155.
43. jk90, "Is This Guy Gay?" January 27, 2004, *IMDb* Message Board for Victor Salva, accessed October 26, 2004, http://www.imdb.com/name/nm0759207/board/flat/5877131?d+6531609#6531609.
44. Kaagaard, "Is This Guy Gay?" March 5, 2004, *IMDb* Message Board for Victor Salva, accessed October 26, 2004, http://www.imdb.com/name/nm0759207/board/flat/5877131?d+6531609#6531609.
45. Gypsywitch84, "Roman vs Victor War of the Pedos," April 18, 2004, IMDb Message Board for Victor Salva, accessed October 26, 2004, http://www.imdb.com/name/nm0759207/board/nest/7889805.

CHAPTER 13

SEED OF CHUCKY: TRANSBIOLOGY AND THE HORROR FLICK

JUDITH (JACK) HALBERSTAM

IN AN AGE WHEN MASSIVE DEBATES ABOUT THE MEANING OF LIFE take place across representative ambiguous forms of embodiment—the embryo as neither baby nor simply protobaby, the cyborg as human and machine, the comatose Terri Schiavo as vegetative, the family pet as companion and irreducibly other, the human partner as both family pet and symbiotically the same—the horror film has become and remains a fabulously rich site for imagining and working out the relations between the human and its others, or the nonhuman and its queering of the site of embodiment. In earlier eras, the horror film theatricalized the unstable relation between inside and outside, or it located the inhuman as already part and parcel of the human, or it scrambled the gendered relations between sexed bodies. Indeed, the slasher film has always been a site for alternative configurations of embodiment, belonging, family, desire, and identification.

The monsters conjured by contemporary horror tread a thin line between animal, human, and machine and could be classified as "transbiological." This term originates in Donna Haraway's work but is developed by Sarah Franklin.[1] Franklin builds upon Haraway's theorization of the cyborg in her infamous "Cyborg Manifesto," and she returns to earlier work by Haraway that concerned itself with biogenetic extensions of the body and of the experience of embodiment. Franklin explains,

> I want to suggest that, in the same way that the cyborg was useful to learn to see an altered landscape of the biological, the technical, and the informatic, similarly Haraway's "kinding" semiotics of trans can help identify features of the postgenomic turn in the biosciences and biomedicine toward the idioms of immortalization, regeneration, and totipotency. However, by reversing Haraway's introduction of *trans-* as the exception or rogue element (as in the *transuranic* elements), I suggest that *transbiology*—biology that is not only born and bred, or born and made, but *made and born*—is indeed today more the norm than the exception.[2]

In this chapter, I want to examine the narrative and visual transbiological leaps that we have made in our understandings of terms like "heterosexuality" and "homosexuality," "male" and "female," "individual" and "community," in an age of artificial insemination, transsexuality, and cloning. I also want to propose that popular culture has already imagined multiple alternatives to male and female, masculine and feminine, family and individuality, and that contemporary popular culture, specifically horror film and animation, can provide a rich archive for an alternative politics of embodiment, reproduction, and nonreproduction. Such alternatives are important to visualize and recognize if only because what Franklin and Haraway term as the "transbiological" is all too often absorbed into new formulations of the same old notions of kinship, relationality, and love. The porous boundary between the biological and the cultural is quickly traversed without any sense of rupture whatsoever, and the biological, the animal, and the nonhuman are simply recruited for the continuing reinforcement of the human, the heteronormative, and the familial. In other words, while it is true that reproduction and kinship relations become more and more obviously artificial, the concept of the "human" tends to absorb the critique of the natural that inevitably follows because we reinvest so vigorously and so frequently in the scaffolding that props up our flailing humanity.

What Sarah Franklin refers to in her work as the legacy and the future of "transbiology,"[3] or rather "the contemporary reorganization of living matter,"[4] takes place not only in the laboratories she studies and surveys but also in the incorporation of the new technologies of artificial insemination, cloning, and regeneration into new narratives about the horror of human embodiment. While studying science can tell us about our dreams of transformation, studying horror can lead us to contemplate our fears and misgivings about the human, the posthuman, the unhuman, and deliberately nonhuman. One horror film series, *Child's Play,* starring a reanimated doll Chucky and his animated bride, Tiffany, exemplifies the power of the neo-splatter film, not only its ability to dismantle the so-called real world, or men and women and repro-heteronormativity, but also its peculiar talent for imagining true alternatives in the queer social relations and counterpublics that the films imagine and call into being.

In what follows, I discuss the fifth film in the series, *Seed of Chucky*. The teaser trailer opens with an image of an embryo suspended in the womb and a voice-over intones: "With every new life, with every new generation, comes the hope that they will make the world a better place . . . to kill! Deliver us some evil." As if riffing on Lee Edelman's acid-tinged polemic against the child in *No Future,* where he argues that the heteronormativity of the political realm is guaranteed by the use of the metaphor of the child as a symbol of hope for a better tomorrow, this trailer upends our expectations about parental ambition. The humanist hope that seeks to find the present extended in the future and the narcissistic wish structure that demands that the child repeat the sins of the parents come to a grim and bloody end in *Seed of Chucky*. Chucky's parents—the match made in Hell of Chucky, the reanimated Good Guy doll and his hideous bride, Tiffany—have brought their union to unholy fruition in the fourth installment, and reproduction, natural, unnatural, and downright queer becomes the central drama in this hilarious episode. But the *Chucky* series also refuses Edelman's flat rejection of the child as a place of resistance and it builds its hope, very differently, around the body of the unsexed and ambiguously gendered child.

For Sarah Franklin, hope plays a role in the new embryology as infertile couples deposit sperm and eggs and embryos in science labs. When they give reproductive material to science, as Franklin says, "couples therefore *trans-substantiate* their embryo from being 'their own' to becoming an anonymous, publicly funded medical-scientific embryonic cell line that, rather than being a specific entity, becomes part of a shared, collective commitment to scientific progress—a value that is almost inextricable from hope." But hope for what? Hope for the extension of life by another ten years? Hope that more wealthy parents with fertility issues can reproduce themselves? Hope that the continuing trend of a steep decline in the number of babies born to white families in the United States and Europe and Australia will not be outpaced or eclipsed completely by the steady rise in populations of color? Hope, as Edelman suggests, goes hand in hand with repro-normativity and can be, must be, countered by "the negativity of the queer," which allows us to "refuse the insistence of hope itself as affirmation, which is always affirmation of an order whose refusal will register as unthinkable, irresponsible, inhumane."[5]

In place of hope, life, and affirmation, Edelman offers the antisocial theory of negativity, impossibility, and the death drive. The death drive, the counterintuitive but insistent limit to all imaginings of an ever-extended body and the endpoint to survivability itself, inscribes itself over and across the annoyingly buoyant scientific dreams of forever, of the end of disease, and of regeneration. And the death drive, in the end, is as important to transbiological imagination as the seemingly altruistic, but actually simply corporate, desire for extended life.

Horror film is the home of the death drive and *The Seed of Chucky* is transbiology in the unmaking. *Bride of Chucky,* the fourth film in the *Child's Play* series, ended with a horrific scene of birth from death—Tiffany has been pulverized and stabbed by her loving husband Chucky but she gives birth while seemingly on her deathbed. The sequel, inevitably, explores the outcome of the birth of Tiffany and Chucky's "seed," and it extends the search by Tiff and Chucky for human bodies into which they hope to transubstantiate their souls in order to leave their plastic casings behind once and for all. *Seed of Chucky* refuses the sentimental or altruistic narrative of child rearing and, like the other films in the *Chucky* series, it offers some fantastic scenes of alternative and queer modes of nonreproduction and transbiology laden with critiques of the human and of normative gender. If, as Franklin suggests, transbiology "carries its own politics, and they are, as Haraway insisted so rightly, fundamentally sociological,"[6] then we must look for the ripple effects of those unpredictable, sometimes queer and sometimes all too normative politics, in the stories we tell ourselves, in all seriousness and with heaps of irony about "unnatural" and engineered reproduction. The extracorporeal embryo, Franklin's work proposes, is not any longer an exceptional feature of human kinship; it is now part of the postmodern family and it interjects its own convulsive and sinister politics of hope and human improvement into otherwise sad and dreary narratives about reproductive failure. And so, while the spectacle of the cyborg embryo in another historical moment represented an altered and potentially queer vision of human progress and transformation, today the cyborg embryo merely extends the "naturalness" of family and the rightness of reproduction.

In Mary Shelley's *Frankenstein,* Shelley created a fantasy of scientific control of reproduction and she imagined both the freeing up of women from the burden of childbirth and the horror of assigning the responsibility of birth to the scientific lab. The queer potential of nonhuman reproduction came to life in the monster and was eradicated in the same gesture as Dr. Frankenstein seeks to eradicate his creation. The *Chucky* series thematizes and keeps alive the queer effects of making reproduction and sex into laboratory techniques. Shelley's monster eclipses its maker, kills his master's human chances of love, romance, and heteroreproduction, and creates a new pairing of maker and monster, which triumphs over the heterosexual couple. In the *Chucky* series, the dolls see humans as inferior life-forms, as fleshly pods for the incubation of their own seed, and heterosexuality is completely outmoded.

There are three scenes/figures for transformative and queer embodiment in *Seed of Chucky*: first, Tiffany and Chucky's child and his or her ambiguous gender; second, the technology of doll animation and its interaction with ideologies of humanism; finally, the use of a human female, Jennifer Tilly, in the film as a surrogate mother for Chucky's babies. Each figuration offers a critique of the human, exposes the relations between human and normative gendering and reproduction, and offers an alternative formulation of embodiment, desire, and identity. I want to close this chapter with a brief description of these three transbiological moments in the film.

No Gender

Tiffany and Chucky are reanimated in *Seed of Chucky* by their own offspring, who gives birth to his parents rather than the other way round. When he finds them in a props studio, with cables coming out of their backs, the oddly melancholic doll child recognizes his parents by the "made in Japan" stamp on their wrists, identical to the one he bears on his own. Chucky and Tiffany have ended up in a film about Chucky and Tiffany and so the whole film within a film becomes a reflection on the production of spirals of discursive truth in the realm of transbiology. Confronted with the strange figure that has reanimated them, Tiffany and Chucky are horrified by the ugliness of their savior. However, when he claims to be their child, both parents rush to claim him and name him. At this point, the question of gender arises and Tiffany calls him Glenda while Chucky names him Glen (riffing on Ed Wood's hilarious B movie, Glen/da). Glen/da turns out to be anatomically incorrect and in a hilarious scene of the construction of sex, the proud parents stare at the naked crotch of their child and both claim to "see" the genitals they want to see. Glen's gender is resolved only at the film's conclusion when he kills his father to save his mother—it is the social and oedipal act that genders him. In this brilliant intersexual thematic, gender legibility is shown to be important for the parents, not the child, and the film foregrounds the ways in which normative identity requires stable gender. In refusing to be either Glen or Glenda and in insisting on being both, Chucky and Tiffany's kid focuses our attention on the horrific effects of heteronormativity and turns attention away from the monstrosity of the ambiguously gendered body.

No Human

Just as hetero–homo seems like an afterglow of an earlier discursive structure, so the human in this film fades to black and leaves the Chucky doll in its place. While the *Chucky* films seem like "child's play," as the subtitle of the series implies, actually, they are masterful creations of cyborg technology and each doll requires about seven or eight puppeteers or human technicians. Each doll has two neutral heads and one screaming head, multiple arms, and several bodies. The three main bodies for each doll include *positionable, floppy,* and *stunt.* These three body types might best describe the fate of the body in the laboratory of transbiology: through discourses of science, nature, and reproduction, we become *positionable* and we perform within an arc of prescribed motions and responses. In the *floppy* mode, discourse makes the body and unmakes it often in the same gesture: what makes us perform a gender say also implies some kind of floppiness; it implies that we are performed *by* gender. In the *stunt* mode, the body does something that is seemingly impossible and in its survival, a new understanding of the body is born. In Chucky's case, Chucky desires a permanent move from his limited doll body to a real live human body. But after watching the spectacle of human childbirth, courtesy of the Jennifer Tilly character, Chucky decides he actually is better off in his positionable/floppy/stunt body.

Transbiology

After the bloody birth of Chucky Jr., Tiffany announces that she is done with reproduction and she decides that Chucky must donate sperm to impregnate a human with their babies. This way Glen/da will have a human body to transubstantiate himself into. Two hilarious scenes follow: one in which Chucky masturbates to a horror magazine in order to provide the seed; and another "lesbian" scene in which Tiffany uses a turkey baster to impregnate Jennifer Tilly. Here IVF leaves the purity of the lab. Franklin explains, "Like the cyborg, transbiology is also made up out of the complex intersection of the pure and the impure, where quality and biological control are literally merged to create new kinds of organisms, but this purity is hedged about by pathology of various kinds," and also like the cyborg, "the transbiological is not just about new mixtures, playful recombinations of parts, or new assemblages: it is fundamentally defined by the effort to differentiate these dirty descent lines into functional, safe, and marketable human biology."[7] Or, the transbiological emerges in the gothic imaginary as the very pathological fringe described here by Franklin as the "dirty descent lines" which are rejected in favor of "marketable human biology." The plastic and lesbian scene in which Tiffany impregnates Jennifer Tilly with Chucky's sperm to produce human babies parodies the entire IVF project and its barely submerged eugenic trajectory and hope for the improvement of the species.

Obviously, I am not locating the *Chucky* narratives in the same relation to IVF technologies that *Frankenstein* occupied in relation to early nineteenth-century fears of population control and the dangers of childbirth and the hope for new technologies of contraception . . . but then again, why not? The animated dolls, with their constructability, manipulability, plasticity, and queer gendering are particularly well suited to tell another story of transbiology—one in which the meaning of human, gender, body, reproduction, failure, hope, life, and death have been remade; one in which art and biology nestle alongside each other; a transbiology, in other words, that finds the body remade not merely in genetic experimentation but in the reimagining of the body, the human and its others in film, in the so-called natural world and in art. The world of animation, ultimately, distorts, manipulates, and messes with human form in a way that makes humanist ideals like heterosexual love and individualism seem creepy and that elevates posthuman, stunt subjectivity from revolting animation to animating revolt.

NOTES

1. Sarah Franklin, "The Cyborg Embryo: Our Path to Transbiology," *Theory, Culture and Society Annual Review* 1, no. 1 (Autumn 2006): 167–188.
2. Franklin, "The Cyborg Embryo," 171.
3. Franklin, "The Cyborg Embryo," 170.
4. Franklin, "The Cyborg Embryo," 171.
5. Lee Edelman, *No Future: Queer Theory and the Death Drive* (Durham, NC: Duke University Press, 2005), 4.
6. Franklin, "The Cyborg Embryo," 178.
7. Franklin, "The Cyborg Embryo," 176.

Section V

Criminology, Law, and Teratologies: Between the Real and the Reel

CHAPTER 14

STAGE FOUR: VIRULENCY (EXTRACT)

LONNIE H. ATHENS

THE SUBJECT HAS NOW SCORED HIS FIRST MAJOR VICTORY OR VIOLENT FEAT during a physical altercation, often only after experiencing many draws and "no decisions," several minor defeats, and even possibly some major ones at the hands of various protagonists. He has now finally prevailed decisively over a protagonist whom he has grievously injured in physical combat. He takes a certain amount of personal satisfaction at having kept his earlier resolution to attack people physically who overly provoke him with the serious intention of gravely harming them. Although he feels temporarily filled with a sense of personal satisfaction at having proven his resolve, the notable violent performance which the subject has given will not *by itself* have any lasting and significant impact upon him. Before the performance can have such an impact, its full significance must be impressed upon the subject's mind. The job of impressing the subject with the full significance of his successful violent action is gladly performed by other people who, for whatever reason, always seem to take a perverse interest and pleasure in violence—all the more so when they know the offender or victim.

In the aftermath of the recent violent performance, many people may come to know of the subject's violent feat. Members of his primary groups such as his brothers and sisters, neighbors, close friends, as well as members of secondary groups such as acquaintances, school officials, the police, prosecutors, and judges may come not only to know of it, but to take an active interest in it. The opinions formed about his violent action by members of the subject's primary groups, especially friends, almost always ultimately have a far greater weight in the subject's shaping of his own opinion about his actions than those drawn by secondary group members, such as official authorities. However, the two are not always independent or at odds with each other. The opinions of secondary groups may often serve to support and reinforce those of primary groups and vice versa.

In any event, the subject becomes conscious that other people's opinions of him have suddenly and drastically changed in the wake of his violent feat. They no longer see the subject as they did before his latest violent performance, but they see him as a very different person. Somewhat to the subject's amazement, he is now seen as an authentically violent individual, instead of a person who was not violent or only possibly capable of violence only a few short days or even hours earlier.

At least some of the people in the subject's primary groups see him not only as violent, but to his great astonishment, as *mentally unbalanced* as well. For the first time in his life, he hears people describe him in complete seriousness, rather than in a jocular vein, as a "violent lunatic," "violent maniac," "violent crazy man," "madman," or "insane killer." The subject may be cast in these terms without the benefit of an official diagnosis from a mental health professional. However, such terms are not always pejorative, since acting crazily may only demonstrate that one has real daring and pluck, which to members of some primary groups, is a positive rather than negative attribute, but only if not taken to extremes. Nevertheless, when the subject hears these colloquial epithets being seriously used to describe him, he may at first find it somewhat difficult to understand and slightly discomforting, if not outright alarming. Although the subject has no reservations at all about being known as having pluck, he may for a short while have true misgivings about being known as really "crazy." The subject may also be more than slightly puzzled as to why some primary group members whom he had always previously presumed strongly supported acting violently towards one's protagonists now suddenly begin hedging their support in the face of his recent violent feat in which he did this very thing.[1]

Moreover, the apparent reason why these primary group members see the subject as mentally unbalanced stems from the degree to which he injured the antagonist. They may truly believe that the antagonist deserved to be hurt, but did not deserve to be hurt as badly as the subject hurt him. Thus, their conclusion that the subject is mentally off balance is drawn from the excessive amount of violence that he chose to use rather than from the decision to resort to violence *per se*. Stated more colloquially, they believe that "he went way too far." This explains the apparent paradox of why some primary group members, including those formerly serving as his violent coaches, may react with shock and dismay after learning about the subject's violent feat.

Because the subject is seen by others as violent and possibly mentally unbalanced, he is treated much differently now than before. People treat him as if he literally were *dangerous*. They act toward him much more cautiously, taking particular pains not to offend or provoke him in any way. Primary group members, as well as secondary group members, take such precautions in the subject's presence. For the first time, the subject keenly senses genuine trepidation when he approaches people whom he knows, or more precisely, whom he is aware know of him. Of course, the irony is that the feeling of trepidation which the subject now senses others feeling toward him is the same feeling the subject himself felt only a short time ago while in the presence of certain other people. The subject's sensing of trepidation towards him on the part of other people marks both the climax to the subject's experience of violent notoriety and the dawning of a new experience: *social trepidation*.

The subject has now reached the critical point in his violence progression where he has experienced violent notoriety and the social trepidation which it brings. Although the notoriousness and others' trepidation which the subject has only recently experienced were not entirely of his own making, the subject must now decide whether to embrace or reject this personal achievement of sorts. The answer to this question presents the subject with a paradox. On the one hand, notoriety denotes being well known for something bad. On the other hand, it is sometimes better to be well known for something which most people think is bad and few think is good than not to be known for anything at all. Although the advantages may not be well recognized, being known as dangerous does have its advantages. The subject is afforded greater power over his immediate social environment. Since other people begin to think twice before provoking him, the subject can freely interact with other people without worrying as much about provoking them, so that for the first time he may feel liberated from the violent oppression of others. Moreover, painful memories of feeling powerless and inadequate originally aroused during his brutalization and later his belligerence experiences still linger in the back of the subject's mind.

This cannot help but make his newly discovered sense of power almost irresistible. Thus, the subject's answer to the question of whether to embrace or reject the violent notoriety is virtually a foregone conclusion. He only too gladly accepts his violent notoriety and the social trepidation that comes with it.

Upon the subject's decision to embrace his newly gained notoriousness, he undergoes a drastic change. The violent notoriety and the trepidation which it generates in others reverberates loudly in the subject's mind. As a result of these reverberations, he becomes overly impressed with his violent performance and ultimately with himself in general. Filled with feelings of exultancy, he concludes that since he performed this violent feat, there is no reason why he cannot perform even more impressive violent feats in the future. The subject much too hastily draws the conclusion that he is now invincible.

Blown up with a false sense of omnipotence, the subject becomes, in a manner of speaking, impervious to all later opinions and sentiments about his violent actions and, by inference, about himself that are not congruent with those he has already heard and wants to continue to believe. The ecstasy produced by his recent experiences certainly renders him incapable of seeing himself in less than sanguine terms, and furthermore, it renders others incapable of making him see himself this way as well. His pugnaciousness has swiftly grown to the point where he will without the slightest hesitation strongly rebuke anyone who would foolishly criticize him. Proselytizing him now would prove especially risky, since he could perceive the attempt as sufficient provocation for his taking violent action.

From the lofty heights of this new psychic plateau, the subject makes a new violence resolution which far surpasses the one made before the latest violent feat. He now firmly resolves to attack people physically with the serious intention of gravely harming or even killing them for the slightest or no provocation whatsoever, whereas before he had resolved to do this only if more than minimally provoked by someone. In making this later violent resolution, the subject has completely switched his stance from a more or less defensive posture to a decidedly offensive one. The subject is determined not to tolerate any provocation from other people, and, should the whim strike him, to provoke other people. He has suddenly been emboldened and made venomous at the same time.

With this last development, the experience of malevolency, the ultimate irony surfaces in the subject's life: he has now gone full circle from a hapless victim of brutalization to a ruthless aggressor—the same kind of brutalizer whom he had earlier despised. The subject, who is once again revelling in thoughts of his now proven courage and prowess, is blind to this ironic turn of his life. If the subject were suddenly to become aware of this irony, there is little likelihood that it would move him in any way to change his present path. He now relishes far too much the idea of being truculent, eagerly looking forward to the opportunity to treat others in the same brutal fashion as he was earlier treated. The subject has what is described in common parlance as "broken bad" and, as a result, has become a dangerous menace to others.

With the achievement of malevolence, a social segregation process begins. The primary groups in which the subject previously traveled gradually and significantly change. Many of his former companions and even some relatives begin to avoid the subject so they do not have to endure feelings of physical intimidation while in his presence, whether or not they, in particular, need feel this way. Meanwhile, the subject may find that he is now a welcome and desired companion among malevolent groups for whom having violent repute is a social requirement. However, until this happens, social isolation may result. The subject may find that he is being shunned by some of his former primary groups and not readily accepted by new ones. Without new primary groups to fill the void created by the loss of former groups, the subject becomes the proverbial violent outcast and loner so often read about in the popular press.

The manner in which subjects undergo virulency is illustrated in the . . . case that follow[s]. [. . .]

[. . .]

CASE 30

> Within three days, everybody in my neighborhood had heard that I fucked up somebody bad . . . . I had gotten an instant reputation.
>
> After that, I noticed a big change in people . . . . People were just too scared to get me mad because they thought I was really a violent lunatic and would do anything to anybody. [. . .]
>
> Although I knew a lot of people didn't think what I did was right, I said to myself, "Fuck what they think. I'm proud of what I did." I was glad that I stabbed that guy after the way everybody else acted . . . . I was ready to go after people and slice them wide open with my blade. I was ready to cut a person up in a minute.

[. . .]

NOTE

1. The very fact that some of the subject's fellow primary group members not only express reservations about his violent feat, but also raise questions about his mental balance, has an important theoretical implication. It casts doubt upon any theory of how people become dangerous violent criminals based upon the idea of violent values, such as the subculture of violent theory developed by [Marvin E. Wolfgang and Franco Ferracuti in their *The Subculture of Violence* (London: Travistock, 1967)] and described in Chapter 2.

CHAPTER 15

PROFILING THE TERRORIST AS A MASS MURDERER (EXTRACT)

CAROLINE JOAN (KAY) S. PICART AND CECIL E. GREEK

[. . .]

[T]HE TERRORIST HAS CURRENTLY REPLACED THE SERIAL KILLER as the most monstrous of all criminals. Among the current proliferation of Gothic discourses, the global terrorist is characterized as an exotic, religious fanatic with affinities to the male serial killer, but one motivated by a death drive, unlike the domestic male serial killer, who seems to want to escape, though he does leave clues behind for his pursuers to find and interpret. In comparison, the suicidal terrorist may be seeking recognition and reward promised beyond the grave, while leaving behind only shards of his explosive rage.[1] [. . .]

[. . .]

GOTHIC DISCOURSES AND TERRORISM

[. . .] If we think of terrorists as representatives of killing organizations, some similarities to the serial killing phenomenon become apparent. First, there is a repetitive patterned nature to the attacks, something we have noted in the serial murderer. While security agencies cannot seem to predict where or when the next attack will occur, targets often are chosen to have maximum political impact and timed so that the efforts appear relentless. Second, efforts to capture and eliminate the core of the terrorist organizations themselves prove to be ineffective. Like serial killers, terrorists avoid detection and capture, at least for a time. Two U.S. wars in response to 9/11 only seem to have strengthened support for the terrorists' view of the United States as murderer of innocent civilians, and allowed Americans abroad, including the military, to be put in greater danger than before 9/11. [. . .]

[. . .]

[. . .] The phenomenon of global terrorism combines Gothic themes from both traditional terror and horror; in fact, terrorists use the creation of real horror to bring nightmares to life. Thus, the tactics used to carry out the strategic objectives of modern global terrorism are themselves Gothic. A major objective of terrorism is to create a feeling of hopelessness among the population. That is why terrorist perpetrators attack symbolic targets in a horrific manner, as the psychological impact will exceed the physical damage of the strike. The repertoire of horrific tactics used includes bombings, arson, assaults, hijackings, kidnappings and taking and executing hostages. Both weapons of mass destruction and cyber-terrorism are expected to be used in the future, thus broadening the impacts and increasing panic among the populace.[2] Horrifying video footage is either filmed by journalists who arrive soon after the carnage, or home-made, like the rape-torture-murder from *Henry: Portrait of a Serial Killer* (1986), and offered to media organizations for broadcast or announcement on Web sites. None of this is senseless violence, as targets and methods of killing are chosen that will maximize the mixture of drama and dread, and create acute feelings of insecurity within targeted countries and populations. As Kegley states, terrorism "presents people with a danger that seems ubiquitous, unavoidable and unpredictable."[3] Besides attacking symbols of government authority or American global capitalism, terrorists also choose to launch vicious indiscriminate attacks at normally tranquil urban locations that citizens visit (e.g., markets, cafes, public transit, tourist sites) to create a "paralyzing sense of foreboding among the public."[4] If anything can happen to anyone at any time, who is safe? The 9/11 attacks were successful initially in the sense that immediate fear-based changes were introduced . . . . While Bush called upon Americans to return to their normal everyday lives, he simultaneously employed a rhetoric and a set of policies aimed at the opposite.[5] Besides signifying that we now live in a state of permanent fear, Bush's speeches resulted in a simplified "us" versus "them" mentality and an inability to comprehend the complexity of terrorist motivations. In a March 19, 2004 speech, Bush (2004) declared: "There is no neutral ground-no neutral ground-in the fight between civilization and terror, because there is no neutral ground between good and evil, freedom and slavery, and life and death." Bush's rhetoric was notable for its repeated use of the word "evil," which implicitly argued for only one political solution: extermination.[6] Ultimately, since Bush's notion of "evil" was not a metaphysical abstraction that transcended gender, race, class and nationality but a specific profile: usually male, Arabic, usually poor and middle-Eastern—set apart from the rest of the races that constitute America and its friendly allies, his rhetoric was plagued by the same anxieties as the postcolonial Gothic. Haunted by the specters of lethal foreign pollution and contamination as the Orientalist Gothic, Bush's rhetoric struggled against its darker underside.

One finds embedded in the rhetoric of President George Bush not only a Gothic interpretation of world events, but also a number of the theories about terrorism frequently cited but often rejected by criminologists. These theories include the perspective that terrorists can be explained either as nihilists out to destroy all of humanity, criminal social deviants motivated by base instincts, or uncivilized barbarians out to destroy civilized society for the sake of destroying it.[7] [. . .]

[. . .]

Even Condoleeza Rice resorted to a Gothic metaphor in her defense of the Bush administration's policies in stating that "there was no silver bullet that could have prevented the 9/11 attacks."[8] What was implied in her succinct statement was that the terrorists . . . are far more difficult to kill than the mythical werewolf, who, like the terrorists, has a dual identity. [. . .]

TERRORISTS IN FILM

[. . .]

[. . .] In contrast, t]he films that feature global terrorism offer both a number of theories regarding the root causes of terrorism as well as a number of suggested American responses . . .

The Siege, though it was made in 1998, was eerily prophetic of what would happen in New York City and Iraq only a few years later, and also foresaw the coming of the Patriot Act. Weaving across the cinematic coding of fact and fiction, *The Siege* began with President Clinton on television in the wake of the Somalia bombing, warning that "America takes care of its own," intercut with video footage of the devastated Federal Building in Oklahoma.[9] Scarred and grainy, the raw actuality of these images created a jarring contrast with the portentous dialogue and glossy production values to come. Footage of Clinton's speech, mediated by television is followed by a fictional action scene depicting a Middle East terrorist being kidnapped by the CIA. [. . .]

[. . .]

However, *The Siege* neither blamed terrorism on Muslim extremism, nor espoused setting aside the Constitution or global human rights to stop the attacks. Ultimately, we learn that the U.S. has trained and armed those who later would become members of these terrorist cells when they were still living in Iraq, part of the effort to bring down Saddam Hussein after the first Gulf War. [But] after training them, the U.S. abandoned them to be slaughtered by the dictator rather than support them with military back up. Their terrorist actions are a revenge on America and thus at least partly justified; in Samir's case, the reaction was doubly justified, as it was clear that Kraft's "treachery," as both a lover and a parental figure left deep wounds. Kraft, the film implicitly argued, functioned as a Frankensteinian scientist who went too far in her experiments with the volatile youth of the region; by teaching the young men how to make bombs, and then allowing the majority of them to be slaughtered, she (and the CIA) in effect created these monsters. As such, she deserved to die. [. . .]

In terms of chronology, *Maryam* (2000) was made just prior to 9/11, but covered the era of the Iranian hostage crisis circa 1979. A troubled young Iranian, Ali Armin (David Ackert), comes to live with his uncle's family in New Jersey, while the deposed Shah of Iran is being treated for cancer at a New York City hospital. The young man plots to assassinate the Shah, but lacks the courage to do it, as he is not really a terrorist or a monster. Ali is psychologically wounded because he believes his father was betrayed by the rich uncle who now functions as his foster parent, who had revealed the whereabouts of his brother to the Shah's security thugs, Savak, who killed him. This is compounded by the fact that Ali, as a devout Muslim, is suffering culture shock upon arriving in what he sees as a decadent, godless society.

[. . .]

The moral center of the film is a teenage girl named Maryam (Marriam Parris), who has spent her whole life in the United States. She is too Americanized to ever become a traditional wife for Ali, and is torn between American and Iranian perspectives on the global situation, mirrored in microcosm in her ambivalent relationships with her own family. The film offers no hope for a better future; the best it offers is an escape for Ali back to his own culture and way of life rather than capture by the police and FBI. Technically, the film has few Gothic elements, and is refreshingly different, in that it manages effectively to convey the point of view of a non-American to whom America's sexual permissiveness, apolitical narcissism and indulgence in drugs seems both strange and objectionable. The only clear scene in which Gothic and stereotypic coding of the terrorist is used happens during the scene when Ali, packing a loaded gun he has acquired illegally, and disguised using a doctor's lab coat and his uncle's hospital pass, heads for the heavily guarded room in which the Shah of Iran is convalescing after an operation. The music turns ominous, and Ali is shot predominantly in low key lighting, from a slightly low angle that focuses mainly on his mask-like face. Yet as soon as Ali hesitates, and sanity returns, the music disappears, and Ali once again becomes the vulnerable and deeply wounded human being he is. [. . .]

[. . .]

In 2003, the short film *T for Terrorist* played at a number of major film festivals. The movie's response to film terrorism is to deconstruct the Hollywood image of the Arab as terrorist. The film opens with a moody, Orientalist-coded scene of an Arab terrorist invading a laid back jazz club and pointing his machine gun at a platinum blond singer. The distinction between the light skinned singer representing the white world and the dark-skinned, bearded Arab parallels the way Bram Stoker contrasted the ever whitening Mina and the swarthy Count in *Dracula.*[10] . . . Fear of Easterners, dark others and the earlier, atavistic forms of race and religion mark *Dracula* in the same way that the Hollywood stereotype of Middle Easterners as terrorists has marked global crime films. [. . .]

T for Terrorist, despite its numerous aesthetic flaws, underlines a persistent problematic. Given the current fixation upon global terrorism, our current everyday life world has become itself a Gothic-like universe of fear . . . with its Arabic other as its most dreaded monster.

[. . .]

NOTES

1. Ariel Merari, "The Readiness to Kill and Die," in *Origins of Terrorism: Psychologies, Ideologies, Theologies, States of Mind,* ed. Walter Reich (Baltimore, MD: Johns Hopkins University Press, 1998), 192–209.
2. Jonathan Randall White, *Terrorism: An Introduction,* fourth ed. (Belmont, CA: Wadsworth Publishing, 2003), 16.
3. Charles W. Kegley, *The New Global Terrorism: Characteristics, Causes, Controls* (Upper Saddle River, NJ: Prentice Hall, 2003), 72.
4. Kegley, *The New Global Terrorism,* 73.
5. See William D. Lutz, "The Rhetoric of Fear," September 7, 2003, *NY Newsday,* accessed June 11, 2004, http://www.commondreams.org/views03/0907-06.htm; and Michael Moore, *Fahrenheit 911* (Hollywood, CA: Miramax Films, 2004).
6. "Stanford Psychologist Questions Over-Use of the Word 'Evil'," November 28, 2001, *Business Journal,* accessed June 17, 2004, http://sanjose.bizjournals.com/sanjose/stories/2001/11/26/daily22.html.
7. Kegley, *The New Global Terrorism,* 179.
8. G. Edmonson, "Rice Defends Bush on Terrorism Policy," April 9, 2004, *Rocky Mount Telegram,* accessed June 13, 2004, http://www.rockymounttelegram.com/news/content/shared/news/rice/09rice.html.
9. K. Hollings, "Review of the Motion Picture *The Siege,*" February 1999, *British Film Institute,* accessed June 17, 2006, http://www.bfi.org.uk/sightandsound/reviews/details.php?id=41.
10. Diane Long Hoeveler, "Objectifying Anxieties: Scientific Ideologies in Bram Stoker's *Dracula* and *The Lair of the White Worm,*" *Romanticism on the Net* 44 (2006), http://www.erudit.org/revue/ron/2006/v/n44/014003ar.html.

CHAPTER 16

WHAT MAKES STALKING MONSTERS SO MONSTROUS, AND HOW TO SURVIVE THEM?

ÔRÎT KĀMÎR

INTRODUCTION

What are monsters? Among other things, monsters are un/supernatural creatures that stalk us. They stalk us in our imaginations when we are alone in the dark; they stalk us in our dreams. Stalking is something that monsters do. So much so that it is sometimes considered "monstrous" when performed by human beings. Perhaps stalking can serve as a prism to get insight into monstrosity. To better understand monsters through stalking, we must define what stalking is. Technically speaking, it is a pattern of conduct that consists of following another and lying in wait for him or her. A hunter stalks his prey. But this definition is surely both too wide and too narrow. A toddler following her father around the house, never letting him out of her sight and lying in wait for him when he steps outside would not be considered stalking him. An estranged husband phoning his estranged wife at all times and hanging up without saying a word might be considered stalking her, even if he never follows her about or lies in wait for her. If so, then what *is* stalking and why is it so intimately connected with monstrosity?

One way to reflect on stalking, as well as its monstrosity, is to consider a few familiar and highly influential stories of monstrous stalking. Each of these stories consists of specific, unique elements that are time- and place-specific. Each of them also consists of deep-seated components that seem to reappear in stories of stalking monsters throughout Western culture. The following sections review five such stories and their stalking monsters: Mary Shelley's 1817 literary "Frankenstein Monster"; the Travis character in the 1976 film *Taxi Driver*; the media portrayal of a serial killer who, in 1976, caused panic and anxiety, calling himself "Son of Sam"; the Michael character in the 1978 film *Halloween*; the Alex character in the 1987 film *Fatal Attraction* that gave rise to widespread hysteria. Examination of these monstrous characters and their stalking stories sheds light on some attributes of the course of conduct we associate with stalking while also illuminating monstrosity.[1]

MARY SHELLEY'S *FRANKENSTEIN, OR THE MODERN PROMETHEUS* (1817)

THE STORY

Mary Shelley may have been the first to associate stalking with hideous monstrosity, a linkage now so widely accepted that we have come to take it for granted. Shelley's *Frankenstein*[2] narrates the story of a young scientist, Dr. Victor Frankenstein, who, in his relentless scientific zeal, creates life. But appalled by the ugliness of his creature, he abandons it. Wandering in streets and forests, the agonizing creature observes people from afar, educating itself in their language and manners. In desperate need of family, it attempts to reunite with its creator and asks him for a mate, only to be refused. In his violence, the monster causes the deaths of Victor's father, brother (William), bride (Elizabeth), best friend (Clerval), and an innocent servant girl. It becomes a serial killer. Determined to take the monster's life, Victor chases it to the North Pole, where he dies while telling his story to Walton, a ship-captain; the creature then appears and promises Walton that it will take its own life.

THE MONSTER'S PERSPECTIVE VERSUS HIS TARGET'S POINT OF VIEW

Mary Shelley presents her stalking story in a unique double first-person narration: once by the stalking monster and once by its target. This frame-tale structure furnishes her reader with an awareness of the very different points of view of the monstrous pursuer and of his target's. Only together do these two distinct perspectives convey the full meaning of monstrous stalking. This section begins by introducing Victor Frankenstein's narration of his experience of being stalked by his monster.

Victor first becomes aware that he is being pursued by his monster in Geneva, after his brother William's funeral:

> I perceived in the gloom a figure which stole from behind a clump of trees near me; I stood fixed, gazing intently: I could not be mistaken. A flash of lightning illuminated the object, and discovered its shape plainly to me; its gigantic stature, and the deformity of its aspect, more hideous than belongs to humanity, instantly informed me that it was the wretch, the filthy daemon to whom I had given life. What did he there? . . . The figure passed me quickly, and I lost it in the gloom.[3]

The next time that Victor notices the unwelcome presence, in the village of Chamonix, the monster approaches him, narrates its experiences to him, and finally demands that Victor make him a female partner. Victor obeys, but horrified by the prospect that the couple breed more monsters, he destroys the female, and, in return, the monster murders Henry Clerval, Victor's best friend. Victor returns to Geneva to marry Elizabeth, but the monster kills her on their wedding night. By now Victor knows that he will never be free: "I do not doubt that he hovers near the spot which I inhabit."[4] He determines to spend the rest of his life chasing the monster and ridding the world of it, but dies before the completion of his task.

In Victor's story, the stalking takes place between Man and his self-made shadow, his dark double, his monstrous, externalized other-self. In Victor's own mind, the monster is not clearly distinguishable from Victor, and its predation seems to be an aspect of *Victor's* "dual existence." Victor experiences the stalking as a punitive reminder of his own inherent, inexplicable monstrosity. The monster's persistent presence is, for him, ugly self-reflection of the evil within. It frightens him, paralyzes him, fills him with guilt, shame, and frustrated rage. He perceives his stalking monster as a dreadful secret about himself, which alienates him from the rest of humanity. He feels trapped.

The stalking monster's perspective offers a different story altogether, in which a cruel creator is pursued by his desperate, abandoned creation, which justly seeks acceptance, affection, and reconciliation. The monster's story is as follows: after a short period of happiness in the woods, the monster is forced to flee and, having no companion and nowhere to go, it chooses to go to Geneva, Victor's hometown. There, the monster runs into young William Frankenstein. Learning that this is Victor's brother, and feeling rejected by him, the monster kills the boy. Avenging its own misery, the monster discovers that

> I too can create desolation; my enemy is not invulnerable; this death will carry despair to him, and a thousand other miseries shall torment and destroy him . . . . For some days I haunted the spot where these scenes had taken place; sometimes wishing to see you, sometimes resolved to quit the world and its miseries forever.[5]

And this is the monster's portrayal of his killings of Clerval and Elizabeth:

> After the murder of Clerval, I returned to Switzerland, heart-broken and overcome. I pitied Frankenstein; my pity amounted to horror: I abhorred myself. But when I discovered that he, the author at once of my existence and of its unspeakable torments, dared to hope for happiness; that while he accumulated wretchedness and despair upon me, he sought his own enjoyment in feelings and passions from the indulgence of which I was forever barred, then impotent envy and bitter indignation filled me with an insatiable thirst for vengeance. I recollected my threat, and resolved that it should be accomplished. I knew that I was preparing for myself a deadly torture; but I was the slave, not the master, of an impulse, which I detested, yet could not disobey. Yet when she died!—nay, then I was not miserable. I had cast off all feeling, subdued all anguish, to riot in the excess of my despair. Evil thenceforth became my good. Urged thus far, I had no choice but to adapt my nature to an element which I had willingly chosen. The completion of my demonical design became an insatiable passion. And now it is ended; there is my last victim.[6]

The monster's account of its pursuit of Victor documents the evolution of the stalking monster's motives and emotions. When it first heads toward Victor's hometown, the monster is seeking only a home for itself; it yearns to belong, to break with the intolerable solitude forced upon it, and Victor's is the only home where it can hope to belong. But once in Geneva, the monster is bluntly rejected by young William Frankenstein, and its sorrow is transformed into fury and rage. In killing William, the monster asserts itself as powerful and capable of initiating meaningful action: it proves to Victor and to itself that, if nothing else, it can be as cruel as its creator. But it also hopes to attract Victor's attention and to evoke his compassion. It hopes to bring Victor to Geneva, so as to at least see him from afar. Following its creator across Europe, the creature joins its "father" as a secret traveling companion. At the same time, it also reinforces its mastery over Victor's consciousness. It longs to be a part of Victor's life, and by keeping Victor constantly aware of its potentially dangerous presence nearby, it ensures that Victor can never stop thinking of it. By forcing itself upon Victor's mind, the monster will never again be completely alone.

The monster becomes violent when Victor refuses to acknowledge it as part of his life, when he disclaims it and refuses to assume responsibility for it. Killing William is the monster's only means to rejoin Victor, who has abandoned it "at birth." The killing of Clerval is in response to Victor's refusal to assume responsibility for the monster's happiness and to supply it with a female partner. Elizabeth is murdered to prevent Victor from pursuing his own happiness without the monster. The message is, "if you don't make sure I am happy—I'll make sure you are not," combined with "if I cannot have you—nobody will."

The monster seeks Victor's attention, and obtains it in full by stalking him and his relatives. Elizabeth's death provokes Victor to dedicate the rest of his life to chasing his shadow: "[m]y first resolution was to quit Geneva forever . . . And now my wanderings began, which are to cease but with life . . . . I pursued him, and for many months this has been my task."[7] Victor thus becomes the stalker of his monstrous image.

In conclusion, if Mary Shelley's monster is monstrous, it is because it was neglected, rejected, and misunderstood. Its monstrosity is a human psychological response to unfair social treatment. Its stalking is a manifestation of deep pain and unattended emotional need. The stalking monster's target is its closest kin; its other self; its creator, the man who represents the monster's abandonment and rejection. It is from him that the monster demands what it considers justice: acknowledgment, acceptance, and painful sacrifice.

Yet, at the same time, as Victor Frankenstein's narrative testifies, the stalking monster is a ghastly, unnatural and inhuman thing. It is a vampiric, blood-lusting living dead. The monster itself further admits that it is possessed by inexplicable, awesome dark forces and serves them. It is doomed to follow a compulsive obsessive pattern of destructive behavior. "I was the slave, not the master, of an impulse, which I detested, yet could not disobey," it admits.[8]

In Mary Shelley's novel, Victor, who is explicitly associated with Adam/"everyman" and with Faust/"over-reaching scientist," is responsible for vampiric, monstrous, fatal stalking. Its victims experience it as being performed by an undead monster, who is Victor's (i.e., Man's/Scientist's) dark mirror image. Victor's (Man's/Scientist's) overreaching scientific zeal is individualistic, vain, irresponsible, loveless, and, therefore, vampirically, monstrously fatal. His loveless passion to Know begets his monstrous vampire self that destroys his closest kin. Monstrosity is the murderous, unnatural, and inhuman manifestation of Man's dark, egotistical zeal to Know. It turns on Man, targeting him and causing havoc all around.

Mary Shelley's story of monstrous stalking clarifies the distinction between a stalking monster's target and its victims. The monster's predation is a manifestation of Victor's split existence: Victor's dark self targets its distinguished self. In this monstrous stalking game, Man and his shadow, monster and target, are the only real players. Victor's brother, his fiancé, and his best friend are not subjects of the monstrous stalking in their own right: they are merely victimized as part of the shadow's targeting of its creator. Dr. Jekyll and Mr. Hyde come to mind, as well as their numerous contemporary literary and cinematic manifestations. These stories all narrate how Man begets Monster, and how they target and stalk each other in a love–hate bonding game that demands the lives of innocent victims.

The Stalking Monster from Fiction to Reality to Fiction (1976–1978)

Taxi Driver

In 1975, psychologist Herb Goldberg published his widely read *The Hazards of Being Male*. In this book, he defined an identity crisis among American men, whom he calls tormented "zombies" and "sleepwalkers," "machinelike," "dehumanized things," and "role robots." Observing that "castrated men" would explode if they did not reclaim their masculinity, he claimed that modern man must embrace his "underlying rage toward the endless, impossible binds under which he lives."[9] Referring to the defeated, antiheroic postwar mood, Ray Raphael related this crisis in the experience of masculinity to the unhappy conclusion of the Vietnam War. He argued that the war had been "an abortive rite of passage for an entire generation of American males, even for those who stayed behind."[10]

In this cultural context, people feared Vietnam War veterans, the young men who had returned frustrated and disoriented from "the heart of darkness." These men seemed to mirror the deep crisis of American masculinity and to reflect men's collective, castrated state: they represented their generation's failure to pass from childhood into manhood. It is little wonder that the film *Taxi Driver* received abundant attention.

In 1976, Martin Scorsese and Paul Schrader introduced the American public to Robert De Niro's Travis Bickle: a shy, lonely Marine veteran, trapped in the meaninglessness of his alienated life as a New York taxi driver. Unable to sleep, he drives his taxi every night, ceaselessly prowling the city. From his taxi window, "Bickle understands the city solely as a place of corruption, filth, violence, dread—an open sewer, filled with garbage and inhabited by human vermin. Only pimps and pushers and prostitutes walk the streets; . . . it is a city of dreadful night and the night's creatures."[11] He documents the city's moral guilt, awaiting supernatural intervention that will cleanse it from the filth. He becomes a ticking bomb of frustrated rage waiting to explode.

Developing an infatuation with a fair, virginal political campaign worker, Betsy (Cybil Shepherd), Travis follows her and succeeds in attaining her attention for a short while. When she rejects him, he purchases three guns, drills himself in their use, changes his appearance into a head-shaven punk, and stalks the presidential candidate for whom she works, in an attempt to assassinate him. Failing in this, he takes on another mission, that of saving an underaged prostitute (Jodie Foster) from her pimp. In the execution of his mission, he shoots and kills three men. These avenging murders turn him into a media celebrity and allow him to reenter his previous life on the ugly streets and resume his original appearance and personality.

On one level, Travis's stalking monstrosity is explained in the context of his delusional, pathetic infatuation with an unattainable, virginal, love object. It is she who rejects (and castrates) him, thus "creating him," in his own mind, as an obsessive, frustrated, raging bully. She is, thus, his target, and it is in his attempt to impose himself on her life that he pursues her, while also stalking and killing others. For Travis, Betsy represents American society. In this sense, society at large created Travis and is responsible for his condition. Like Frankenstein's monster, Travis rages against what he perceives as Betsy/society's unjust rejection. In his stalking he calls for attention as well as takes his revenge.

But on another deeper level, Travis's monstrous features are all manifestations of his "veteran character"; that is, it is his doomed, hopeless existential state as a contemporary American man that renders him vampiric, monstrous, and Hyde-like. He is the community's Hyde in that he is its innate dark, shadowy mirror image set loose. In this sense, his monstrous stalking represents the community's stalking of itself.

On one level, then, Betsy/American society is the cause of Travis's misery, obsession, monstrosity, and stalking. The war, the rejection, and the meaninglessness are to blame. But at the same time, stalking monstrosity is simply inherent in him as a Vietnam veteran, the shadow of the American man.

"Son of Sam": Reality Mimics Fiction

The same year that the fictional Travis first stalked America on-screen (1976), a real predator was stalking it on the streets of New York City. "Son of Sam," as he called himself, shot thirteen people, killing six and wounding seven, in seven shooting incidents that occurred between July 1976 and June 1977. He usually attacked young couples in parked cars late at night. Most of his victims were young women with long brown hair. In his sixth shooting, a note was found. In part, it read:

> I am the "Monster"—"Beelzebub"—the Chubby Behemoth. I love to hunt. Prowling the streets looking for fair game—tasty meat. The women of Queens are prettiest of all . . . I live for the hunt—my life. Blood for papa.[12]

The assassin also sent letters to a *New York Daily News* reporter, Jimmy Breslin, one containing the following passage:

> I am deeply hurt by your calling me a women hater. I am not. But I am a monster. I am the Son of Sam . . . . Sam loves to drink blood. "Go out and kill", commands father Sam. Behind our house some rest. Mostly young—raped and slaughtered—their blood drained—just bones now . . . . Papa Sam keeps me locked in the attic . . . . I feel like an outsider. I am on a different wavelength than everybody else—programmed to kill.[13]

One of the letters was signed "Sam's creation."

His notorious actions made "Son of Sam" a contemporary of Jack the Ripper. His letters explicitly portrayed him as a hunter, a vampire's slave, and a Frankensteinian monster. It was almost inevitable that both the public and the media would associate him with the fictional Travis Bickle. Two common speculations that appeared in the newspapers were that "Son of Sam" was a veteran and that he drove a taxi. The list of "Son of Sam's" victims was relatively short, and his deeds were not half as gruesome as those committed by other serial killers, but the combination of the killer's teasing, chilling letters, his self-description as a vampiric monster, and his popular association with the murderous protagonist of a powerful film touched an open nerve. The press described and analyzed his exploits relentlessly. The American public was obsessed and fascinated. "Son of Sam" became a household name and a national celebrity.

When he was finally caught, the media portrayal of "Son of Sam" (David Richard Berkowitz) confirmed the popular suspicion that he was a "Travis come true." Berkowitz was described as a "well-mannered, 24-year-old postal worker who lived alone. His apartment was filthy . . . and the walls were scratched with graffiti"[14]—just as in *Taxi Driver*. This army veteran's "main character trait seemed to be that he was introverted and liked to roam the streets alone at night."[15] Like Travis, he was a keen consumer of pornography and owned two guns (his notorious .44 and a machinegun). Like the taxi driver, he documented his exploits in writing and was fascinated with the newspaper coverage of his escapades.

In the public imagination, as orchestrated by the media, "Son of Sam," the real stalking monster, was the tragic victim of the war, of social alienation and the meaninglessness of life, of loneliness and neglect in contemporary America. He was also inherently Other: a veteran; a blood-lusting vampire; a deranged monster. The killer himself claimed that he is possessed by evil forces that he cannot control, and that "[A]lmost everyone else is like me, for we commit numerous perverted sexual acts in our minds day after day." He constituted himself as society's innately evil Hyde.

HALLOWEEN: FRANKENSTEIN'S MONSTER BECOMES AN EVER-RETURNING SLASHER

Two years later, in 1978, John Carpenter directed a low-budget film that became a fad: *Halloween*. In this fictional narrative, Travis and "Son of Sam" were stripped, or abstracted, of social contextualization and reinstituted, in the character of Michael, as the paradigmatic, universalistic stalking monster: Frankenstein's creature. In *Halloween*, society and psychiatry are responsible for Michael's monstrous stalking; yet at the same time he is also evil incarnate, with no reason or cure—pure malevolence. As in Mary Shelley's text, only combined do these two perspectives capture the essence of this film's stalking monster.

Halloween opens with a murder committed on Halloween night by a 6-year-old Michael wielding a kitchen knife. The victim is the boy's teenage sister, who had spent the evening with a boy in the parents' bedroom. Fifteen years later, one night before Halloween 1978, Michael escapes (in a thunderstorm) from the mental institution where he has been confined and heads back home. He spends Halloween day stalking Tommy, a young boy who looks much as Michael himself did 15 years earlier, and Laurie, the teenager who is to babysit Tommy that night. While Michael is stalking, wearing a mask, his psychiatrist, Dr. Loomis, roams the little town, hunting for his patient and trying to warn the unbelieving authorities that evil has returned to their jurisdiction. He declares, "I spent 8 years trying to reach him and another 7 trying to keep him locked up, because I realized that what was living behind that boy's eyes was purely and simply evil."

Slaughtering two of Laurie's friends, Michael attempts to murder her as well. In the final scene, the monster is shot by his psychiatrist, who finally arrives on the scene. But although Dr. Loomis shoots Michael six times, the monster walks away and disappears, only to return in sequels released in 1981, 1983, 1988, and 1998. Michael's monstrous slasher-stalking image has reappeared in many subsequent horror films, establishing itself as an essential component of our collective imagination.

Much like Frankenstein's monster, Michael returns home, to bond and wreak havoc. Much like Victor Frankenstein, Dr. Loomis, Michael's "scientist father image," chases Michael in an attempt to kill him and contain the danger he poses to innocent bystanders. Like Frankenstein, Dr. Loomis refers to Michael as "it," stressing that despite appearances, Michael is more monster than human. The doctor declares that the creature is "simply evil." Indeed, Michael, whose face we never see and who never utters a single word, is portrayed as a diabolical, blood drinking, stalking living dead creature. This portrayal mimics Victor Frankenstein's view of his monstrous creation.

Yet Michael is also very much a Frankensteinian monster as presented through that creature's tormented perspective. Halloween does not give Michael a voice to tell of his misery, but it does portray him as lonely, abandoned, and unloved, seeking his family and desiring revenge. Despite Michael's own muteness, the film does offer the view that family, society, and the psychiatric profession are all responsible for having created this monster. Deserted and rejected by family and society, abandoned to years of institutionalization and psychoanalytic treatment, Michael, like Frankenstein's monster, becomes a vengeful, ruthless murderer. He returns home to bond with the only "family" he has (Tommy and Laurie), and to empower himself by causing them pain and suffering. He will not let the others enjoy their lives without him. He is obsessed by a deadly power that he cannot control—much like Frankenstein's monster.

The Female Stalking Monster: *Fatal Attraction* (1987)

In the conservative Reagan–Bush era, *Fatal Attraction*'s protagonist Dan (Michael Douglas) is a married man whose fair wife is a perfect homemaker and attentive mother to their daughter. When his wife and daughter are away for a weekend, the naive Dan is seduced by the independent professional Alex (Glen Close), who promises that no strings would be attached to their liaison. When, starting the following day, she insists on continuing a relationship, he feels trapped, helpless, and terrified. She appears constantly—in his office, by his car, and even in his home—demanding his recognition and affection. Feeling mistreated, she resorts to violence and even kills (Dan's daughter's pet rabbit). She attempts suicide to arouse Dan's compassion, is frequently seized by extreme fits of hysteria, and rapidly deteriorates into destructive, uncontrolled lunacy. Dan's terror peaks when she notifies him of her pregnancy, and when, eventually, she enters Dan's home and attempts to murder his wife. Ultimately, the good wife prevails.

Dan is the prototypical new man; he is the ideal type of the tormented, "politically correct" American man of the 1980s and 1990s, who, although not faultless, nevertheless invites sympathy and understanding. Alex is the backlash-inspired image of the dangerous feminist: the independent career woman, who is emotionally unstable and a threat to family values.

Alex is a 1987 female version of a Frankensteinian monster and the year's most notorious stalking monster. She feels unjustly abandoned by the man who, she claims, made her into what she has become. Lonely and tormented, she accuses Dan of rejecting her, of abandoning her, and of refusing to assume responsibility for her suffering. She desperately stalks him as a means of calling his attention, bonding with him, and punishing him. She stalks and hurts the people most dear to him. Her message to Dan is, "if you don't make sure I am happy—I'll make sure you are not," combined with "if I cannot have you—nobody will."

At the same time, like Frankenstein's creation, Alex too is a deranged, raving monster; an uncontrollable "thing," possessed by an obsession she cannot control. As such, Alex is a hellish female demon of the occult-horror, as well as a reincarnation of *Halloween*'s Michael character. Her persistent returns to Dan's life, sometimes shot from her peeping perspective outside his window, associate her with Michael. This is particularly clear in the final scene. In Dan's new family home in the country, Alex ambushes his wife in the shower and tries to kill her with a large kitchen knife. When, in the nick of time, Dan comes to the rescue, he and Alex battle fiercely, until he manages to drown her in the bathtub. Alex's dead eyes are fixed on the tormented Dan for a very long time. And then, just when the tension begins to fade, Alex returns from death, leaping on Dan like a demented vampire armed with a knife. Luckily, the good wife arrives on the scene to shoot the ghastly demon down.

The public, in both America and abroad, was preoccupied, if not obsessed, with *Fatal Attraction*. *Time* magazine noted that "people just can't stop talking about this movie." Peter Van Gelder notes in *That's Hollywood: A Behind the Scenes Look at 60 of the Greatest Films of All Times* (1990) that

> The gross in North America had topped $150,000,000 by the end of the year, and it broke box office records in Britain, taking 1,000,000 pounds in the first week. In analyst-ridden New York it was reported that 70% of patients with marital problems were claiming to be obsessed with *Fatal Attraction*.[16]

Judging by surveys of audience response, the film seems to have aroused in male viewers strong feelings of anxiety, hatred (toward the woman-stalker), and revenge.[17] Similarly, Susan Faludi notes in her book *Backlash* (1991) that "A headline in one supermarket tabloid even dubbed the film's single-woman character the MOST HATED WOMAN IN AMERICA."[18]

Stalking Monsters

So what are stalking monsters, and what is it that makes them "monstrous"? Judging by Frankenstein's monster, as well as some of its notorious contemporary descendants (*Taxi Driver*'s Travis, "Son of Sam," *Halloween*'s Michael, and Fatal *Attraction*'s Alex), stalking monsters combine two distinct characterizations. On the one hand, they are tormented by what they perceive as their abandonment and neglect, and stalk to bond with those whom they perceive as their tormentors, as well as to hurt them and avenge themselves on them. They desperately attempt to prevent their would-be-tormentors from enjoying their lives without them. Each monster constructs his or her alleged tormentor as a close family member, such as a parent figure or a lover. The relationship with this "family member" is experienced by the monster as primary, eternal, and inevitable. In the monster's mind, the "relative" is in some sense the monster's creator, responsible both for its existence and for its suffering. In turn, the monster is in some sense the "relative's" shadowy Hyde double. The monster does everything in its power to convey these feelings to its target, that is, to the monster's "relative"/creator/double image, and make the target adopt the monster's perspective.

In this characterization, the monster's stalking is an act of desperate pain, reaching out and acting out in the face of cruel denunciation; it is a response to provocation; a reaction to a cause. Since the bond between monster and "relative" is so deep, the rejection and abandonment are of monumental dimensions, the pain is unbearable, and the passion for vengeance—enormous. In this narrative, the stalking monster's endeavor, subjectively, from its perspective, is to achieve justice: to (re)enforce a relationship that was "meant to be" on a beloved who seems to be indifferent, uncooperative, or trying to break away.

On the other hand, in the parallel characterization, stalking monsters are inhuman, deranged Others, who are possessed by murderous lust for blood which they cannot control. They are pure evil that cannot be explained, understood, or treated. Their stalking is almost mechanical. There is no hope of communication, negotiation, or reasoning with them. The monsters are unreachable foes.

The unnerving fusion of familiarity, closeness, anguish and vengeance, guilt and pity with the raw, innate, unfeasible evil is gruesome and disorienting. These monsters are us—and also not us; they are "close kin"—and alien strangers; they are creatures we can relate to, take pity on, feel guilty toward—yet they are also completely estranged to us, inaccessible. As they stalk us, we want to pacify them; however, we know that they are possessed by powers we cannot grasp.

Similarly, stalking monsters transgress additional fundamental boundaries that we rely on, blurring distinctions that are crucial to our ability to make sense of reality. "Living dead," they are both dead and alive, as well as neither. They are human and inhuman; victims and predators; sufferers and aggressors. They are independent—but also "shadow images" of their creators and inseparable from them. As they stalk us, they are both there and not there, present and absent. They undermine the basic distinction between past, present, and future by always already being there. Their repeated reappearances create both the feeling of multitude "visits" and that of perpetual presence. The repetitive returns also constitute a sense of circular time that unites the monster and its target in a closed, seemingly eternal, unbreakable cycle. Yet the target also feels time in a very linear sense: time is running out, and every moment the stalking monster seems to be ever closer.

These stalking monsters are impossible by any human standard, yet many of us experience them as very much in our pursuit. They invade our privacy, disregard our will and free choice, deny our right to self-determination and undermine us. They jeopardize our freedom, individuality, and autonomy and change us despite ourselves. They blur every distinction we rely on, confusing all the familiar categories that make up our world. They threaten to suffocate us, to devour us. The chilling paralysis caused by the stalking monster is the deep significance of its monstrosity.

PRELUDE: ANTISTALKING VERSUS ANTIMONSTERS LEGISLATION

ANTIMONSTERS LEGISLATION

The first antistalking statute was legislated in California in 1990, after the murder of actress Rebecca Schaeffer by a fan who was presented by the media as a "Travis-Hinckley"/ "Travis-Michael" character, that is, a "serial-killer type." A great number of press items and law review articles describing the legislation of California's antistalking law associated it with *Fatal Attraction*. Similar "Anti Travis/Michael/Alex Laws" were quickly legislated in all states. When, in January 30, 1992, State Representative Dianne Byrum introduced the bill that eventually became Michigan's stalking law, she explained her motivation to the press in the following manner:

> In recent years, the most sensational stalking cases have involved celebrities... Rebecca Schaeffer was brutally killed by a man who stalked her across the country.
>
> But the usual stalking victim is an average woman who is terrorized by a vengeful ex-husband or boyfriend, and in some cases a man who is pursued by a woman with a "fatal attraction."

The association of antistalking legislation with *Fatal Attraction* became so strong that in the following years antistalking laws were sometimes referred to as "Fatal Attraction laws."

California's legislation was intended to protect the public from the threat allegedly posed by this "profile" of stalkers, that is, from stalking monsters. No attempt was made to investigate and analyze the *real* social phenomenon of stalking. Addressing monstrous images rather than social reality, the legislature did not adequately conceptualize the prohibited behavior and the "panicky" drafting rendered an imperfect law that is almost inapplicable to most situations of stalking. Most states followed suit and adopted California's formulation. Some legal scholarly literature added insult to injury by explicitly associating the prohibited behavior with the cultural images of stalkers.

AntiStalking Legislation

Statutes are legislated to prohibit and prevent well-specified, damaging conduct. They cannot and should not attempt to prohibit types of people (or creatures). They are inadequate to cope with monsters, nor should they try to. What laws must do is define, in great precision, which concrete stalking actions are not legitimate; they must distinguish such actions carefully from socially acceptable ones. Based on the experiences of women and men who felt damaged and injured by human stalking, I suggest that the legal prohibition of stalking should contain three components:

1. *A course of conduct directed at the targeted person.* The course of conduct may involve repeated or continual unwelcome following, lying in wait, surveillance, trespassing, peeping, physical proximity, harassment, communication, vandalism, or threatening. It must be defined as including only behaviors that are not a part of the stalker's legitimate lifestyle, or part of his or her professional and/or lawful practice;
2. *A specific intent.* This intent may be one to establish, reestablish, maintain, or reinforce a nonconsensual, personal relationship with the targeted person; or, with no lawful justification, to control the targeted person, or to punish him or her, or to prevent him or her from creating, pursuing, or continuing a relationship with another person, or to severely frighten or terrorize the targeted person, or to undermine her or his sense of personal security, or to severely harm him or her bodily or mentally;
3. *The stalker's actual or normative knowledge, that is, his or her awareness of the likely consequences of his or her behavior.* The law may require that the stalker knew, or should have known, that the ensuing course of conduct was sufficiently severe or pervasive to significantly alter the targeted person's conditions of life and to create for her or him a hostile, abusive, or personally insecure environment.

Such legislation offers protection from "regular" stalking, which is usually performed on women by controlling partners or ex-partners. It also prohibits stalking perpetrated by serial killers as prelude to their murders. It does not address stalking monsters, monstrosity, and deep-seated supernatural anxiety.

SURVIVING STALKING MONSTERS

Laws must address real-life people who perform such stalking. Enforcement agencies must detain such individuals and protect us from their stalking and its damaging effects. But laws must not fool us to believe that they can shield us from or cure us of the paralyzing anxiety that stalking monsters sometime instill in us. This anxiety can only be addressed by unpacking sentiments of intimacy, identification, guilt, longing, or supernatural bonding we may harbor toward ghosts that stalk us in the depth of our souls. This anxiety can only be cured by overcoming the overwhelming fear that evil, pure evil, lurks inside us manifesting itself as our murderous Hydes. Symptoms of guilt and insecurity, which breed our stalking monsters, can only be treated by far more delicate tools than the law.

NOTES

1. This chapter relies on the research published in Ôrît Kāmîr's book *Every Breath You Take: Stalking Narratives and the Law* (Ann Arbor, MI: Michigan University Press, 1991). For a full discussion of stories of stalking, references, and legal analysis, see *Every Breath You Take*.
2. Mary Shelley, *Frankenstein, or The Modern Prometheus* (London: Penguin, 1817/1992).
3. Shelley, *Frankenstein*, 73.
4. Shelley, *Frankenstein*, 193.
5. Shelley, *Frankenstein*, 138–139.
6. Shelley, *Frankenstein*, 212.
7. Shelley, *Frankenstein*, 195–196.
8. Shelley, *Frankenstein*, 212.
9. Herb Goldberg, *The New Male: From Macho to Sensitive But Still All Male* (New York: Signet, 1975/1979), 5.
10. Ray Raphael, *The Men from the Boys: Rites of Passage in Male America* (Lincoln: University of Nebraska Press, 1988), 146–147.
11. Jay Martin, *Who Am I This Time?: Uncovering the Fictive Personality* (New York: W.W. Norton & Co,. 1988), 46.
12. Jimmy Breslin and Dick Schaap, *44* (New York: The Viking Press, 1978), 143.
13. Breslin and Schaap, *.44*, 143.
14. Eric W. Hickey, *Serial Murderers and Their Victims* (Pacific Grove, CA: Brooks/Cole Publishing Company, 1991), 172.
15. Hickey, *Serial Murderers and Their Victims*, 172.
16. Peter Van Gelder, *That's Hollywood: A Behind the Scenes Look at 60 of the Greatest Films of All Times* (New York: Harper Perennial, 1990), 92.
17. Susan Faludi, *Backlash* (New York: Doubleday, 1991), 113; Gelder, *That's Hollywood*, 92.
18. Faludi, *Backlash*, 117.

CHAPTER 17

RACE AND SERIAL KILLING IN THE MEDIA: THE CASE OF WAYNE WILLIAMS

CAROLINE JOAN (KAY) S. PICART

INTRODUCTION

In an iconic scene from the 1995 movie *Copycat,* criminal psychologist Helen Hudson (played by Sigourney Weaver) is giving a lecture on serial killing. She first requests all males in the room to stand up, explaining that serial killing is principally a male trait. Then, she asks all African American and Asian males to sit down. Those who remain, the white men, become the iconic image of serial killers. The popular misconception or media fallacy that arises from this cinematic depiction is that all serial killings are done by white males.

This chapter is not about profiling serial killers racially. It is about analyzing media myths in relation to serial killing, against the backdrop of the interaction between popular culture and the criminal justice system.[1] Ultimately, the chapter's moral compass relies upon returning the focus to the victims, who are often forgotten in the media circus that follows highly publicized violent crimes. In specific, this chapter is about analyzing monstrous media myths and remembering the principal lesson from this case: that racially stereotyping serial killers can have dangerous consequences, especially for a group vulnerable to victimization.

Most black serial killers are relatively unknown. Unlike Ted Bundy and Jeffrey Dahmer, Coral Watts, Milton Johnson, Calvin Jackson, and Alton Coleman are not household names.[2] One of the well-known myths, as illustrated in the *Copycat* scene earlier, is that nearly all serial killers are white males; yet, the reality is that one in every five serial killers is black, and nearly 16 percent of all serial killers are female.[3] The main exception to the relative media obscurity of black serial killers is Wayne Williams, a then-23-year-old African American music promoter.

Williams, popularly dubbed by the mainstream media as "America's first black serial killer," was arrested as the killer of over 20 black children, though he was formally charged and convicted of murdering just two of his victims.[4] The case increased the media visibility of serial killers and drew attention to the fact that there are non-white male serial killers and that even children could be targets (as the stereotype was again that adult women were the group most in peril).[5] Technologically, fiber evidence was a key feature of the prosecution's case against Williams; but profiling was a new investigative technique, which also featured prominently in both the arrest and eventual media coverage of Williams's arrest.[6]

The questions this chapter seeks to explore are the following:

1. Generally, why are black serial homicide cases not given as much media coverage as white serial–killer cases?
2. In particular, why was the case of Wayne Williams different from the general media pattern of ignoring black serial killers?
3. What does the case of the Atlanta youth murders tell us about how whites and blacks perceive the media coverage of the trial of Wayne Williams and the criminal justice system?
4. Is there a relation between media narratives concerning race and serial killers, and media coverage of racial hoaxes?

Method

This chapter finds its center of gravity in the focus on media constructions of blackness and whiteness in relation to serial killing, as found in the case of Wayne Williams. The analysis relies principally upon the approaches of two well-established legal theorists and law professors. First, law professor and criminologist Katheryn Russell-Brown focuses on "how the racialized images of black skin have become embedded within the American fabric."[7] Russell-Brown's work focuses both on racialized contemporary popular cultural constructions as spawned by media depictions and on the operation of the criminal justice system.[8] She covers both the historical genealogy and the influence of race in the formation of the criminal justice system, from the slave codes to Jim Crow legislation.[9] Given the limitations, I will not be able to have the depth Russell-Brown has in her book, but I am indebted to her for the clarity of the analytical methods she uses, which are both empirical and qualitative.

The second law professor I rely on is Kimberlé Crenshaw. Acknowledging the complexity and mobility of racial construction in relation to power, Crenshaw proposes an "intersectional" approach: one that takes into account how race, gender, and class, for example, are not isolated indicia of personhood and privilege, but operate as concrete foundations of power, which interact much like variables.[10] Crenshaw's focus is less on whiteness and identity politics than on one of its counterparts, the experiences of violence lived by poor African American women, who are institutionalized through an accretion of norms.[11] Although I look more at constructions of masculinity rather than femininity in this chapter, one thing to draw from Crenshaw is a recognition of the reductive quality of identity politics and its failure to grapple with lived power differentials, institutionalized through legal practices and social norms. Crenshaw argues that the problem with identity politics is that, at a basic level, it "frequently conflates or ignores intragroup differences," which in turn "contributes to tension *among* groups."[12]

However, this chapter also grows out of a prior project, which is crucial to my analysis, and in specific, my focus on the use of monstrous metaphors, and how these monstrous metaphors function rhetorically in media narratives.[13] Drawing from Stanford Lyman's "Gothic sociology,"[14] Cecil Greek, a professor of criminology and criminal justice, and I, a social and political philosopher, used a Gothic criminological approach to analyze how Gothic metaphors and imagery rhetorically work to describe crime, as depicted by the media.[15] Yet the objective was less to show that media myths are simply "fiction."[16] Rather, our focus was on the complex interaction between the "fact" of public policy and the "fiction" of media depictions that constitutes lived reality, such that one realm cannot be absolutely demarcated from the other.[17] This is not to say that there is no such thing as "fact," or that "fact" and "fiction" are the same thing; rather, it is to point out that fact and fiction do not form a simple binary, especially in media depictions.

To some extent, it is precisely the dynamic that contributes to the complex unfolding of the story of the Atlanta youth murders, in so far as the "Monster" of the narrative, as told by the prosecution and the media, was a fair-skinned black man who identified so much with whites that he hated his own race and remorselessly killed off those whom he deemed unworthy of life. This narrative exploded into widely varying reactions from predominantly white and black communities.

THE ABSENCE OF BLACK MALE SERIAL KILLERS IN THE MEDIA

EXAMPLES OF BLACK MALE SERIAL KILLERS

While they are not the majority of serial murderers, there are black male serial killers. Eric N. Hickey,[18] a criminologist, did a recent study, identifying black male serial killers to comprise about 23 percent of the serial murderer population, while white males occupy 72 percent of the population.[19] To name a few recent examples of black male serial killers, Henry Louis Wallace raped and strangled at least nine African American women from 1993 until his capture in 1996 (though he confessed, to his psychiatrist, to raping between 35 and 100).[20] Maury Travis was apprehended in 2002 and subsequently hanged himself in his jail cell; Travis had built a secret torture chamber in his basement, where the police found bondage equipment, videotapes recording his rape and torture sessions, and clippings covering police investigations of his murdered victims (most of whom were prostitutes and crack addicts).[21] Derrick Todd Lee, arrested in 2003, was convicted of killing seven women by strangulation.[22] More recently, Anthony Sowell, a convicted sex offender, was charged with killing 11 black women in Detroit in 2010.[23]

What is puzzling is why the mainstream media, in general, does not pay as close attention to these stories, as they do to white male serial killers. One could argue that these men have not killed as many as Ted Bundy (20-plus victims)[24] or John Wayne Gacy (33).[25] But there are other white male serial killers, with a comparable victim body count who have been more thoroughly covered, such as David Berkowitz (6)[26] and Ed Kemper (9).[27] One could also conjecture that it is because these lesser known serial killers were neither as violent nor as savage in their attacks. Yet Coral Watts/the Detroit "Sunday Morning Slasher," a sexually motivated serial killer whose exploits made him "comparable to Ted Bundy" remains relatively unknown.[28]

THE "MARKETABILITY" OF STORIES ABOUT BLACK SERIAL KILLERS

Philip Jenkins, a criminologist who has done extensive work on serial killers, poses two compelling reasons why there is less coverage of black serial killers. First, Jenkins shrewdly points to publishers' attitudes regarding how "newsworthy" or "saleable" the story will be.[29] Precisely because the popular perception is that psychopathic serial killers are white, there is a prevailing assumption that books on black serial killers will be relegated to the "Black Studies" sections of bookstores and never have a mass appeal.[30] To illustrate his point, Jenkins compared the very similar cases of Gary Heidnik and Harrison "Marty" Graham.[31] Both men imprisoned and murdered several victims in their houses in poor urban areas, and the hideous details of both crimes (involving sex slavery) were initially heavily reported upon by the media.[32] Heidnik achieved notoriety: he is the subject of a book-length study;[33] in 1991, he was interviewed on *60 Minutes;* his profile was partially used to create the *Silence of the Lambs*'s Buffalo Bill, who trapped women in his basement.[34] By contrast, save for some coverage in Philadelphia, Graham sunk into obscurity.[35] The only difference between the two men: Heidnik is white; Graham is black.[36]

THE RACE AND CLASS OF THE VICTIMS

Second, Jenkins points to a well-known phenomenon among criminologists, social scientists, and lawyers, among others. If the victims the serial killer chooses are poor and black, their deaths are less likely to be seen by law enforcement, as part of a serial-killer pattern.[37] For example, Albert Fish, a white man who predatorily molested and killed black children in Washington, D.C. and New York from 1910 to 1935 remained at large for a quarter of a century because of his victim choice.[38] In his final confession, he stated that the police simply did not care about poor, "colored" children and were not as vigilant when they died or disappeared.[39] Significantly, Fish got caught only when he murdered the child of his white, middle-class neighbors.[40] The *Fish* case illustrates the important interactions between race and class (i.e., that race could not be isolated from class, in terms of Fish's choice of victims) and shows the analytic power of Crenshaw's intersectional approach.

Along a parallel track, the Baldus study shows that black defendants who kill white victims have a 22 percent chance of getting the death penalty, as opposed to 1 percent for black defendants killing black victims,[41] showing that black deaths caused by black violence are punished less rigorously. Similarly, James W. Clarke arrives at a similar indictment of the criminal justice system, which, in his view, replaced the slaveholders' authority.[42] He states that the "warped criminal justice system" has three destructive and enduring consequences: (1) it granted an "immunity for crimes committed against black victims";[43] (2) it condoned black-on-black violence as a way of settling disputes;[44] and (3) it "contributed directly to disruption, disunity and rising rates of violent crime within the black community and, not incidentally, black families."[45] Jenkins concurs and goes even further, in terms of serial killing and blackness:

> Discriminatory police attitudes go some way toward explaining the low priority attached to African-American murder victims, and this benefits any offender who chooses to pursue minority victims. As homicide is primarily an intra-racial crime, this would mean that African-American serial killers would be far more likely to escape detection. Racial attitudes here are profoundly linked to social stereotypes . . . .[46]

Thus, Jenkins conjectures, if a killer of "moderate intelligence" were to plant money, drugs, or even gang insignia at the scene of the crime, the crime would likely be viewed as simply urban homicide rather than serial killing.[47] Particularly if the means of killing were subtle (such as suffocation), the murderer would probably go undetected for years.[48]

MONSTROUS METAPHORS AND SERIAL-KILLER STEREOTYPES

Convincing as Jenkins's theses are, the Atlanta youth murders are in direct contradiction to the patterns Jenkins outlines. In spite of Wayne Williams's blackness, the story of the Atlanta youth murders produced documentaries, television interviews, fictional films (see Figure 17.1), and numerous books; in 2010, Soledad O'Brien conducted an updated interview with the incarcerated Williams.[49] The victims, whose decomposing bodies were dumped in poor neighborhoods, the woods, or the Chattahoochee River were predominantly poor black children, and the accused was a black man. Using the patterns Jenkins drew, this case should also have eventually been forgotten. But there is something about this case that continues to touch a very raw nerve at the heart of the American psyche.

There is a third reason Jenkins touches on briefly and tentatively. Speaking of why there have been no black *Psycho* films, for example, Jenkins remarked that filmmakers are "anxious to avoid being accused of depicting crude or controversial racial stereotypes";[50] nevertheless, it is curious that in many other areas, the media's depictions of black skin with criminality are

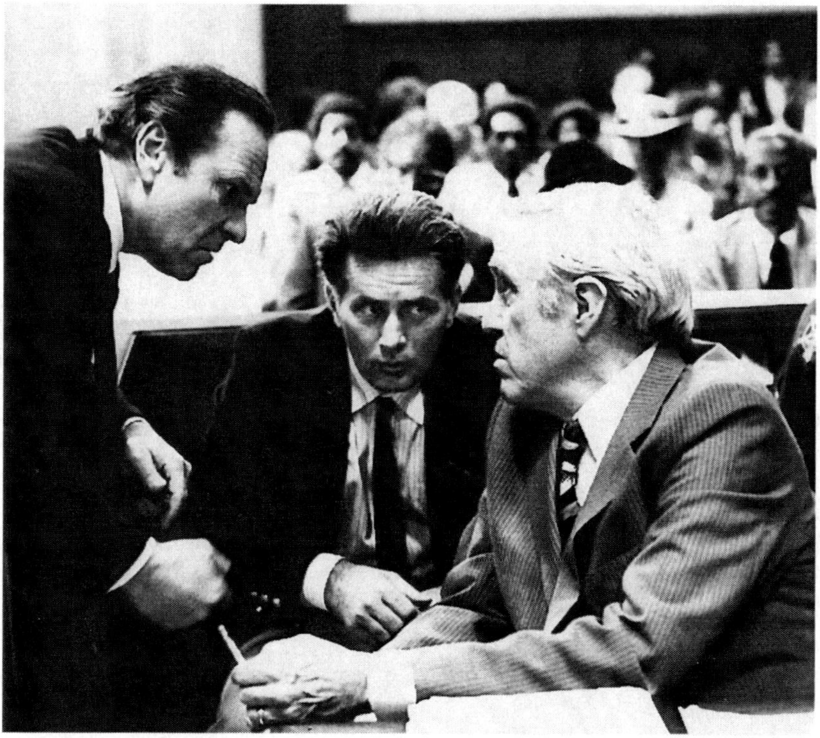

Figure 17.1 Jason Robards (Alvin Binder) plays opposite Martin Sheen (Chet Dettlinger) and Rip Torn (Lewis Slaton) in the television miniseries *The Atlanta Child Murders* (1985), starring Calvin Levels as Wayne Williams. (Courtesy of Finnegan/Pinchuk Productions/Columbia Broadcasting System.)

ubiquitous. While I think this thesis may be simplistic, there is a heuristic value to tracking or mapping the rhetorical framing of how the "Atlanta monster" was detected and convicted, and from whose point of view these narratives were constructed. Thus, I analyze metaphors of monstrosity that abound, in relation to the narrative of the Atlanta youth murders. That is, since the stories concerning Williams either depict him as a psychopath or another victim diverge so strikingly, it is important to track how such wildly different interpretations of the "monstrous" emerge. Finally, applying Russell-Brown and Crenshaw's methods, the chapter will track how race, class, gender, and sexuality are connected in the vastly different white and black narratives that emerge concerning Williams, in retrospect. The value of this exercise to me is less about taking sides, than simply documenting both points of views and grounding them rhetorically, in order to reveal what lies underneath the monstrous metaphors. To do so, I analyze the logic behind the narratives concerning race, monstrous metaphors, and the criminal justice system.

The Case of the Atlanta Youth Murders: General Facts

For 22 months, from the summer of 1979 to the spring of 1981, Atlanta residents lived in increasing fear and outrage as 30 victims, mostly poor black children (28 males and 2 females), were killed. The ages of the victims ranged from 7 to 28, and most were youths of a similar build; they were all black. Some of the victims were shot or strangled; others were stabbed, bludgeoned, or suffocated.[51]

Though Atlanta authorities were initially reluctant to believe these deaths were linked, partly because of the activism of the mothers of the missing or dead children, they eventually conceded that perhaps these deaths were part of a pattern, and a special task force was formed.[52] Because all the victims were black, some speculated that this was part of a white supremacist plot to systematically kill all black children.[53] Others conjectured that the culprits were Satan worshipers, blood cultists, or even copycat murderers.[54] The Ku Klux Klan were placed under surveillance, but there were no clear links that could be established between the KKK and the increasing deaths.[55] Bernard Headley paints a clear picture of the atmosphere of fear that suffused the city.

> Some believed, for instance, that the murders were the handiwork of white supremacist groups like the Ku Klux Klan. Others held that an agency of the federal government was carrying out the killings. Or that one government agency, like the FBI, had been in conspiracy with another—say, the Central Intelligence Agency (CIA) or the Atlanta-based Centers for Disease Control (CDC)—to commit mass murder. Or worst of all, the FBI and CIA were in diabolical cahoots with the Klan to murder black male children, whose bodies the CIA needed for penile experimentation . . . .[56]

As the tension mounted, Atlanta became a city under siege. In a startling newscast, the mayor offered $150,000 reward money, stacked high invitingly, for tips leading to the trial.[57] Boxing legend Muhammad Ali donated $400,000.[58] Sammy Davis Jr. and Frank Sinatra raised more money through a benefit concert.[59] Then-President Ronald Reagan appointed then-Vice President George Bush Sr. to coordinate efforts.[60] As the turmoil rose, Atlanta's convention dollars sank.[61]

It was at this point, when nude bodies began showing up at the Chattahoochee River (as if in response to news reports that police were gathering trace fiber evidence from the bodies of the victims) that the police conducted a three-week stakeout of bridges over the river.[62] On May 22, 1981, shortly before 3 A.M., Robert Campbell, Atlanta police recruit, was approximately eight feet from the water under the James Jackson Parkway Bridge when he heard a "loud splash." In Campbell's testimony, as narrated by Jack Mallard (the prosecutor), Campbell, the former lifeguard, accustomed to hearing the sound of human bodies hitting the water, said that the "splash" he heard sounded different from the sound of beavers diving in. He used a flashlight to follow the ripples in the river when he looked up at the bridge and saw car lights come on "right there above where the splash originated."[63] Campbell called Freddie Jacobs, another Atlanta police recruit, who was also on stakeout in the bushes above the rail. Jacobs testified that he saw a station wagon close to the rail, as it came across the bridge from a parked position very slowly. After crossing the bridge, the vehicle turned around and came across the bridge; patrolman Carl Holden and FBI agent Gregg Gilliland stopped the station wagon at I-285.[64] When Wayne Williams, the driver, stepped out of the car, Williams inquired into what "this [was] all about."[65] When Gilliland responded that he couldn't tell Williams at this time, Williams remarked, "I know this must be about those boys."[66]

According to FBI records, Williams then "voluntarily consented" to a routine search of his station wagon.[67] According to patrolman Holden, when he was interviewed by Soledad O'Brien during a recent CNN interview,[68] a flashlight, a pair of dirty gloves, and a nylon cord were on the front passenger seat. In the same documentary, Williams vehemently denied that there had been a nylon cord, and said that if there had been, it would have shown up later. According to Headley, there were also a knapsack of men's clothing, a large open bag of women's clothing, and a white bedspread with a black and green design; in addition, the car was a "mess" because it looked like it had been used to "transfer animals."[69] Williams admitted that his parents' 14-year-old German Shepherd had been in the car a number of times.

Despite the disagreements, the accounts concur that Wayne Williams was detained for about an hour and a half, as he was questioned about why he was on the bridge at that hour.[70] Wayne's story, at that time, was that because he was a musical talent scout, he had an early appointment with a woman called Cheryl Johnson; he claimed he was simply trying to check out the neighborhood to find her address, purportedly at the Spanish Trace Apartments in Smyrna.[71] Unfortunately, no such woman ever turned up, despite the intense media coverage of Williams's activities before he was officially charged.[72]

Though there was not enough evidence to hold or charge Williams at that time, word leaked to the press.[73] The *New York Post* went straight for the racial button with the headline: "Atlanta Monster Seized; Police Nab Black Suspect."[74] A three-week media circus ensued, which Williams partially helped generate by handing reporters a five-page resume of himself during a "news conference" he held at his parent's home;[75] Williams also liked leading the police who were tailing him on 80-mph wild goose chases down one-way streets.[76]

On June 21, 1981, Wayne Williams was arrested for the murder of Nathaniel Cater.[77] Eventually, Williams was indicted for the murders of Jimmy Payne and Nathaniel Cater.[78] The forensic fiber evidence pointed to a link between Williams and ten of the homicides.[79] Judge Clarence Cooper ruled the evidence admissible.[80] A jury of eight blacks and four whites found Williams guilty of the two murders, and the judge sentenced Williams to two consecutive life sentences.[81] On March 1, 1982, two days after Williams's guilty verdict, law enforcement officials declared, via a "preponderance of incriminating forensic evidence," that Wayne Williams was responsible for murdering Alfred Evans (13); Yusef Bell (9); Eric Middlebrooks (14); Christopher Richardson (12); Aaron Wyche (10); Anthony Carter (9); Earl Terrell (10); Clifford Jones (12); Charles Stephens (10); Aaron Jackson (9); Lubie Geter (14); Terry Pue (15); Patrick Baltazar (12); Curtis Walker (13); Joseph "Jo-Jo" Bell (15); Timothy Hill (13); Eddie Duncan (21); Larry Rogers (20); Michael McIntosh (23); John Porter (28); William Barrett (17), Jimmy Payne (21); Nathaniel Cater (27).[82]

ANALYZING METAPHORS OF MONSTROSITY

MONSTROUS METAPHORS IN THE PROSECUTION'S PROFILE

Profiling as a New Investigative Tool

The prosecution's fiber evidence, then a relatively new forensic technique, was and continues to be much touted as circumstantially airtight by those who believe Wayne Williams to be the Atlanta youth murderer. Conversely, detractors impugned and continued to reject the evidence, especially the fibers derived from bodies in the river, as open to too much contamination to be credible. Yet what lies underneath the disagreement regarding the credibility of the fiber evidence is something more fundamental and can be found in the monstrous metaphors that lurk in what appear as purely rational discourses.

At the height of the crisis, the "big city super-cops," and a new breed of crimefighters, profilers, were called in to assist the Atlanta police.[83] The Atlanta youth murder investigation was the "first major test" for profiling.[84] The profile they produced was that the killer not only had to be intelligent but also black, because he could move around comfortably in these neighborhoods and get these children into dangerous circumstances without detecting attention.[85] He was a con-man (someone charismatic, who inspired trust in his victims), and who probably had an obsession with the police and police work and was media-savvy (as the killer seemed to be responding to leaks about the fiber evidence the police were collecting by throwing the nude bodies of the victims into the river, to wash away any fiber evidence).[86]

Table 17.1 The FBI Theoretical Profile Compared with Wayne Williams' Actual Profile

Profile	Wayne Williams
Intelligent but with unfulfilled dreams	Virtual child prodigy (ran an amateur radio station); dropped out of Georgia State University
Tried to impersonate the police	Arrested for impersonating police when he was 18
Prone to exaggerations	Resume filled with exaggerations
Prone to deception	Failed polygraph testa
News-savvy; kept close watch on police	Had police scanners in his car, which he used to take photos of fires during the overnight beat for a local news organization
Could lure poor street-wise kids	Posted ads for auditions to aspiring young musicians or dancers, aged 11–21, all over the Atlanta housing project, without any financial benefit to himself

Source: Paraphrased from *American Justice—The Atlanta Child Murders*. (A&E Television Networks, 2000/2001.)

After Williams was apprehended at the bridge, the police began collecting information on the self-proclaimed music promoter and freelance photographer. They found a large degree of convergence between the profile of the unknown killer and Williams. Table 17.1 reveals a tabulated summary of the convergences between the profile and Williams's biography.

A Black Man Who Hated Blackness

Yet the profile, to be persuasive enough to make the circumstantial evidence compelling and to convince a predominantly black jury of Williams's guilt, needed one thing: a motive. To be credible, such a motive would have to be powerful enough to rhetorically conjure the most hideous of monsters. The profilers predicted a black man filled with an intense loathing for poor members of his own race; a man who was "racist with his own kind" and out to "terminate them."[87] And indeed, despite Williams's vehement denials, there appear to be several sources that independently corroborate Williams's contempt for poor, black kids, whom he saw as "dragging down his race."[88] For example, Bernard Headley, a professor of criminology and criminal justice, extensively documented some of the corroborating evidence.

> Wayne often expressed negative feelings toward blacks; he frequently did so to the white emergency workers around whom he freelanced. He seemed "resentful of being black," recalled one white police officer. White ambulance driver Bobby Toland said "it was common knowledge that Wayne was not crazy about the black race." Another emergency worker said Wayne often would portray black people as a "sorry lot—the way they lived, the way they acted, leeching off the government" . . . .
>
> Once when the entire nation seemed genuinely affected by the mysterious youth slayings and disappearances, an associate of Wayne's recalled him "putting down the idea" of people raising money for victims' families. Wade Marcus would remember mentioning to Wayne in January or February 1981 that he was considering sending money to assist in the investigation of the Atlanta murders. Wayne, Marcus recalled, told him not to waste his money because the kids were "just prostitutes hanging around all night long" . . . .[89]

"Drop Shots"

Additionally, the profilers predicted that given the psychopathic and narcissistic qualities of the killer, Williams would most likely crack after extensive cross-examination.[90] After two days of intense cross-examination, Williams exploded, calling the police "goons" and the prosecutor a "fool."[91] That sudden change in character, from composed to combative, seemed to be a decisive factor in the jury's belief that Williams was guilty; it was as if underneath a civil and "normal" exterior, a creature of anger and unnatural appetites had lurked, and been unmasked, to the shock and horror of the principally black jury.

Furthermore, Jack Mallard, the prosecutor, picked up on a derogatory term Williams had used in relation to Ken Kimbro and his friend, young black males who lived in the projects (like the other street kids Williams had referred to in his "June 4 News Conference").[92] Mallard asked if the term referred to people who live in the projects; Williams denied that and transferred the epithet to Mallard, calling him a "drop shot."[93] Mallard did not know the meaning of the term until a few years later, when Assistant Prosecutor Chuck Clay of Cobb County came across the genealogy of the term.[94] Quoting *The Story of Georgia and The Georgia People,* Williams cited the definition:

> A large plantation was a little kingdom. The overseer was in charge, a black driver was under him, there were hoe-hands, plowmen, quartermasters, cooks, gardeners, blacksmiths, carpenters, shoe-makers, a midwife, nurses, dairy maids, spinners, weavers, seamstresses, chicken-and-turkey raisers, and even a gang of little negroes, called the "drop-shot gang," who carried water and food to the hands in the field.[95]

Despite the fact that the true meaning of the term did not emerge until later, there was a striking resonance between the prosecution's profile of Williams as the killer and the derogatory meaning of the term. "Drop shots" were the "little negroes" at the bottom of rung on the plantation, who were only worthy of carrying water to those even lower than themselves in the hierarchy: the field hands.[96]

Men Who Eat Their Own

Thus, the prosecution painted the monstrous image of a man who hated the color of his own skin so much that he killed others who reminded him of his own self-loathing.[97] District Attorney Lewis Slaton did the closing arguments: he portrayed Williams as "doing away with inferiors as Attila the Hun, Adolf Hitler, Idi Amin from Uganda . . . ."[98] For the most part, it is this monstrous picture that is accepted by most whites, and has entered criminology textbooks and the mainstream culture.

METAPHORS OF MONSTROSITY IN CRITIQUES OF THE TRIAL

The Legal Lie of the One Drop Rule

James Baldwin, a well-known African American author and civil rights activist, responded to the prosecution's profile of both Williams and his victims, with eloquent fury:

> The imagination is poorly equipped to deal with this action because self-hatred is so common, and takes so many forms . . . [G]iven the bottom-line realities of life in these so ambiguously United States, the missing, menaced, murdered children were menaced by color and locality: they were—visibly Black, which, in this Republic, is a kind of doom, and actually poor—which condition elicits from the land of opportunity and the work ethic a judgment as merciless as it is defensive.[99]

Baldwin recounted that "half-breeds" or "mulattoes," using the "elegant" terms of the "Civilized," were "legal creations"—fair-skinned blacks who were pale enough to "hope to be treated as white."[100] Thus, what was principally monstrous, for Baldwin, was the lie strictly demarcating black blood from white blood: "Underlying the tremendous unwillingness to believe that a Black person could be murdering Black children was the specifically Southern knowledge and experience of how much Black blood is in White veins—and how much White blood is in black veins."[101]

In addition, to Baldwin, the black survival strategy of "passing" became appropriated as a (white) profiling tool to trap a murderer "dark enough to pass unnoticed in Black neighborhoods."[102] That is, instead of a fair-skinned black person passing as white in an environment dominated by privileged whites, the picture the profile painted, which the mainstream media adopted, was of a monstrous fair-skinned black man passing as a normal black man in poor black neighborhoods. To Baldwin, that was a monstrous appropriation of a black survival strategy.

The Criminal Justice System as Juggernaut

The next monstrous metaphor that lurks in Baldwin's book is that of a system that like a juggernaut, levels inconsistencies in order to maintain its self-perpetuating hierarchy. In conjunction with this metaphor of the system-as-monstrous, the view that Williams was simply a scapegoat for authorities under intense pressure is a common one,[103] as was the peculiarly Southern knowledge that "Atlanta policemen had to join the Ku Klux Klan if they ever hoped to become accepted members of the force."[104]

Indeed, there seems to be evidence that Lubie Geter, one of the victims, was killed by a Klansman, Sanders.[105] In addition, a witness claimed that he saw another victim, Clifford Jones, being sexually tortured and strangled by a white man, Jamie Brooks, who was later seen in a hooded robe, carrying something "heavy wrapped in plastic," and who reportedly walked to a further dumpster to drop off the heavy load.[106] Unfortunately, the witness, Freddie Cosby, was not deemed credible because he was mentally retarded.[107]

Williams as Another Victim

The results from years of fruitless appeals have led,[108] until possibly recently, many to view Williams as simply another victim, alongside the murdered Atlanta youths, especially Clifford Jones, whose death, like Emmett Till, raised the hue and cry. "Jones, like Emmett Till, in 1955 . . . was an out-of-state visitor from . . . the North. Had he been a 'Mississippi boy,' his bones might yet be irrecoverable at the bottom of the river . . . ."[109] Baldwin's reference to Emmett Till is another civil rights–related battle cry. This allusion becomes even more potent because it juxtaposes images of the mutilated body of a young boy, whose image is burnt into public memory, alongside the numerous, violated bodies of the Atlanta youth murder victims. If the violence inflicted on Emmett Till's body could stoke such national indignation, Baldwin's juxtaposition seemed to imply, how much more righteous anger could the virtual Holocaust of discarded bodies of Atlanta youth murder victims awaken?

The Monstrous Within

Yet Baldwin's ultimate metaphor of monstrosity is less something "out there" such as a racist criminal justice system. For Baldwin, the most ghastly of monstrosities is not some external order or superhumanly evil person. That ultimate metaphor of monstrosity resides within, complicit with an unjust and racist order.

> The author of a crime is what he is—he knows it, can make no more demands, nor is anything more demanded of him. But he who collaborates is doomed, bound forever in that unimaginable and yet very common condition which we weakly suggest as *Hell*. In that condition, and every American should know it, one can never again summon breath to cry *let my people go*![110]

THE UNIQUENESS OF THE MEDIA COVERAGE OF THE ATLANTA YOUTH MURDERS

To this day, Williams's conviction as the Atlanta youth serial murderer remains controversial and continues to generate a steady stream of updated documentaries. Part of the rhetorical uniqueness of the case is tied up with the sheer proliferation of Gothic tropes used in conjunction with its coverage. For example, the prosecution used another monstrous metaphor I did not discuss: that of being a homosexual pedophile. Similarly, the monstrous specter of a KKK plan to start a race war has refused to be dispelled, and remains a persistent feature of the media coverage of this story. Additionally, experts of various sorts either praise or criticize the trilobal fiber evidence and the criminal profile, resulting in either a laudable judgement of justice or of hideous injustice, keeping the case in the national spotlight.

Hypothesizing on why this case received as much media coverage as it did, perhaps Wayne Williams's case became nationally noteworthy because before the profile had been created, there was rampant suspicion that the killer was white; the media thus initially treated it as such. Additionally, probably because the activism of the victims' mothers created such a powerful grassroots movement, the resultant public visibility (combined with the effect on the city's tourist-oriented economy) forced local and federal authorities to respond to their cries for justice. Finally, perhaps the case was as heavily covered because the Atlanta youth serial murders took place in the aspiring "jewel of the south," showcasing the drama of an upwardly mobile black administration pitted against its poor black constituents, in a city where racial tensions were high and the political balance of power could tip.

What is clear is that Atlanta youth murders touched a raw nerve, in relation to race relations, perceptions of the criminal justice system, and rhetorical constructions of monstrosity. And what has been lost in the media parade of monstrous metaphors are the quiet voices of the victims, seven of whose cases remain officially unsolved. In analyzing the monstrous metaphors at work in the sensationalization of the Atlanta youth murders, the moral fulcrum of this chapter has been to help prevent attacks on victims with the same profile that made them easy marks: being poor and black.

LOOKING BEYOND THE ATLANTA YOUTH MURDERS: MEDIA DEPICTIONS OF FACT AND FICTION IN RELATION TO RACE AND SERIAL KILLING

Recent criminological data has begun to document black serial killers. For example, Professor of Criminal Justice Anthony Walsh compiled data on approximately 90 African American serial killers and the time periods and states in which they committed their crimes.[111] Walsh concludes,

> Based on these figures, there were approximately five times more African American serial killers operating in the 1980s than there were from 1945 to 1979. Likewise, the 13-year period between 1990 and the first half of 2004 revealed 32 African American serial killers—an average of about 2.3 per year.[112]

Walsh's figures correspond with Hicks's findings in finding that black serial killers make up about 21.8 percent of his study of black and white serial killers. An earlier study by criminologists Michael Newton and Judy Ann Newton in 1991 came up with a 16 percent estimate of the number of blacks in the serial murderer category.[113]

While it is clear that white males remain the majority in the serial murderer category, recent studies have begun to document the existence of black male serial killers. The value of studies, such as these, is to demystify racist cultural myths, one of which is the view that serial killers are "white and brilliant, thus alluding that Black aren't smart enough to carry out organized murder."[114] Such a myth has a long history, starting with Samuel Morton's *Crania Americana*.[115] In brief, Morton claimed that there was a direct correlation between intelligence and the size of the skull/brain.[116] He also claimed a correlation between intelligence and race, with whites at the top of the pyramid and blacks at the bottom.[117] The derogatory racist implication is that only white males are "brilliant" enough to plan and commit serial murders. However, legal scholars and historians, such as Russell-Brown[118] and Schiebinger,[119] have also demystified this cultural fallacy concerning intelligence dressed in a pseudoscientific veneer.

The history of the negative stereotyping of African Americans and the resultant harmful social, legal, and political consequences of these cultural myths are well documented. Serial killing, a particularly violent form of homicide, is one area where stereotypes imply a different type of stereotyping. Though criminologist Walsh attributes this relative media reluctance to cover stories of black serial killers to a liberal fear of being labeled "racist," (which he compares to the situation of untenured assistant professors afraid to publish anything explosive that could get them fired),[120] I believe the situation is more complex than that.

For example, there is a striking affinity between the narrative patterns yielded by the Atlanta youth murders and racial hoaxes, as analyzed by Russell-Brown.

Russell-Brown described a racial hoax as occurring when:

(a) someone fabricates a crime and blames it on another person because of his race or

(b) an actual crime has been committed and the perpetrator falsely blames someone because of his race.[121]

Among other findings, Russell-Brown found that white-on-black hoaxes (where whites blame blacks for real or imagined crimes) are perpetrated based on the myth of the "criminalblackman"—an aberrant individual capable of random acts of violence with "menacing, demonlike details."[122] By contrast, black-on-white racial hoaxes, such as the cases of the Duke lacrosse team and Tawana Brawley (though Brawley has never recanted), usually appeal to a different type of narrative: one bound up with a conspiracy bound up with white privilege or white supremacy.[123]

Similarly, in the Atlanta youth murders, for example, the prosecution's racial profile of Wayne Williams, as a self-hating light-skinned black man who preyed on the poor black kids whom he regarded as society's scum, corresponds with the racial narrative characteristic of white-on-black hoaxes. In other words, it is the narrative of the criminalblackman, writ large. It is this story of the Monstrous Black Man that a mostly white community and the mainstream media propagated, miming the rhetorical patterns of a white-on-black hoax. By contrast, a predominantly black community then believed that the murders of the poor black children were tied up in a KKK conspiracy to kill one black child every month in order to spark a race war. This rhetorical pattern corresponds with the general narrative form of black-on-white hoaxes.

In other words, the mainstream media coverage of the Atlanta youth murders constructed the story, not as a typical/normal "black-on-black" assault, but as something more akin to a "white-on-black" assault, writ Monstrously large. As journalist and author John Perazzo writes regarding popular media representations, "*white*-on-black transgressions are testaments to racism, while *black*-on-black offenses are meaningless."[124] This differed radically from the black community's reaction to the media coverage.

Furthermore, in keeping with a Gothic criminological approach, the spheres of "fact" and "fiction" in relation to race and the criminal justice system, as reported in the media, are complexly intertwined. Empirically, there is a rough correlation between the proportion of whites to blacks in Newton and Newton's,[125] Walsh's[126], and Hickey's[127] studies of serial murderers (between 16 and 23 percent black and 72 percent white) and Russell-Brown's findings on the proportions of the reported cases of white-on-black hoaxes (20 percent) and black-on-white hoaxes (67 percent).[128] That is, the racial breakdown of the serial killer population, based on the factual accounts gathered by criminologists, roughly corresponds with Russell-Brown's racial breakdown of hoaxes (thus "fictional" accounts). What this simply shows, in my view, is the media's choices regarding what "deserves" coverage, reinforcing racial stereotypes, as well as reflecting their influence.

Though these statistical racial correspondences may be coincidental, what is clear is that cultural myths (often simplistically labeled "false") and "factual reality" (often simplistically characterized as "truth") are not related in a simple oppositional binary. Often, it is the media that shapes how perceptions of "truth" and "lie" interrelate, and popular perceptions, in turn, influence public policy, which flow back to affect trends in media representations and cultural stereotypes.[129] As Raymond Surette, professor of criminal justice and legal studies, noted, "We live in a multimedia web that has resulted in the common practice of media content looping... Real events migrate to entertainment media and the public sees fictional events as real. The... prevalence of *Frankensteinian* as an adjective... and the trope of being a bloodsucking vampire as a political description are all examples of content looping in the multimedia web and the associated ascension of the popular version of Gothic criminology."[130]

The racial dimension of such narratives is particularly crucial to document because as journalist Jared Taylor states,

> In our multiracial society, race lurks just below the surface of much that is not explicitly racial. Newspaper stories about other things—housing patterns, local elections, crime, antipoverty programs, law-school admissions, mortgage lending, employment rates—are also, sometimes only by implication, about race. When race is not in the foreground of American life, it does not usually take much searching to find it in the background.[131]

And given that one of the cultural myths is that black-on-black violence does not matter, and its correspondent factual reality is that poor black youths are the most vulnerable to violent crime, it is important to address the popular cultural racial (mis)perceptions about serial murderers. The popular stereotype of the serial killer being a white male is, as criminologist Jenkins argues, as "inaccurate and as pernicious as any of the more familiar racial slurs."[132] Perhaps ultimately destroying this simplistic stereotype may help prevent the often invisible perpetration of violence against these types of victims. As Walsh soberly conjectures, "one wonders how many additional victims have been lost because law enforcement succumbed to the stereotype and concentrated their efforts on White males."[133] Ultimately, the greatest danger of silencing stories concerning non-white serial killers is, as Jenkins points out, the possibility that "[u]nderestimating minority involvement in serial homicide can thus lead to neglecting the protection of minority individuals and communities who stand in greatest peril of victimization."[134]

Of course, these types of stories must be treated with caution, as they could be sensationalized to further the already harmful stereotype of the "criminalblackman" so prevalent in other media narratives. But that is a risk well worth taking, given what the price of silence demands, of those victims chosen because they are most likely to go unnoticed and forgotten, by both the media and the criminal justice system.

Summary of Findings and Conclusion

In summary, this chapter has explored the following theses, in relation to the questions it posed in the Introduction.

First, generally, black serial homicide cases are not given as much media coverage as white serial killer cases because of three principal reasons: (1) publishers do not think stories about black serial murderers will prove as commercially successful as stories about white male serial killers, so they usually choose not to cover it; for example, even though Gary Heidnik and Marty Graham committed comparable crimes (sexual enslavement and murder in their urban homes) in Philadelphia at roughly the same time, Heidnik achieved media immortality, while Graham is now virtually unknown; (2) if the victims are poor and black and the suspect is also black, the police are less likely to view the case as a serial murder; (3) the media, like untenured professors, are afraid of publishing and perishing, because the conjunction of monstrous metaphors with a black man leave them open to the charge of racism.

Second, in particular, the case of Wayne Williams was different from the general media pattern of ignoring black serial killers partly because of the prevalence and severity of monstrous metaphors in the coverage and reactions to the story, as evidenced in the rhetoric used by the predominantly white prosecution and the predominantly black civil rights community in relation to a mysterious fairer skinned black man. Yet there were other factors as well that contributed to the "newsworthiness" of the story: the initial suspicion that the killings were associated with a KKK-inspired plot to spark a race war; the political activism of the victims' mothers who ignited a grassroots movement; the detrimental effect of the stories on Atlanta's economy; the spectacle of a progressive city with a black mayor and a black police chief pitted against poor black constituents, in a city where racial tensions were rampant and the balance of power was tenuous.

Third, for the most part, whites tended to identify with the prosecution's narrative concerning Wayne Williams, while blacks tended to be skeptical. Both sides engaged in a battle of warring monstrous metaphors. For the prosecution/predominantly white community, Wayne Williams was the same kind of creature as Attila the Hun, Adolf Hitler, and Idi Amin. For the predominantly black civil rights community, the Monsters were the racist criminal justice and legal systems that produced the lies of one drop rule; the "half-breeds" who could hope to be treated as white; and the mentality of complicity with these institutional structures and cultural myths.

Fourth, factual media narratives concerning race and serial killers and media coverage of racial hoaxes seem to intersect in two ways: (1) In this particular case, the mainstream coverage of the prosecution's arguments resembled the narrative pattern of white-on-black hoaxes, focusing on the monstrosity of the criminalblackman; by contrast, the coverage of those opposed to the prosecution rhetorically mimed the narrative pattern of black-on-white hoaxes, emphasizing the monstrosity of white supremacy and/or white privilege. (2) More generally, the proportion of blacks to whites in the male serial killer population as reported by criminologists (20:72) roughly corresponds with the proportion of black-on-white hoaxes compared with white-on-black hoaxes (20:67), as analyzed by Russell-Brown. Thus, the realm of "fact" as reported by criminologists, in some ways, statistically mirrors the "fiction" of hoaxes, and vice versa; this is not to conflate fact with fiction, but to show the complexity of their relationship, especially when refracted through the prism of media depictions, which often reinforce and attest to the strength of racial stereotypes.

Ultimately, this chapter on the media depictions of race and serial killing constitutes one attempt to grapple with the effects of racism and white privilege. Thus, to achieve a more effective engagement with racism and white privilege and their influence on media accounts of what is "real," what is necessary is a structural and political critique that is sensitive to the power of metaphors and the rhetorical construction of reality. To borrow from Robert Jensen, a professor of journalism:

> The fundamental frame for pursuing analyses of issues around race, ethnicity, gender, sexuality and class should not be cultural but political, not individual but structural. Instead of

> talking about diversity in race, class, gender, and sexual orientation, we should critique white supremacy, economic inequality in capitalism, patriarchy and heterosexism. We should talk about systems and structures of power, about ideologies of domination and subordination—and the injuries done to those in subordinate groups, and the benefits and privileges that accrue to those in dominant groups.[135]

Crucial to such an analysis would be a study of how the rhetorics of monstrosity interact with the institutional and political factors that create the matrix of power in which we all partake and participate.

ACKNOWLEDGMENTS

This study was originally awarded the Book Award for a seminar on Race, Law and Justice, taught by Professor Katheryn Russell-Brown in Fall 2010 at the University of Florida Levin College of Law. I am indebted to Professor Russell-Brown for her insightful comments on earlier drafts and generosity with her time. I also wish to thank Professor Michael Seigel for his excellent instruction on Criminal Law, and Professors Lani Guinier and Raymond Fleming for their acute mentorship on Critical Race Theory.

NOTES

1. Criminologists Ronald M. Holmes and Stephen T. Holmes recount a dinner conversation with Tom Harris, the author of *Red Dragon* (1981) and *Silence of the Lambs* (1989). Harris's books were the source of the cinematic myth of Hannibal Lechter as "dark knight" and hyperintelligent savage iconized by Anthony Hopkins's performances in *Silence of the Lambs* (1991) and *Hannibal* (2001). When Ronald's wife and Stephen's mother remarked that they did not read Harris's books because they "scare the hell out of [them]," Harris, smiling over the rim of his wine glass, responded, "They scare the hell out of me, too!" Ronald M. Holmes and Stephen T. Holmes, *Serial Murder,* third ed. (Thousand Oaks, CA: Sage Publications, Inc., 2010), 7, 9.
2. Philip Jenkins, "African-Americans and Serial Homicide," in *Contemporary Perspectives on Serial Murder,* ed. Ronald M. Holmes and Stephen T. Holmes (Thousand Oaks, CA: Sage Publications, Inc., 1998), 17.
3. Eric W. Hickey, *Serial Murderers and Their Victims,* fifth ed. (Florence, KY: Carnegie Learning, 2010), 5.
4. Hickey, *Serial Murderers and Their Victims,* 2.
5. Hickey, *Serial Murderers and Their Victims,* 1–2.
6. Hickey, *Serial Murderers and Their Victims,* 2.
7. Katheryn Russell-Brown, *The Color of Crime,* second ed. (New York: New York University Press, 2008/2009), 3.
8. Russell-Brown, *The Color of Crime,* 3–4.
9. Russell-Brown, *The Color of Crime,* 35–52.
10. Kimberlé Crenshaw, "Mapping the Margins: Intersectionality, Identity Politics, and Violence Against Women of Color," in *Critical Race Theory: The Key Writings That Formed the Movement,* ed. Kimberlé Crenshaw, Neil Gotanda, Gary Peller, and Kendall Thomas (New York: The New Press, 1995), 350.
11. Crenshaw, "Mapping the Margins," 358.
12. Crenshaw, "Mapping the Margins," 357.
13. Caroline Joan (Kay) Picart and Cecil Greek, "Introduction: Toward a Gothic Criminology," in *Monsters In and Among Us* (Madison, NJ: Fairleigh Dickinson University Press, 2007), 11. In *Monsters In and Among Us,* Cecil Greek, a criminologist, and I collaborated on examining the plethora of books and films connecting violence, fear, visualizations of the "monstrous," and Gothic modes of narration in popular culture, academia, and even public policy. Using an interdisciplinary approach, and a variety of essays from invited specialists in film criticism, media studies, and rhetoric, as well as

communication, criminology, and sociology, we analyzed contemporary visualizations of the Gothic and the monstrous in film and media. Contributors included media and film specialists Edward Ingebretsen, Jason Grant McKahan, and Pat Gill; rhetoricians Davis Houck and Thomas Benson; and sociologist-criminologist Raymond Surette. The "media monsters" we chose to focus on were the pedophilic homosexual priest (Ingebretsen's essay); the hypermasculinized rogue cop (Houck and Greek's essays); the masculinized mother (Benson's essay); the drug addict (McKahan's essay); the white-collar criminal (Gill's contribution); the serial killer (Picart and Greek's essay); and the terrorist (Picart and Greek's essay). See Picart and Greek, "Introduction," 5, 13.

14. Stanford M. Lyman, "Rereading Robert E. Park: Toward a Gothic Perspective on Capitalism and Imperialism," in *Explorations: The Age of Enlightenment,* ed. M. W. duQuesnay (Lafayette, LA: University of Southwestern Louisiana Foundation, 1990), 29–108. See generally, Stanford M. Lyman, *The Seven Deadly Sins: Society and Evil* (New York: St. Martin's Press, 1978).
15. See Picart and Greek, "Introduction," 11–12.
16. Picart and Greek, "Introduction," 12. Ultimately, we also found that the class, gender, and sexuality of the serial killer resulted in different Gothic metaphors: Hannibal Lecter, the hyperintelligent, classy white male heterosexual cannibal was associated with the glamorous vampire. By contrast, in the case of Wuornos, reputedly "America's first female serial killer," instead of the powerful and glamorous vampire, we found the pitiful and ugly outcast of the Frankensteinian monster. Wuornos was depicted as white trash eternally in search of companionship and love; tragically, she did everything for the lover who eventually betrayed and abandoned her. Caroline Joan (Kay) Picart and Cecil Greek, "When Women Kill: Undead Imagery in the Cinematic Portrait of Aileen Wuornos," in *Draculas, Vampires & Other Undead Forms: Essays on Gender, Race and Culture,* ed. John Edgar Browning and Caroline Joan (Kay) Picart (Lanham, MD: Scarecrow Press, 2009), 93, 94, 102.
17. Picart and Greek, "When Women Kill," 13–14. In the case of the celebrity of the *Hannibal* films, for example, Surette argued that the media-induced frenzy over the menace of serial killers funneled more funding for the special FBI Behavioral Science Unit featured in *Silence of the Lambs* and fostered crucial criminal justice policy changes, boosting the image of profilers as modern-day heroes. Raymond Surette, "Gothic Criminology and Criminal Justice Policy," in *Monsters In and Among Us,* ed. Caroline Joan (Kay) Picart and Cecil Greek (Madison, NJ: Fairleigh Dickinson University Press, 2007), 220–221.
18. Hickey, *Serial Murderers and Their Victims,* 192.
19. Hickey, *Serial Murderers and Their Victims,* 5.
20. Hickey, *Serial Murderers and Their Victims,* 196–197.
21. Peter Shinkle, "Serial Killer Caught by His Own Internet Footprint," *St. Louis Post-Dispatch,* June 17, 1992, http://www.rense.com/general26/serial.htm.
22. Holmes and Holmes, *Serial Murder,* 45.
23. Paul Lindsay, "Anthony Sowell, Alleged 'Cleveland Strangler': Is Race a Factor in Serial Killer Probe?," *Crimesider,* April 14, 2010, http://www.cbsnews.com/8301-504083_162-20002361-504083.html.
24. Holmes and Holmes, *Serial Murder,* 156–157.
25. Holmes and Holmes, *Serial Murder,* 68.
26. Holmes and Holmes, *Serial Murder,* 96.
27. Holmes and Holmes, *Serial Murder,* 2.
28. Jenkins, "African Americans and Serial Homicide," 17, 25. Of course, one could also point out that some cases, regardless of the race of serial killer, remain of purely regional interest, such as the case of Danny Rolling, the "Gainesville Ripper," whose name does not even appear in Hickey's book. Hickey, *Serial Murderers and Their Victims,* 5. Rolling is briefly mentioned in Holmes and Holmes, *Serial Murder,* 46.
29. Holmes and Holmes, *Serial Murder,* 26–27.
30. Holmes and Holmes, *Serial Murder,* 27.
31. Holmes and Holmes, *Serial Murder,* 27.
32. Holmes and Holmes, *Serial Murder,* 27.
33. Ken Englade, *Cellar of Horror* (New York: St. Martin's Press, 1988).
34. Jenkins, "African Americans and Serial Homicide," 27.

35. Jenkins, "African Americans and Serial Homicide," 27.
36. Jenkins, "African Americans and Serial Homicide," 27.
37. Jenkins, "African Americans and Serial Homicide," 28.
38. Jenkins, "African Americans and Serial Homicide," 28.
39. Jenkins, "African Americans and Serial Homicide," 28.
40. Jenkins, "African Americans and Serial Homicide," 28.
41. McCleskey *v.* Kemp, 481 U.S. 282, 275 (1987). See also Eric Monkkonen, "Racial Factors in New York City Homicides, 1800–1874," in *Ethnicity, Race and Crime: Perspectives Across Time and Place,* ed. Darnell F. Hawkins (Albany, NY: State University Press of New York, 1995), 101, 110–111.
42. James W. Clarke, *The Lineaments of Wrath: Race, Violent Crime and American Culture* (New Brunswick, NJ: Transaction Publishers, 1998), 210. See also Stephan Thernstrom and Abigail Thernstrom, *America in Black and White: One Nation, Indivisible* (New York: Touchstone 1997/1999), 54.
43. Clarke, *The Lineaments of Wrath,* 210.
44. Clarke, *The Lineaments of Wrath,* 210.
45. Clarke, *The Lineaments of Wrath,* 210.
46. Jenkins, "African Americans and Serial Homicide," 28.
47. Jenkins, "African Americans and Serial Homicide," 29.
48. Jenkins, "African Americans and Serial Homicide," 29.
49. "CNN Documentary: The Atlanta Child Murders," *CNN,* June 1, 2010. See also "CNN Viewers: Williams 'guilty' in Atlanta Child Murders," *CNN Justice,* June 11, 2010, http://articles.cnn.com/2010-06-11/justice/atlanta.murders.poll.ireport_1_atlanta-child-murders-two-life-sentences-killings/2?_s=PM:CRIME.
50. Jenkins, "African Americans and Serial Homicide," 24.
51. Hickey, *Serial Murderers and Their Victims,* 192.
52. Hickey, *Serial Murderers and Their Victims,* 192.
53. Hickey, *Serial Murderers and Their Victims,* 192.
54. Hickey, *Serial Murderers and Their Victims,* 192.
55. The hypothesis of a federal cover-up of evidence implicating the KKK because of fear of a race war within the United States is the animating idea of the fictional film, *Echo of Murder. Echo of Murder* (Showtime Entertainment 2001).
56. Bernard Headley, *The Atlanta Youth Murders and the Politics of Race* (Carbondale, IL: Southern Illinois University Press, 1998), 2. The Tuskegee study on syphilis, where black men were used like guinea pigs to study the onset and progression of the disease, while denying them the cure (penicillin), was exposed in July 1972. See Headley, *The Atlanta Youth Murders and the Politics of Race,* 219, n3.
57. Headley, *The Atlanta Youth Murders and the Politics of Race,* 98.
58. Headley, *The Atlanta Youth Murders and the Politics of Race,* 98.
59. Headley, *The Atlanta Youth Murders and the Politics of Race,* 98.
60. Headley, *The Atlanta Youth Murders and the Politics of Race,* 106.
61. Headley, *The Atlanta Youth Murders and the Politics of Race,* 123.
62. Headley, *The Atlanta Youth Murders and the Politics of Race,* 130.
63. Jack Mallard, *The Atlanta Child Murders: The Night Stalker* (Charleston, SC: BookSurge Publishing, 2009), 96.
64. Mallard, *The Atlanta Child Murders,* 97.
65. Headley, *The Atlanta Youth Murders and the Politics of Race,* 132.
66. Headley, *The Atlanta Youth Murders and the Politics of Race,* 132.
67. Headley, *The Atlanta Youth Murders and the Politics of Race,* 132.
68. "CNN Documentary."
69. Headley, *The Atlanta Youth Murders and the Politics of Race,* 132.
70. Headley, *The Atlanta Youth Murders and the Politics of Race,* 132.
71. Headley, *The Atlanta Youth Murders and the Politics of Race,* 147.
72. Headley, *The Atlanta Youth Murders and the Politics of Race,* 132.

73. Headley, *The Atlanta Youth Murders and the Politics of Race,* 149.
74. Headley, *The Atlanta Youth Murders and the Politics of Race,* 149.
75. Headley, *The Atlanta Youth Murders and the Politics of Race,* 150–151.
76. Headley, *The Atlanta Youth Murders and the Politics of Race,* 163.
77. Headley, *The Atlanta Youth Murders and the Politics of Race,* 165.
78. Headley, *The Atlanta Youth Murders and the Politics of Race,* 169.
79. Headley, *The Atlanta Youth Murders and the Politics of Race,* 183–185.
80. Headley, *The Atlanta Youth Murders and the Politics of Race,* 178–179.
81. Headley, *The Atlanta Youth Murders and the Politics of Race,* 197.
82. Headley, *The Atlanta Youth Murders and the Politics of Race,* 197.
83. *A&E: American Justice—The Atlanta Child Murders* (A&E Television Networks 2000/2001).
84. *A&E: American Justice.*
85. *A&E: American Justice.*
86. *A&E: American Justice.*
87. *A&E: American Justice.*
88. *A&E: American Justice.*
89. Headley, *The Atlanta Youth Murders and the Politics of Race,* 141–142.
90. *A&E: American Justice.*
91. *A&E: American Justice.*
92. Mallard, *The Atlanta Child Murders,* 293–294.
93. Mallard, *The Atlanta Child Murders,* 293.
94. Mallard, *The Atlanta Child Murders,* 293.
95. Mallard, *The Atlanta Child Murders,* 294, citing George Gillman Smith, *The Story of Georgia and the Georgia People, 1732 to 1860* (Baltimore, MD: Genealogical Publishing Co., 1901/1968), 350.
96. Mallard, *The Atlanta Child Murders,* 294.
97. *A&E: American Justice.*
98. Mallard, *The Atlanta Child Murders,* 294.
99. James Baldwin, *The Evidence of Things Not Seen* (New York: Henry Holt and Co., LLC, 1985), 6.
100. Baldwin, *The Evidence of Things Not Seen,* 6.
101. Baldwin, *The Evidence of Things Not Seen,* 8.
102. Baldwin, *The Evidence of Things Not Seen,* 8.
103. *A&E: American Justice.*
104. Headley, *The Atlanta Youth Murders and the Politics of Race,* 17.
105. *A&E: American Justice.*
106. Mark Mori, *Wayne Williams and the Atlanta Child Murders,* for *Court TV* (Single Spark Pictures, Inc. 2010).
107. Mori, *Wayne Williams and the Atlanta Child Murders.*
108. Additionally, on September 26, 1990, Williams's new defense team filed a 184-page Amended Petition for writ of habeas corpus. One of the major issues raised was that Williams's counsel was denied access to a secret independent investigation of the Ku Klux Klan in relation to the Atlanta child murders. On July 10, 1998, Superior Court Judge Hal Craig denied the defense petition, effectively ruling that the KKK probe had not yielded any evidence relevant to the outcome of the Williams's trial, and that its exclusion from Williams's trial did not constitute harmful error. See Headley, *The Atlanta Youth Murders and the Politics of Race,* 345, 349.
109. Baldwin, *The Evidence of Things Not Seen,* 40.
110. Baldwin, *The Evidence of Things Not Seen,* 125.
111. Anthony Walsh, "African Americans and Serial Killing in the Media: The Myth and the Reality," *Homicide Studies* 9, no. 4 (2005): 271, 278.
112. Walsh, "African Americans and Serial Killing in the Media: The Myth and the Reality," 271, 278.
113. Michael Newton and Judy Ann Newton, *Racial and Religious Violence in America: A Chronology* (New York: Garland 1991), 40.
114. Carol Chehade, *Big Little White Lies: Our Attempt to White-Out America* (Kearney, NE: Nehmarche Publishing, Inc., 2001/2003), 2.

115. Samuel George Morton, *Crania Americana; or, A Comparative View of the Skulls of Various Aboriginal Nations of North and South America: To which Is Prefixed an Essay on the Varieties of the Human Species* (Philadelphia: J. Dobson, 1839).
116. Morton, *Crania Americana.*
117. Morton, *Crania Americana.*
118. Katheryn Russell-Brown, *Protecting Our Own: Race, Crime and African Americans* (Lanham, MD: Rowman & Littlefield Publishing, 2006), 23–24.
119. Londa Schiebinger, *Nature's Body: Gender in the Making of Modern Science,* second ed. (Piscataway, NJ: Rutgers University Press, 2004), 135.
120. Anthony Walsh, *Race and Crime: A Biosocial Analysis* (Hauppauge, NJ: Nova Science Publishers, Inc. 2004), 42.
121. Russell-Brown, *The Color of Crime,* 100.
122. Russell-Brown, *The Color of Crime,* 107.
123. Russell-Brown, *The Color of Crime,* 111–112.
124. John Perazzo, *The Myths That Divide Us: How Lies Have Poisoned American Race Relations,* second ed. (Briarcliff Manor, NY: World Studies Books, 1999), 49.
125. Newton and Newton, *Racial and Religious Violence in America,* 40.
126. Walsh, *Race and Crime,* 278.
127. Hickey, *Serial Murderers and Their Victims,* 5.
128. Russell-Brown, *The Color of Crime,* 105.
129. Picart and Greek, "Introduction," 11.
130. Surette, "Gothic Criminology and Criminal Justice Policy," 222.
131. Jared Taylor, *Paved with Good Intentions: The Failure of Race Relations in Contemporary America* (New York: Carroll and Graf Publishers, Inc. 1992/1993), 10.
132. Jenkins, "African-Americans and Serial Homicide," 30.
133. Walsh, *Race and Crime,* 287.
134. Jenkins, "African-Americans and Serial Homicide," 30.
135. Robert Jensen, *The Heart of Whiteness: Confronting Race, Racism, and White Privilege* (San Francisco: City Lights Books, 2005), 78.

Section VI

The Biological Monstrous and Gender: The Human-Animal-Machine Divides

CHAPTER 18

"NATURE ABHORS NORMALITY": THEORIES OF THE MONSTROUS FROM ARISTOTLE TO *THE X-FILES* (1993–2002)

KATHLEEN LONG

FOR ALL OF THE DISTANCE BETWEEN MODERN REPRESENTATIONS OF MONSTROSITY and their ancient and medieval precursors, the resonance between these two bodies of material is striking. In the most general terms, the longstanding tension between fundamentally Aristotelian notions of monstrosity as defect or excess and the Augustinian notion of monstrous forms as signs of the power of God (or Nature) still plays out in the combined horror and fascination with which monsters are represented in popular culture. In Aristotle's work, monstrosity is the ground for a discussion of the interplay between individual and familial identities in their narrowest and broadest senses; according to Augustine, monstrosity is the sign of infinite diversity in God's creation (and thus, monstrosity is potentially inherent in each individual, who differs from all others in some way). The Aristotelian and Augustinian versions of the monstrous complement rather than contradict each other, and Augustine's ideas can be seen as a logical extreme of the Aristotelian notion of the monstrous as that which is simply different from the paternal norm.

After Pliny's accounts of monstrous races,[1] the notion that groups of monstrous humans who do not resemble "us" (in this case the Romans, but later this concept is recycled by Europeans colonizing the New World) exist somewhere on the periphery of the civilized world spawns a complex taxonomy of monstrous types that will return incessantly in Western culture. One of these types, the Wild Man, comes to dominate European culture at the end of the Middle Ages, raising the question of human exceptionalism. By the early modern period, the taxonomies of the monstrous are replaced by theorizations of their origins, ranging from theological to teratological explanations. At some point, the inferiority of the monstrous, already suggested in Aristotle and Pliny, becomes moralized, and the monster is presented as threatening and possibly evil. This thread is already present in the representation of the Wild Man (Grendel) in *Beowulf,* and resurfaces in the early modern period in the form of ogres and other cannibals. But the interest in monsters primarily as curiosities dominates this period, and it is only much later that the threat of the monster becomes the primary concern of Western literature. A dichotomy arises at the dawn of the modern era as freaks replace curiosities, as objects of fascination and vampires, werewolves, and zombies haunt our nightmares. Now, we are faced with the attractive vampires of *Twilight* and the self-created monsters of somatechnics, even as various disability rights movements redefine difference as simply that, rather than as some form of monstrosity. At every turn, the fundamental question is one of identity and difference, the extent to which resembling others is essential to acceptance as normal, and what this fairly circular definition of the normal might actually mean.

The TV series *The X-Files* ran from 1993 to 2002, and is considered the iconic series for the 1990s. The premise of the series was that a pair of FBI agents, Fox Mulder, a profiler with a penchant for the supernatural, and Dana Scully, the rational scientist brought on board to debunk Fox's theories, were to investigate cases that defied rational explanation and that thus seemed to invoke the paranormal. That these roles would shift over the course of the seasons seemed natural, given the complex relationship between these two characters. The running storyline of the series was a complex narration about alien abduction; this storyline was frequently punctuated with "one-off" or "monster of the week" episodes.

These monster episodes reference a broad range of knowledge of canonical monsters; for example, several episodes allude to *Beowulf* (the torn-off arm in "The Jersey Devil,"[2] the hoard of bodies in "Detour," 5.4), while others tap into demonology (possession or demonic behavior in "The Walk," 3.7, "Grotesque," 3.14, "Small Potatoes," 4.20, "Elegy," 4.22, "Demons," 4.23, and "Terms of Endearment," 6.7, among others). Almost never did Mulder and Scully solve the mystery; in fact, most frequently either the monster escaped entirely (as in "GenderBender," 1.14, "El Mundo Gira," 4.11, "Detour," 5.4, "Bad Blood," 5.12, and many other episodes), gave itself up (as in "Pusher," 3.17), or was caught by sheer dumb luck (in "The Post-Modern Prometheus," 5.5, which presents itself as a comic-book fantasy). In episodes such as "Hell Money," 3.19, and "El Mundo Gira," the agents' inability to speak another language (Chinese and Spanish, respectively) and their ignorance concerning the culture impede their ability to solve the crimes.

In many of the monster episodes, then, our protagonists come across as "ignorant rubes" (as they are called in "Humbug," 2.20), who are trying to piece together the narration of events before they can even begin to solve the mystery. This aspect of the series is particularly evident in "Bad Blood," where Mulder and Scully each tell a different, very gendered, version of the story, in "El Mundo Gira," where various narrations are revealed to be misunderstandings or imaginative elaborations (several narrations of the story are also staged in this episode), and "Field Trip" (6.21), where an hallucinogenic fungus replaces actual events with fantasies based on thoughts already present in the protagonists' minds.

The level of "monster literacy" in various episodes is impressive, nowhere more so than in "Humbug," the homage to circus sideshow performers and to the Tod Browning's *Freaks* (1932). In fact, this show is haunted by the cultural history of monstrosity, revealing fragments of various moments in the history of monstrosity even as it presents monstrosity as a vision of difference seen in a series of funhouse mirrors (a theme that runs throughout the episode). Rather than focusing on the vagaries of narration, as other episodes, cited earlier, do quite prominently, "Humbug" plays games of perspective to suggest that our perception guides or misguides our interpretation of events, and that that perception can change from one individual to another and according to the context in which it takes place. As a result, the episode is full of visual games and exchanged gazes as characters scrutinize each other and misperceive various events. Attitudes as far distant as Aristotle's formulations of monstrosity, as well as Saint Augustine's more tolerant views, lurk at the edges of the narrative, even as eugenics and freak shows are prominently discussed and displayed. This multitude of historical perspectives, combined with the use of mirrors and other perspectival devices in the episode, suggests that monstrosity is a way of seeing, rather than an actual state of being, thus placing the *X-Files* in the camp of Augustinian tolerance, as we shall see.

"Humbug" offers a *summa* of theories and representations of the monstrous, from Aristotle to the film *Freaks,* and beyond to the dwarf power movement of the 1980s. The episode refuses to settle on a particular view of monstrosity, moving between various theories of what this means, and oscillating from the very beginning between notions of the monster as a cultural creation and as a genuine threat. In this episode, Fox Mulder and Dana Scully, the two FBI agents who are the protagonists of the series, go to Gibsonton, Florida, where they find a community of current and former circus sideshow performers. They have been sent there to investigate the latest in a series of gruesome murders. In this case, one of the performers, the Alligator Man, has been disemboweled. As they interview various possible witnesses to the crime, they engage with individuals or situations that evoke the history of monstrosity. The entire episode is framed by the remark "Imagine going through your whole life looking like that," initially made by Scully in response to a photograph of the Alligator Man. Generally Scully, as the scientist, represents the neo-Aristotelian, post-Enlightenment view of the monstrous as something that is outside of the natural order of things, but can be explained. Mulder, with his motto "The Truth Is Out There," represents a more Augustinian view of the monster as a sign of the unknown. In this episode, they switch roles repeatedly, suggesting the symbiotic nature of these two perspectives.

From the opening sequence, this episode plays with the various notions of monstrosity. It begins with a shot of a frightening monster, hideously deformed, with obviously scaly skin. He is hiding in the bushes, spying on two children playing in a swimming pool; then he jumps out at them and scares them. They yell, "Dad!" and he sends them in to bed. And so, the monster is instantly normalized. Suddenly, another monster is stalking the first one; it jumps into the pool as well, and attacks. The monster thus retakes its places as an evil threat. The episode will continue to shift from one perspective to another as the story unfurls, leaving us with the notion that the concept of monstrosity itself is a funhouse ride (a central image of the episode), complete with distorting mirrors and shadows that obscure any clear view of the monster. At the end of the opening sequence, the camera pans to a truck, with a sign painted on the side: Jerrold Glazebrook, The Alligator Man. Credits roll.

The Aristotelian notion of monstrosity as excess or lack[3] is evoked by two characters who are also close friends, Mr. Nutt, a dwarf, and Lennie, a man with what seems to be a parasitic twin extending from his abdomen. But the situation is much more complex than this, and evokes Aristotelian ideas in entangled ways. Lennie's relationship with his twin, Leonard, echoes Aristotelian notions of monstrosity in a particularly complex fashion. Aristotle's treatise on the *Generation of Animals,* which contains one of the earliest and most influential theories of monstrosity, manifests deep concern with issues of identity. While the Aristotelian theory of the causes of monstrosity is frequently summarized as the excess or lack of matter in the production of offspring, the relevant passages from this treatise suggest a complex interplay between resemblance and difference:

> The same causes must be held responsible for the facts that some children resemble their parents, while others do not (some being like the father and others like the mother, both in the body as a whole and in each part); and that they resemble their parents more than remoter ancestors, and resemble those ancestors more than any chance individual; and that males rather resemble their fathers, females their mothers; and that some, though resembling none of their relations, yet do at any rate resemble a human being, but others are not even like a human being, but a monstrosity. For even he who does not resemble his parents is already in a certain sense a monstrosity; for in these cases nature has in a way departed from the type. The first

departure indeed is that the offspring should become female instead of male; this, however, is a natural necessity.[4]

Any departure from the (male) parental type is already seen as a monstrosity, thus leaving a broad range of potential monsters, and a very narrow definition of what might not be seen as monstrous. The continuation of this discussion, however, complicates matters:

> If the generative residue in the menstrual fluids is properly concocted, the movement imparted by the male will make the form of the embryo in the likeness of itself.... Now the peculiar and the individual has always more force in generation. Coriscus is both a man and an animal, but his manhood is nearer to what is peculiar to him than is his animal-hood. In generation both the individual and the class are operative, but the individual is the more so of the two, for this is the substance. And the offspring is produced indeed of a certain quality, but also as a certain "this," and this latter is the substance.[5]

The individual is always connected to a broader web of identity (ancestors, humanity, animalhood), but is better situated in this web the more precisely it resembles a particular male (the father). Thus, Aristotle acknowledges the connections among humans, and between the human and the animal, but still posits particularity (e.g., the particular Greek male citizen Coriscus) as the highest manifestation of identity. The level of monstrosity increases the more an individual departs from a particular type (Coriscus, Coriscus's family, human, animal . . .).[6]

In short, monstrosity is that which calls into question the conformity of the individual to a type. But the more particular the type, and the more closely the individual conforms to it, the less monstrous he will be. This definition creates a tension between particularity and universalism; at what point does the particularity of the type press against the limits of the nonmonstrous? Already, the female is designated as monstrous, even if she fits a fairly generally recognized type. And finally, if a certain "monstrosity" occurs frequently enough, and in a way that can be explained, it is not so monstrous after all. Thus, within the discourse of the *Generation of Animals* remains the possibility of normalizing the monstrous. Arguably, this can take place when the monstrous form becomes a "type" of its own, as is the case with monstrous races:

> For the monstrosity belongs to the class of things contrary to nature, not any and every kind of nature, but nature taken as what holds for the most part; nothing can happen contrary to nature considered as eternal and necessary, but only in those cases where things generally happen in a certain way but may also happen in another way. In fact, even in the case of monstrosities, whenever things occur contrary indeed to the established order but still always in a certain way and not at random, the result seems to be less of a monstrosity because even that which is contrary to nature is in a certain sense according to nature, whenever, that is, the formal nature has not mastered the material nature.[7]

Aristotle then equates monstrosity and deformity, an equation that will determine the treatment of deformed and disabled individuals for millennia: "The account of the cause of monstrosities is very close and similar in a way to that of the deformed; for monstrosity is actually a kind of deformity."[8] Finally, as he cites the Democritean theory of monstrosity arising from an excess of matter, he returns to the issue of identity, but from a different angle. He discusses the frequent occurrence of double eggs in bird species:

> In such double eggs, when the yolks are separated by the membrane, two separate chickens are produced with nothing abnormal about them; when the yolks are continuous, with no

> division between them, the chickens produced are monstrous, having one body and head but four legs and four wings.[9]

In a later passage, Aristotle ponders how to determine whether such a double creature is one being or two, and concludes that "that which has one heart will be one animal."[10] As recent discussions of conjoined twins reveal,[11] the answer is not really that simple. In the course of his discussion of double beings, Aristotle declares that "both deficiency and excess are monstrous."[12]

Following Aristotle's pronouncements, Mr. Nutt is monstrous because of his size, which would signal a lack of material. Lennie/Leonard is monstrous because of his excessive nature, with extra limbs and a second trunk extending from Lennie's body. But Lennie/Leonard is also monstrous because he does not fit into a broader type; this not a case of conjoined twins, or even of a typical parasitic twin, as we discover. Leonard can detach himself from Lennie, and has his own heart and head (which would make him a separate individual, according to Aristotle), and his own will. He cannot remain separate from Lennie, as he apparently cannot eat and is dependent on an umbilical-like connection to his brother. This makes Lennie additionally monstrous, as he has internal characteristics similar to those of women, thus further not fitting into the normal male "type." Paradoxically, Leonard, with his diminutive stature, can be seen as a monster of lack even though when joined with his brother he is an Aristotelian monster of excess. Furthermore, he is also a monster of type inasmuch as he is frequently compared to the Fiji mermaid, a hybrid of monkey and fish that never really existed, but was on display in the nineteenth century. Leonard never speaks (he screams), cannot feed himself or walk, and so is never seen as fully human.

Lennie/Leonard thus embody many qualities of the monstrous "type"—if there can in fact be such a type. They do not fit into the broader category of normal humans as they not only are typically male and share some aspects of their identity but also are two separate individuals in most ways. They are thus excessive in a number of ways, eluding most categories that would enable them to be included in the realm of normal humanity. The symbiotic relationship between Leonard and Lennie, which is essential to their unique but joint identity, also evokes the Kristevan idea of the abject as both the distance and connection between the self and the other, a point where individual identity, based on the other as object, is called into doubt.[13] This resonates with the identity politics of the Aristotelian model of the nonmonstrous human as both a particular individual and inextricably linked to a paternal type.

The setting for "Humbug" evokes Pliny's descriptions of monstrous races, from the seventh book of his *Natural History*, in which radical bodily difference is relegated to the periphery of the Roman Empire. While Pliny seems at first to focus on how difference is distant from us, many of his examples of Romans show diverse individuals who do not fit into a type (he prefers to discuss the exceptional examples, rather than the uniform ones); thus, monstrous races (or "types") and monstrous individuals coexist already in the ancient world. The isolation of the sciopods (one-footed or umbrella-footed people), the panotii (a race of people whose ears hang to their feet), the monoculi (Cyclops), and other such races is echoed by the isolation of the Gibsonton community. But this isolation turns back upon supposedly normal interlopers who arrive in town. There is apparently so little contact between this town of "freaks" and the rest of the world that "normals" are received like curiosities or monsters in their own right.

Monstrous races dominate the Middle Ages, although individual monsters such as werewolves—originally also a race in Pliny, but later seen as exceptional individuals—do also exist. As John Block Friedman points out, various taxonomies of monstrous races are produced.[14] Augustinian theories of the monstrous, as influential as those of Aristotle for medieval thought in particular, present monsters as signs of the diversity of creation, of God's power. Augustine's discussions of the monstrous are frequently contrasted with those of Aristotle. His description of the monstrous races, based to some extent on Pliny's *Natural History*, leads him to declare:

> For God is the Creator of all things: He Himself knows where and when anything should be, or should have been, created; and He knows how to weave the beauty of the whole out of the similarity and diversity of its parts. The man who cannot view the whole is offended by what he takes to be the deformity of a part; but this is because he does not know how it is adapted or related to the whole.[15]

Thus, our belief that an individual is monstrous is derived from our own lack of understanding, our limited knowledge of the world. We cannot possibly understand God's plan from our limited human perspective. Monsters thus become a symbol of the limits of human knowledge and the transcendence of the divine.

Rather than emphasizing the ways in which monsters depart from a type, Augustine underscores the universal humanity of all men:

> Again, who could call to mind all the human infants who have been born very unlike those who were most certainly their parents? It cannot be denied, however, that these derive their origin from that one man, Adam; and the same is therefore true of all those races which, by reason of their bodily differences, are said to have deviated from the usual pattern of nature exhibited by most—indeed, by almost the whole—of mankind. If these races are included in the definition of "human," that is, if they are rational and mortal animals, then it must be admitted that they trace their lineage from that same one man, the first father of all mankind: if, that is, what we are told of the diversity of those races, and their great difference from one another and from us, is true.[16]

The suggestion is that everything is different; that difference is part of existence itself. As Mulder and Scully enter the community of Gibsonton in the wake of the murder that prompted their investigation, they are introduced to a town full of diverse individuals. The camera pans around the site of Glazebrook's burial, and takes in his widow (the bearded lady), Lennie, with his parasitic twin, the armless minister who turns the pages of the bible with his foot, a giant, a dwarf, and others. Each individual at the funeral is presented as unique, rather than part of a particular group or type. They also represent the range of performers who would have been part of a "freak show" in the nineteenth and twentieth centuries, so, ironically, they can be seen as representative "types."[17] The ground shakes, and Dr. Blockhead, another circus performer with a "normal" physique, bursts out of the ground and pounds a spike into his chest. The other attendees yell "Freak!" and run away, the irony being that Dr. Blockhead is a "normal" and therefore only a fake freak. Mulder and Scully find themselves in a sort of world turned upside-down, where the "normals" are unusual and the object of the intrigued gaze, while the "freaks" are the norm, and no two people look quite alike.

The Augustinian notion of radically different human beings as nonetheless human will later become a basis for tolerance and even acceptance of different bodies as divine in origin. But this divine origin is a double-edged sword, a sign that can be read negatively as a sign of God's wrath as well as positively as a sign of God's power. Monsters' status as signs becomes particularly important for Augustine and for subsequent medieval theorists of monstrosity:

> Therefore, just as it was not impossible for God to create whatever natures He chose, so it is not impossible for Him to change those natures which He has created in whatever way He chooses. This is why there has sprung up so great a multitude of those marvels which are

> called "monsters," "signs," "portents," or "prodigies." If I chose to recall and mention them all, would this work ever come to an end? The word "monster", we are told, clearly comes from "to demonstrate" [*monstrare*], because monsters are signs by which something is demonstrated. "Sign" [*ostentum*] comes from "to show" [*ostendere*]; "portent" from "to portend", that is "to show in advance" [*praeostendere*]; and "prodigy" from "to speak of what is far away" [*porro dicere*], that is, to foretell the future.[18]

Once again, Augustine expresses skepticism as to whether men can read these signs adequately, even as he urges his readers to interpret them as signs of God's ability to perform miracles, such as raising the dead. Monstrosity becomes the expression of that which escapes the human grasp and resides only in the realm of the divine.

This skepticism is further developed by Christian Neoplatonic thought in the wake of Pseudo-Dionysius, as David Williams points out:

> Just as Christian Neoplatonism asserted the superiority of negation in theology and philosophy, so, too, in its epistemology it followed the *via negativa,* and once again the sign of this superior form of unknowing was the deformed.[19]

The deformed or monstrous, as something incomprehensible, becomes a symbol of the divine and of the failures of human systems of thought. Williams asserts this as the symbolic aspect of monstrosity, in contrast to the literal aspect. Both of these aspects coexisted throughout the Middle Ages[20], and well into the sixteenth century in the form of monstrous races and extraordinary creatures, which often served double-duty as symbolic figures of the unknowable divine and objects of early scientific inquiry.[21] The Rebis, or double being, was thus a symbol of Christ's mystical double nature or of alchemic perfection,[22] and the conjoined twin, its human homologue, was studied in the attempt to understand the natural causes of such deformities.[23]

Katharine Park and Lorraine Daston recognize the overlapping constructions of the monstrous in the early modern period, and propose three modes of interpretation with three "associated emotions—horror, pleasure, and repugnance."[24] The religious aspect of monsters as prodigies is still omnipresent in the sixteenth century, accompanied by the emotion of horror. The pleasurable aspect of monsters is evident in their display, whether at local fairs or in cabinets of curiosities. The repugnance arises in medical treatises that represent monsters as errors of nature. These three categories echo to some extent the three traditions concerning the monstrous delineated by Jean Céard: the Aristotelian theory of monsters as natural phenomena; the Ciceronian one of monsters as prodigies or signs sent by the gods; the Augustinian model of monsters as marvelous signs of God's power.[25] These categories coexist and are even joined in the work of authors such as Michel de Montaigne, who, in his essay "On a Monstrous Child," associates the pleasurable with the prodigious.[26] He sees a child with a parasitic twin being displayed at a fair, and offers an interpretation of it as a prodigy, finally rejecting the notion that this child is monstrous by alluding to Augustine's insistence that our view of unusual beings as monstrous is merely a sign of our own ignorance. The religious, scientific, and entertaining aspects of the monstrous also coexist in Ambroise Paré's *Des Monstres et prodigies,* along with a new category, that of the morally monstrous, or the transgressor of the law, embodied in the supposedly monstrous beggars. It should also be noted that, in Paré, the prodigy might evoke horror, but it can also elicit awe; the teratological anomaly might evoke repugnance, but it can also give rise to sympathy; the "curiosity" might elicit amusement, but it can also call up any of the emotions associated with the other categories listed by Park and Daston.[27] As Céard points out in his study of monsters and prodigies, the early modern period is not one where categories arrange themselves neatly.[28] And it is somehow fitting that the monstrous defies such clear categorization, as Jeffrey Jerome Cohen points out.[29] These categories are also present in the rhetoric of the freak show, as Bogdan points out,[30] and are echoed in "Humbug" in the final confrontation between Dr. Blockhead and Scully.

In the course of the early modern period, taxonomies of monstrous races are replaced by theorizations of the origins of monstrous individuals. This is the dawn of teratology, the study of abnormal fetal development. To some extent, this represents a return to Aristotelian theories, and a move away from moralizations. But the moralizing versions of the monstrous still exist in relation to depictions of different races as monstrous, particularly in the case of the "cannibals" in the Western Hemisphere. In a reversal of their usual roles as advocate of the paranormal and scientist, Mulder offers scientific explanations and Scully recoils in horror at the sight of the monstrous. As they prepare to go down to Gibsonton to investigate Glazebrook's murder, Scully looks at the file and is shocked by the picture of Glazebrook. "What happened to him?" she asks. "Nothing you can ascertain from those photos," Mulder replies. Glazebrook had ichthyosis, which made his skin scaly. Mulder focuses on the 48 similar murders that have taken place over many years, but Scully still focuses on the pictures of Glazebrook: "Imagine going through your whole life looking like this." To Scully, the scientist, the Alligator Man is an unacceptable deviation from the norm, an object of horror, almost a prodigy. To Mulder, he is a scientific anomaly, but one that carries with it a rational explanation for its appearance. So, when Mulder explains to Scully that Glazebrook's condition was ichthyosis, a hereditary condition which causes scaly skin, he is the heir to a long period of medicalization of bodily difference.

Physical variations are natural and can be seen as normal in certain contexts. At the same time, the causes of these physical variations are never entirely comprehensible; there is always something about nature that eludes our grasp, our understanding. In this case, the modern mystery that demands to be solved touches upon the medieval mystery, which signals the unknowable divinity and thus is itself unsolvable. Human limitations cause our misunderstanding, and thus cause us to label certain things as monstrous, because they elude our grasp. The misunderstanding caused by our limited human perceptions is emphasized from the beginning of "Humbug." As has been stated, when we first see Glazebrook, before the opening credits, spying in some children in a pool and breathing harshly, we assume he is the monster. When he jumps out at the boys and they scream "Dad!" we realize that he is not a monster, as he is now linked to "normal" humans in a recognizable fashion. When he sends them in, and is himself spied upon by another creature, we don't really know what to think any more—even as he is attacked by the monster.

Two scenes at the center of the episode emphasize these shifting perspectives and the unsteady ground on which notions of the monstrous are founded; both scenes use mirrors to disorient the viewer and to suggest that monstrosity may simply be a perspectival distortion. In the Gibsonton Museum of Curiosities ("Freaks Free: All Others, Please Leave Donation"), Scully learns more about freaks and sideshow performers. At first, the museum keeper is only visible to us in a distorting mirror; it is hard to tell whether his features are normal or anomalous until partway through the scene, when he puts a deformed hand on Scully's shoulder. He tells the story of Chang and Eng, ending with an account of how Eng died of fright when he realized that Chang was dead. He explains that blockheads are skilled performers, while geeks are "merely unseemly." He explains gaffes or fakes (conjoined twins are always identical, but he shows a picture of conjoined twins who clearly are not). He then gives her a pamphlet about Jim-Jim the Dog-Faced Boy. He sends her to see a P. T. Barnum exhibit, which is really an empty chest (when she opens it, the exit door opens). The movement of his presentation from genuine curiosities (Chang and Eng) to complete fraud suggests the unstable nature of the freak show; one can never be quite certain of what one is seeing. Even if there are "true" anomalies, at the center of this show is "humbug" or fraud; the empty chest stands in for absent knowledge just as the monster stands in for the unknowable divine in the post-Augustinian mystical version of the monstrous.

Later in the episode, Scully and Mulder chase Leonard into the funhouse, where they only see him briefly or in distorting mirrors. When Scully tries to shoot him, she merely shatters the mirrors. In a previous scene, in which Leonard murdered Hepcat, we see him and the event only in the distorting mirrors in Hepcat's workshop. These scenes call into doubt the existence of the monster, and suggest that it is merely a reflection of our own fears or even of ourselves. This in turn echoes the scene where Hepcat explained that the picture he painted on a dinner menu is of P. T. Barnum's Fiji Mermaid, which was really a monkey head and torso sewn to a fish tail. This curiosity was billed as a "genuine hoax." Hepcat remarks, "That's the beauty of it: you never know where the truth ends, and the humbug begins." All of this suggests that, in a world of shifting perspectives, the truth remains "out there" as Mulder's motto, visually present throughout the series, suggests. These shifting perspectives are not created by the circus sideshow performers, but merely reflected by them, like images in a mirror.

This bizarre game of distorted reflections is echoed by the episode's narrative. Now that Scully and Mulder have found out that the town sheriff (Hamilton) used to be Jim-Jim the Dog-Faced Boy, they become suspicious. They spy on him as he buries something under a full moon, and then try to dig it up. As they do so, they acknowledge that they might be jumping to conclusions, after all "Hypertrychosis does not denote lycanthropy." Still, they keep digging, and the sheriff walks up behind them. "May I ask what you are doing?" Scully starts to explain that many serial killers are attracted to law enforcement, but Mulder cuts to the chase: "We discovered that you used to be the dog-faced boy." He shows Sheriff Hamilton the pamphlet, and the sheriff laughs at how much hair he had. He explains that he became sheriff of Gibsonton when he started to lose his hair, and could not continue to make a living on the sideshow circuit. He also explains that he was burying a potato to cure warts, and asks "Investigation isn't going too well, is it?" The sheriff is sympathetic to Scully and Mulder, but a little condescending because of their initial arrogance in the investigation and their relative ignorance concerning the world of circus sideshow performers. While they are not (yet) monsters, the two FBI agents are objects of pity and curiosity, and the tables are being turned on them. Just as Sheriff Hamilton transformed from monster to normal human simply by losing his hair, Scully and Mulder are being redefined as monstrous in the land of the monsters; both categories become interchangeable.

This sort of game of perspective/reverse perspective is played throughout the episode. It is particularly evident in the exchanges between Mr. Nutt, the embodiment of the 1970s "dwarf power" movement, and Mulder. They first meet when Mulder and Scully are registering at the motel where he is the owner/manager. Mulder asks Mr. Nutt whether he was ever in the circus, and his response is, "What made you think I ever attended the circus, much less let myself be enslaved by one . . . just because I am a person of short stature." He points out that he has a degree in hotel management. But it is human nature to judge people by their appearance, he adds: "Why, for example, when I consider your all-American features, your dour demeanor, your unimaginative necktie, I guess that you are an FBI agent. But you see . . . I have reduced you to a stereotype." Mulder replies, "But I am an FBI agent," and Mr. Nutt looks disappointed. The fact that sometimes stereotypes hold true closes off the possibility of even negative knowledge, the understanding that certain forms of knowledge must simply be rejected. Later, Mulder finds Mr. Nutt under Scully's trailer, and is suspicious, but Mr. Nutt replies, "Just because I am not of so-called average height does not mean I have to seek my thrills vicariously. Not all women are attracted to overly tall, lanky men such as yourself." Mr. Nutt does not see himself as too short; he sees Mulder as too tall.

Mr. Nutt's militancy can be seen as a sort of "pushing back" on the momentum over the past 200 years toward reshaping humanity into a more regular, idealized form. Lennard Davis analyzes this preference for idealized body types in his essay on "Constructing Normalcy." The eugenicist Sir Francis Galton (1822–1911) transformed the interpretation of statistics from perceiving the average as normal to promoting above-average traits as normal:

> In an "error curve" the extremes of the curve are the most mistaken in accuracy. But if one is looking at human traits, then the extremes, particularly what Galton saw as positive extremes—tallness, high intelligence, ambitiousness, strength, fertility—would have to be seen as errors. Rather than "errors," Galton wanted to think of the extremes as distributions of a trait.[31]

Galton made revisions to his system in order to privilege traits which he deemed superior. Davis considers the effects of these revisions on our concept of normal humanity:

> What these revisions by Galton signify is an attempt to redefine the concept of the "ideal" in relation to the general population. First, the application of the idea of a norm to the human body creates the idea of deviance or a "deviant" body. Second, the idea of a norm pushes the normal variation of the body through a stricter template guiding the way the body "should" be. Third, the revision of the "normal curve of distribution" into quartiles, ranked in order, and so on, creates a new kind of "ideal." This statistical ideal is unlike the classical ideal which contains no imperative to be the ideal. The new ideal of ranked order is powered by the imperative of the norm, and then is supplemented by the notion of progress, human perfectibility, and the elimination of deviance, to create a dominating, hegemonic vision of what the human body should be.[32]

Arguably, this vision of an attainable human ideal is more monstrous than the "deviant" physical forms that it was developed to eliminate; eugenics and Nazism were close companions, a point already suggested before the Holocaust by Tod Browning and made explicit by Dr. Blockhead at the end of "Humbug" and in the most direct homage to Browning's film.

The modern era inherits complex versions of the Aristotelian/Augustinian split, with a large dose of Pliny. Freaks are like the early modern curiosities; exceptional beings displayed because of their unusual nature. Because they are presented as exceptional, they are not linked to any particular social identity. At the same time, they echo the Augustinian notion of the monstrous as sign of universal diversity and of God's power. They are thus marginalized, but also objects of fascination. Purely fictional monsters, vampires, werewolves, and zombies evoke the threat of the monstrous.

In this period, when monstrosity represents difference as marginalization, as a threat, or as both at once, eugenics is proposed as a solution to differences seen as unacceptable.[33] Today, fewer children are born with disabilities because of genetic screening and selective abortion. This is presented as progress, but this "progress" carries with it some very real risks: What if diversity is necessary to our survival and thriving as a species? What if what we see as a deficit or lack (dwarfism, deafness) is not so when seen from a different perspective? What are the potential costs of striving for an entirely uniform body of humanity?

The advent of disability rights movements, represented by Mr. Nutt, and of notions of somatechnics, represented by Dr. Blockhead and the tattooed Conundrum, changes the discussion entirely. For the deaf culture movement, as well as for other such movements, difference does not denote deficit or lack—in fact, in its own domain, difference can denote superiority. This is, in the end, one of the lessons of Gibsonton. Thus, some individuals cultivate difference by transforming their own bodies. Body modification becomes a way of celebrating difference by creating it. Thus, the Conundrum has had his entire body tattooed. He is also a geek, a performer who will eat anything (e.g., crickets, fish). One scene in particular underscores his difference from others. When the Conundrum later pops out of a pot of boiling water, Mulder is startled, "I saw him eating fish." Dr. Blockhead replies, "He knows better than to snack between shows." Mulder quips, "Maybe it was another naked, bald-headed, tattooed man I saw . . . ," again underscoring the unique nature of the monsters in Gibsonton. But the Conundrum has made himself unique, rather than being born that way; he has chosen to mark his difference in defiance of the normalization of humanity.

Dr. Blockhead manipulates his body in other ways, declaring, "I perform astounding acts of body manipulation and pain endurance" as he hammers a nail into his nose. He claims that he is from Yemen, and that he studied with swamis, thus evoking the Plinian monstrous races and their superhuman strength and endurance. But he is also lying, thus echoing the fraudulent nature of many freak show acts. He is a combination of endurance artist, escape artist, and contortionist, and thus becomes a suspect after the bizarre deaths of Hepcat (where someone had to squeeze through a small window) and Mr. Nutt (where someone had to squeeze through a pet door). He is viewed with suspicion by the "natural" freaks in Gibsonton.

The association of body manipulation with fraud evokes some early modern precursors of "somatechnicians"—the beggars in Ambroise Paré's *Des Monstres et prodigies* (chapters 20–24), who feign various illnesses and deformities in order to receive alms at the church door. While Paré does not in fact seem repulsed by humans with naturally occurring deformities, he is incensed by the self-made monsters and declares that their death is not a bad thing.[34] What seems most threatening about these beggars is that they have formed a society apart, one that functions according to its own laws (laws that often seem more fair than those of the French nation, since the beggars share any money they make with those in need) and outside of the established laws of the country in which they live.[35] In their fraudulent activities, the beggars are also associated with demons, presented in chapters 25 through 33, who manipulate human perceptions of the world around them. For Paré, these monsters of misperception or manipulation are the most threatening, because they call into question the grounds upon which our knowledge of the world is based. They violate not only fundamental social laws and laws imposed by the state, but what had been up to that point accepted as "natural laws" that dictated the order of the cosmos. In this, they already touch upon issues that Michel Foucault will associate with the monstrous in his lectures on the abnormal.[36] They also represent the flip side of Augustinian notions of divine mystery, the idea that the knowledge we do have is at best factitious and at worst fraudulent and dangerous.

In embracing their identities as "self-made freaks," Dr. Blockhead (a.k.a. Jeffrey Swain) and the Conundrum seem to anticipate the concept of somatechnics, or body modification with a view to emphasizing difference rather than effacing it. Recent theorizations of the monstrous emphasize the monster as a site where meaning is made;[37] the sort of body modification undertaken by Dr. Blockhead and his companion represents at the very least an attempt to wrest that making of meaning out of the hands of others return it to the control of the "monsters" themselves. This gesture is complicated by the fact that the meaning of the monstrous escapes the grasp of virtually everybody in this episode, in a return to Augustinian mysticism.

The elusive meaning, represented also by the empty chest in the Gibsonton museum, is echoed by the missing monster, Leonard, the murderer who is never directly or clearly seen. At the end of the episode, the Conundrum is taking out the garbage when he is attacked by Leonard. He seems dead at first, but his stomach is gurgling; Leonard is nowhere to be found. The next day, at daylight, Scully and Mulder start to search for Leonard again. The sheriff quips, "Maybe it was the Fiji mermaid" as Mulder grumbles to Scully "Now you know how I feel." The "monsters" are mocking their belief in monsters! Dr. Blockhead and the Conundrum are preparing to leave; they don't want to stay around with the monster on the loose. Scully tells him that the monster was the parasitic twin, Leonard, who had detached himself from Lennie. Dr. Blockhead expresses the hope that he will just crawl back up into his twin, but Scully answers that Lennie died of cirrhosis the previous night. She adds, "I've never seen anything like it." Dr. Blockhead then channels the prologue to Tod Browning's *Freaks,* commenting on eugenics, but adds his own Augustinian twist[38]:

> *Dr. B.*: And you never will gain. Twenty-first century genetic engineering will not only eradicate the Siamese twins and the alligator-skinned people, but you will be hard-pressed to find a slight overbite or a not-so-high cheekbone. I've seen the future, and the future looks just like... [he points to Mulder] HIM! Imagine going through your whole life looking like that. That why it's left to the self-made freaks like me and the Conundrum to remind people.
>
> *Scully*: Remind them of what?
>
> *Dr. B.*: Nature abhors normality; it can't go for very long without creating a mutant. Do you know why?
>
> *Scully*: No, why?
>
> *Dr. B.*: I don't know, either.... Maybe some mysteries are not meant to be solved.

Scully remarks that the Conundrum does not look well; he says, "Maybe it was something I ate" (the only words he says throughout the episode) and smiles. Dr. Blockhead then gets into the car and they drive away, with the murder mystery at the end of the episode also unsolved (if resolved in a singularly monstrous manner).

If "Humbug" can be read as the *summa* of *X-Files* representations of the monstrous, Dr. Blockhead's speech at the end of the episode can be read as the *summa* of the *summa,* neatly returning to a line Scully utters at the beginning, and twisting it back upon her (or rather, upon Mulder). In the land of the freaks, the "normals" (or "rubes" as they are called by another character, Hepcat) are the freaks. The genetic perfection of Mulder is more freakish because of its potentially unnatural origins than the natural genetic imperfections of the freaks themselves. Bodily differences, even anomalies, occur naturally; uniformity does not. For Dr. Blockhead, this is one of the unsolved mysteries of the world, and it was not meant to be solved, meaning both that it was not meant to be understood and that it should not be solved by genetic engineering. His speech brilliantly updates the Augustinian/Pseudo-Dionysian view of monstrosity as both a reflection of God's power and a symbol of human incapacity to comprehend that power.

In a world where genetic engineering is available and used, where the "monsters" can be done away with, the "normals" become monstrous. Thus "Humbug" deftly reverses millennia of monster theory, reflecting our own unease with our technologically but perhaps not ethically advanced culture. When normality can be engineered, it is no longer natural, thus fulfilling one of the categories of the monstrous, that which occurs outside of the realm of nature. In his statement "Nature abhors normality," Dr. Blockhead naturalizes the monstrous and reveals the monstrosity informing modern culture. In so doing, he both reveals and reverses the cultural foundations of knowledge based on divisions such as those between normal and monstrous, leaving the empty and evocative space of mystery where once we thought that knowledge might reside.

NOTES

1. Pliny, *Natural History* (Cambridge, MA: Harvard University Press, Loeb Classical Library, 2006), vol. 7, 512–527.

2. *The X-Files* (Fox Broadcasting Network, 1993–2002), season 1, episode 5 (October 8, 1993). All other references to episodes will give season and episode number (e.g., for "The Jersey Devil," 1.5).
3. The most influential work on monstrosity comes from Aristotle's *Generation of Animals*. See *The Complete Works of Aristotle*, ed. Jonathan Barnes (Princeton, NJ: Princeton University Press, 1984), 1111–1218, in particular book IV, 1187–1196.
4. Aristotle, *Generation of Animals*, in *The Complete Works of Aristotle*, ed. Jonathan Barnes (Princeton, NJ: Princeton University Press, 1984), 1: 1187 [767a.36–767b.1–9].
5. Aristotle, *Generation of Animals*, 1: 1188 [767b.15–36].
6. But if we assign only one form of cause, it is not easy to explain all of the phenomena—the distinction of sex, why the female is often like the father and the male like the mother and gain the resemblance to the remoter ancestors, and further the reason why the offspring is sometimes unlike any of these but still a human being, but sometimes, proceeding further on these lines, appears finally to be not even a human being but only some kind of animal, what is called a monstrosity.

   For, following what has been said, it remains to give the reason for such monsters. If the movements relapse and the material is not controlled, at last there remains what is most universal, that is to say, the animal. Then people say that the child has the head of a ram or a bull, and so on with other animals, as that a calf has the head of a child or a sheep that of an ox. All these monsters result from the causes stated earlier, but they are none of the things they are said to be; there is only some similarity, such as may arise even where there is no defect of growth (Aristotle, *Generation of Animals*, 1: 1191 [769b.1–18]). This rather reasonable explanation of animalistic bodily forms in humans was long neglected in favor of those that featured sexual relations between humans and animals (which Aristotle dismisses based on the impossibility of such relations resulting in reproduction, given differences in gestational periods).
7. Aristotle, *Generation of Animals*, 1: 1192 [770b.9–17].
8. Aristotle, *Generation of Animals*, 1: 1191 [769b.29–30].
9. Aristotle, *Generation of Animals*, 1: 1191–1192 [770a.15–20].
10. Aristotle, *Generation of Animals*, 1: 1196 [773a.9–10].
11. See Alice Domurat Dreger, *One of Us: Conjoined Twins and the Future of Normal* (Cambridge, MA: Harvard University Press, 2004).
12. Aristotle, *Generation of Animals*, 1: 1192 [770b.8].
13. Julia Kristeva, *Pouvoirs de l'horreur. Essai sur l'abjection* (Paris: Seuil, 1980).
14. John Block Friedman, *The Monstrous Races in Medieval Art and Thought* (Syracuse, NY: Syracuse University Press, 2000).
15. Augustine of Hippo, *The City of God Against the Pagans*, ed. R. W. Dyson (Cambridge: Cambridge University Press, 1998/2010), 708.
16. Augustine of Hippo, *The City of God Against the Pagans*, 709.
17. See Robert Bogdan, 'Introduction," to *Freak Show: Presenting Human Oddities for Amusement and Profit* (Chicago: University of Chicago Press, 1988), 1–21.
18. Augustine of Hippo, *The City of God Against the Pagans*, 1063.
19. David Williams, *Deformed Discourse: The Function of the Monster in Mediaeval Thought and Literature* (Montreal: McGill-Queen's University Press, 1996).
20. Williams, *Deformed Discourse*, 11.
21. Lisa Verner discusses this dualism at some length in her book, *The Epistemology of the Monstrous in the Middle Ages* (New York: Routledge, 2005).
22. See Leah DeVun, "The Jesus Hermaphrodite: Science and Sex Difference in Premodern Europe," *Journal of the History of Ideas* 69, no. 2 (2008): 193–218.
23. See Ambroise Paré, *Des Monstres et prodiges*, ed. Jean Céard (Geneva: Droz, 1971), chapter 4, 9–20. For an English translation, see Ambroise Paré, *On Monsters and Marvels*, trans. Janis Pallister (Chicago: University of Chicago Press, 1982).
24. Lorraine Daston and Katharine Park, *Wonders and the Order of Nature: 1150–1750* (New York: Zone Books, 1998), 176.
25. Jean Céard, *La Nature et les prodiges* (Geneva: Droz, 1977), 3.

26. Michel de Montaigne, *Essais,* ed. Pierre Villey (Paris: Presses Universitaires de France, 1978), 1; "Ce double corps et ces members divers, se rapportans à une seule teste, pourroient bien fournir de favorable prognostique au Roy de maintenir sous l'union de ses loix ces pars et pieces diverses de nostre estat" ("This double body and these diverse members, joined in one head, could well furnish a favorable prognostication to the King to maintain under the union of his laws these diverse parts and pieces of our state") and "Ce que nous appellons monsters, ne le sont pas à Dieu, qui voit en l'immensité de son ouvrage l'infinité des formes qu'il y a comprinses" ("That which we call monsters are not so to God, who sees in the immensity of his work the infinity of forms included there").
27. Also useful for considering the categories of the marvelous is Lorraine Daston's article on "Marvelous Facts and Miraculous Evidence in Early modern Europe," first published in *Critical Inquiry* 18 (1991): 93–124 and reprinted in James Chandler et al., *Questions of Evidence: Proof, Practice, and Persuasion Across the Disciplines* (Chicago: University of Chicago Press, 1994), 243–274.
28. *La Nature,* XIII: "les notions de merveille, de prodige, de monstre, etc., que nous étudions sont d'une fluidité telle qu'un exposé par matières aurait contredit à la nature même de son objet" ("the notions of marvel, of prodigy, of monster, etc., that we are studying are of such fluidity that an analysis organized according to categories would have contradicted the very nature of its object").
29. Jeffrey Jerome Cohen, "Monster Theory (Seven Theses)," in *Monster Theory: Reading Culture,* ed. Jeffrey Jerome Cohen (Minneapolis: University of Minnesota Press, 1996), 6.
30. Bogdan, *Freak Show,* 3–6.
31. Lennard J. Davis, "Constructing Normalcy: The Bell Curve, the Novel, and the Invention of the Disabled Body in the Nineteenth Century," in *The Disability Studies Reader*, ed. Lennard J. Davis (New York: Routledge, 2006), 7.
32. Davis, "Constructing Normalcy," 8.
33. For this shift, see Davis, "Constructing Normalcy," 3–16.
34. Paré, *Des Monstres et prodiges,* 73.
35. Paré, *Des Monstres et prodiges,* 74.
36. See Andrew Sharpe, *Foucault's Monsters and the Challenge of the Law* (New York: Routledge, 2010), particularly chapter 2, "Foucault's Theoretical Framework," 21–42. See also Michel Foucault, *Abnormal: Lectures at the College de France, 1974–1975* (New York: Picador, 2003).
37. See Elizabeth Stephens, "Queer Monsters: Technologies of Self-Transformation" in Bulwer's *Anthropometamorphosis* and Braidotti's *Metamorphosis,*" in *Somatechnics: Queering the Technologisation of Bodies,* ed. Nikki Sullivan and Samantha Murray (Surrey: Ashgate Publishing, 2009), 171–186. See also Rosi Braidotti, *Metamorphoses: Towards a Materialist Theory of Becoming* (Malden: Blackwell Publishers, 2002).
38. One justified, however, by Madame Tetralini's line in Tod Browning's *Freaks* (1932): "God takes care of all of his children," implying that even the freaks, just vilified by a horrified groundskeeper who discovers them on his employer's estate, are loved by God, an Augustinian touch in the middle of a film that militantly favors the "freaks."

CHAPTER 19

Monster Spawn of Animal Experimentation in the Early Work of H. G. Wells: On the Containment of Psychopathic Violence as Preliminary to the Onset of the Capacity for Mourning

Laurence A. Rickels

Animal Identification

H. G. Wells's mother staged her inability to mourn her missing daughter Fanny with the next in line, her son Herbert. Dressed up as Fanny (as seen in a photograph included in Wells's autobiography), Herbert gives the address of a work of mourning that lay upon him as an obscure charge but which he brought to completion on his mother's better behalf during his first season of authorship between *The Time Machine* (1895) and *The War of the Worlds* (1898). By all accounts, the mother's participation in the mourning show only went the distance she kept. For Herbert, the maternal environment provisionally bereft of Fanny was that of his own deprivation of goods, the condition, as we shall see, according to D. W. Winnicott that can lead to antisocial tendencies and, via their consolidation through secondary gains, to psychopathy. That the science fiction genre is particularly suited for consideration of the problem and topic of containment and integration of the relationship to psychopathy appears more evident in post–World War II works like Philip K. Dick's *Do Androids Dream of Electric Sheep?* (1968). But that the connection is less historically determined and more genre-specific or intrapsychic can be discerned in the early development of Wells's fiction till the release of the science fiction *The War of the Worlds*.

In *The War of the Worlds,* we are informed that among the lessons learned during mankind's brief sojourn as Martian cattle was the urgency of lessening the suffering of the animals we keep close to us. The loop that opens here begins to close in *Do Androids Dream of Electric Sheep?* where the testable distinction of being human begins with identification with animals. But at its opening, the loop marks the inward turn of this identification as incarnation of the early effort to secure what Melanie Klein theorized as the all-important relationship to the internal good object. Before the totemic animal emerges as mournable under the aegis of father, our first critters are delegates of our unmournables: mother, children, and siblings.

Prior to *The War of the Worlds,* Wells published the liminal science fictions, *The Island of Dr. Moreau* (1896) and *The Invisible Man* (1897), which thematize, under the multi- aegis of deprivation, psychopathy, and monstrous figurations of transference, the work of integration preliminary to the onset of the capacity for mourning. Wells followed *The Time Machine* not with *The Island of Dr. Moreau,* however, but with *The Wonderful Visit* (1895), in which an angel on earth must become human or otherwise adapt to the fallen state. An enabling condition of the sci-fi genre is the alternation at its boundary with the fantasy genre, which signifies the metabolic change required before there can be acceptance of the sci-fi task of expanding the finitude of remembrance. Between *The Island of Dr. Moreau* and *The Invisible Man,* Wells published *The Wheels of Chance* (1896), a comedic novel about cycling and social change—another drop scene inserted within the relay of liminal science fictions that slowed down the identification of Wells's work as science fiction. What *The Invisible Man* posits and pursues as unknown ingredient of a never-before-seen state and change emerges for the first time fully recognizable as techno future from outer space in the 1898 novel that closes this preamble. The summary work at the summit of Wells's psy-fi drive introduces the Martian invasion as interruption of the philosopher-protagonist's treatise on the future while projecting the advance of the threat, as it advances, as gigantic writing machine. Inside the machine, the Martians communicate by telepathy only; on the outside, the machine imposes blackout conditions on the space of legibility: "It would have seemed as if some monstrous pen had flung ink upon the chart. Steadily, incessantly, each black splash grew and spread . . . exactly as a gout of ink would spread itself upon blotting paper."[1] But this extermination-writing machine also clears away the blotting to grasp its progress. "The glittering Martians went to and fro, calmly and methodically spreading their poison cloud over this patch of country and then over that, laying it again with their stream jets when it had served its purpose, and taking possession of the conquered country."[2] The intervention from outer space ultimately returns the philosopher to his writing project, which was as much blocked as interrupted, but in a resetting mutated by internal conditions of the overturning of the extermination-writing machine. The Earthlings, who can't defeat the technologically advanced vampire brains from outer space, nevertheless prevail by dint of their own mortality, the evolutionary milieu that guarantees survival of what Wells names in the title of his autobiography an ordinary brain. The microbial organisms that attack human bodies when they lapse into lifelessness take the Martians for dead and set about disposing of them as corpses while yet alive:

> But by virtue of . . . natural selection of our kind we have developed resisting power; to no germs do we succumb without a struggle, and to many—those that cause putrefaction in dead matter, for instance—our living frames are altogether immune . . . By the toll of a billion deaths man has bought his birthright of the earth.[3]

To be taken for dead while alive and yet to survive is the closing image of the ordinary human bond of relationality that Wells's philosopher-narrator gives as his conclusion. "And strangest of all is it to hold my wife's hand again, and to think that I have counted her, and that she has counted me, among the dead." This surviving acknowledgment of the death wish at close quarters is the intrapsychic counterpart to the victory over the Martians.

These developments follow Wells's biographical blurb that opens with his 1890 degree in zoology and the commencement of his teaching career.[4] Science fiction proper follows Wells's turn to a substitutive economy of transference with the replacement in 1894 of his first wife, the cousin he married in 1891, with his second wife, who was one of his students.[5] That he characterizes his incestuous choice (in *An Experiment in Autobiography*[6]) as unmarked and unmediated by reading brings her that much closer to Weena, the lost object the time traveler must give up, but then lets go as but the memory of pain in a dream. In *The War of the Worlds* we end up with the couple that has internalized conditions of mourning that were still out there, liminally disseminated, as haunting in *The Time Machine,* the opening bookend of Wells's prefatory progress toward science fiction. *The Time Machine* closes upon the nonreturn of the time traveler from the trip he took upon recounting his first episode in the future, the main body of Wells's narrative. Although the loss of Weena returned from that future muted as memory of a dream, the traveler sets out on a suicide mission of identification with loss, one that, after three years have passed, everyone knows has exceeded the two-year period of expectations for his comeback. He ends up, then, back there with ghosts who, however, no longer break through to the present (since he took them with him). Wells's narrative leaves the underworld of the mortally ill and exquisite Eloi behind. Their second deaths, deferred through "more locks" upon the "wells," otherwise control releasing their relationship as cattle to the Morlocks.[7] The span that lands Wells inside science fiction thus begins and ends as contemplation and survival of an aberrant reversal that treats humans as the livestock of aggressors.

The closing sentence of *The War of the Worlds* marking the mutation—the introjection of the death-wish dynamic of mourning—follows the narrator-protagonist's return home: just as he despairs that he is sole survivor he hears his thoughts projected out loud just outside the door: "And there, amazed and afraid, even as I stood amazed and afraid, were my cousin and my wife."[8] While cousin and wife are separated out for the conversation just overheard and the protagonist catches his wife alone in a dead faint in his arms, Wells's cousin-wife in one can also be overheard as named, as well as the wife separated out from that double identity (of cousin-wife), standing up to the acknowledgment of death wishes at close quarters.

What falls to the opposing side of the test for empathy in *Do Androids Dream of Electric Sheep?* would be, by implication and silence on Dick's part, psychopathy or sociopathy. That these terms are loose in the canon of clinical assessment only underscores their uncanny association with untreatability and the failure of interpretation. D. W. Winnicott sought to retrofit what he would rename neurotic analysis to admit the psychopath. For the best treatment outcome, he nipped the budding psychopath by intervening early in the antisocial tendencies of children—disturbances in development prior to the advent of the capacity for mourning, toward which he, in theory, was ushering his clients. "Mourning itself," Winnicott advises and admits, "indicates maturity in the . . . ego of the individual."[9] The antisocial tendencies in young children, which can, once consolidated and rationalized for secondary gain, spawn the psychopath, are symptoms of deprivations in and of the holding environment prior to the egoic maturity set for mourning, but also at an age old enough to be beyond fateful internalization of this environmental fault line. In Winnicott's estimation, there are certain advantages to the industry of the psychopath over the psychotic's playing dead or the neurotic's endless involution of dependency.

According to Winnicott, the child, whose grounds for stealing or acting destructively are as yet unconscious, signals with each delinquent act both the importance of the environment and the return of hope.[10] These two senses or directions of delinquency must be met halfway and held together by analyst and family if testing for love in all the wrong places is to be reversed and the child replaced on the path toward integration and mourning. Winnicott's attribution of hope's expression to the antisocial child's first delinquencies resonates, especially given the importance of the environment these acts simultaneously illuminate, with a sense of hope to which the history of the word tracks back. Preserved to this day as the cognate *verhoffen* in the German "language of hunters,"[11] hope originally designated the startle response that allows animal and human alike to consider, in pulling back before a blockage in the intended path, the alternate directions to take within a suddenly altered environment. The moment of hope thus gives pause for thought or reality testing while marking the spot of identification and prehistory we occupy with the animal.

By implication and passing reference, Winnicott situates the animal relation within the primal maternal provision: for good-enough mothering the mother needs only "a chance to be natural . . . in the way that mothers have . . . since the dawn of human history, and indeed before the evolution of man from mammal."[12] The small creatures Freud identified (e.g., in *Group Psychology and the Analysis of the Ego* [1921]) as carriers of souls of the dead and as representatives of sibling bonds are identified by Klein[13] as scurrying across the struggle to resecure the inner world, the agon of mourning according to her rereading of Freud's "Mourning and Melancholi."[14]

Prior to mourning, however, the resecuring of relations with the internal good object can ground a child's derailment into antisocial tendencies. As cited in Klein's "Infantile Anxiety Situations Reflected in a Work of Art and in the Creative Impulse,"[15] the boy faced with homework in Ravel's opera *L'Enfant et les Sortilèges* (1925) (or rather in Collette's libretto) feels an upsurge of rebelliousness against the stupid lessons: "Want to go for a walk in the park! I'd like best of all to eat up all the cake in the world, or pull the cat's tail r pull out all the parrot's feathers! I'd like to scold every one! Most of all I'd like to put mama in the corner!"[16] When he sticks out his tongue at his mother who comes to inquire about his progress, she promises him dry bread and tea without sugar for his efforts. When she's gone, the boy starts raging. In the interior scene on which the boy's tantrum is set, the caged squirrel he attacks, like the pendulum he wrenches out of the clock, represents the father's penis inside the mother. "The fact that it is the father's penis and that it is in the act of coitus with the mother is indicated by the rent in the wallpaper 'which separates Corydon from his Amaryllis,' all of which it has been said that to the boy it has become 'a rent in the fabric of the world.' "[17] Klein shows here what it takes for the boy to imagine being able to pay the "rent" revealed to him in or as his primal scene and fill in the paternal gap inside the mother and her substitutes.

When he goes outside, chased out of doors by an associate of the clock, the boy is greeted by trees that react not to the most recent tantrum but to a whole phase of his scientific research, which has led him repeatedly to carve wounds in their bark with his knife. Now he feels remorse: doubly so when the dragonfly demands back the companion the boy had netted and then stuck against the wall with a pin. When the animals forget about their complaints in celebration of animal joy, the child feels the process as his elimination: "They've forgotten me . . . I'm alone."[18] Then they forget one another as they unite to fight the boy but then end up fighting each other. They wound one of their own, the squirrel that escaped the child's research cage, but not before the boy in his fit jabbed it with his pen. Now the boy binds the squirrel's double wound and falls back unconscious. Fearing for the child they now praise as kind and wise, as healer, the animals rebroadcast the "Mama" they overheard him call out earlier: it is the magic word promised by the opera's title. Thus the repaired animal relation repairs the boy with his mother.

Monsters of Transference

In both *The Island of Dr. Moreau* and *The Invisible Man,* the datemark of the fictional worlds submitted for their future historicization is vivisection as norm in science and contemporary topic of controversy in society. Prendick, the protagonist-narrator of *The Island of Dr. Moreau,* is witness to the animal experimentation of the doctor and his assistant Montgomery. He doesn't like hearing the puma shriek:

> Yet had I known such pain was in the next room, and had it been dumb, I believe—I have thought since—I could have stood it well enough. It is when suffering finds a voice and sets our nerves quivering that this pity comes troubling us.[19]

When he is reassured that the experiments humanize animals rather than bestialize men—he wasn't willing to abide vivisection of humans, which he came to believe was the crux of the secret experiments—his remaining doubt is the very kernel of speciesism: "They may once have been animals. But I never before saw an animal trying to think."[20]

Only posttraumatic cosmetic surgery has come close to Dr. Moreau's handling of vivisection. Otherwise he inherits a secret practice, as in the medieval fabrication of show-monsters (as described by Victor Hugo in *The Man Who Laughs*) or in the "artistic torture" of the Inquisition, which, Dr. Moreau is convinced, always ultimately allowed "scientific curiosity" to cut in. But the doctor "was the first man to take up this question armed with antiseptic surgery, and with a really scientific knowledge of the laws of growth."[21] The note that closes the narrative wraps the earlier appearance of one of its parts in a magazine as reality effect: "the manufacture of monsters—and perhaps even *quasi*-human monsters—is within the possibilities of vivisection."[22]

That Prendick is hung up on the evidence of pain qualifies him as "materialist" in Dr. Moreau's book. "So long as visible or audible pain turns you sick, so long as your own pains drive you, so long as pain underlies your propositions about sin, so long, I tell you, you are an animal, thinking a little less obscurely what an animal feels."[23] Pain as a medical index that warns and stimulates us is marked like the appendix for evolutionary extinction. "This store men and women set on pleasure and pain, Prendick, is the mark of the beast upon them, the mark of the beast from which they came."[24]

The island is now populated with the experiments Dr. Moreau once deemed successful but then, on second thought, abandoned as botched. "These creatures of mine seemed strange and uncanny to you as soon as you began to observe them, but to me, just after I make them, they seem to be indisputable human beings. It's afterwards as I observe them that the persuasion fades."[25] This fadeout is the disappointment of identification that Dr. Moreau withdraws from the transferential construction of his creatures, which protects him from responsibility for their failed, fallen, and fatal condition. On their own, Dr. Moreau advises, the Beast Folk pursue

> a kind of mockery of a rational life—poor beasts! There's something they call the Law . . . . But I can see through it all, see into their very souls, and see there nothing but the souls of beasts, beasts that perish . . . . There is a kind of upward striving in them, part vanity, part waste sexual emotion, part waste curiosity. It only mocks me.[26]

It is a projection of waste that refers to the doctor's controlling interest in his own resources. Only Prendick, as we will see, indicates a prehistory for this waste management, to which his doubles on the I-land equally belong.

Dr. Moreau's testimony notwithstanding, the totemic environment he establishes is in working order. Montgomery attributes his and the doctor's relative safety in the midst of the monsters to "certain Fixed Ideas implanted by Moreau in their minds which absolutely bounded their imaginations. They were really hypnotised, had been told certain things were impossible, and certain things were not to be done, and these prohibitions were woven into the texture of their minds beyond any possibility of disobedience or dispute."[27] The series of propositions called the Law nevertheless "battled in their minds with the deep-seated, ever rebellious cravings of their animal natures."[28] Thus the Law—of denial—is perpetually repeated and perpetually broken.

From the point of view of relative safety, the gist of the Law was to keep the creatures "ignorant of the taste of blood."[29] The shadow of this law falls on Prendick when it comes to creaturely laughter. "None could laugh," he concludes.[30] But then he discerns that one of the monsters is indeed laughing—at him.[31] And then when Dr. Moreau sends a pack of Law-abiding creatures to seize a Law breaker, Prendick recognizes that the Wolf-Bear is "laughing" into his face "with the exultation of hunting."[32] The inverted world in which we register our problem with food and death, which was tracked specifically with regard to laughter by Henri Bergson,[33] yields a denial of the value of life which is basic to specism (as well as, according to Theodor Adorno,[34] to fascism).[35]

Prendick admits a "strange contradiction" in the face of the creature "distorted with terror." Though the hunted creature crouches "in a perfectly animal attitude," the hunter recognizes in the scared face "the fact of its humanity."[36] A heartbeat earlier, at the gathering of creatures called on to hunt down the transgressor, he wondered, looking at the group, how he "had ever believed them to be men."[37] As is underscored when Dr. Moreau must be buried, the creatures are indeed us, the only mark of their distinction being something akin to transference: they "lived in a fear that never died, fretted by law they could not understand; their mock-human existence began in an agony, was one long internal struggle."[38] And for what, Prendick asks himself. "It was the wantonness that stirred me."[39]

As the realm of Dr. Moreau begins to break down and yields casualties to be buried, the new task of representation as interment strikes Prendick, suddenly, "like a wave across" his mind, as nadir of despair. But "the realisation of the unspeakable aimlessness of things upon the island"[40] also restarts his identification of the creatures as his identification with them. "A strange persuasion came upon me that, save for the grossness of the line, the grotesqueness of the forms, I had here before me the whole balance of human life in miniature, the whole interplay of instinct, reason, and fate, in its simplest form."[41] The defective cornerstone of Moreau's world, however, as issued in the codex of denial, is burial, which the creatures, on the basis of curiosity deemed human, cannot accept as lasting, not the first time around. "The Beast People manifested a quite human curiosity about the dead body," which was being carried to the sea for burial.[42] Part of this curiosity is contained in one of the prohibitions not "to go scratching at the graves of the dead."[43] We break through, then, to the other primal question, alongside: Where do babies come from? Where do the dead go? Where are they kept?

The burial detail does not carry forward an earlier loss but rather a message of meaninglessness and a lack of matching affect. One man's sentimentality is another's affection deficit. Whining about his lot in life in the wake of Dr. Moreau's dying, Montgomery asks Prendick what it all means, in other words: "Are we bubbles blown by a baby?"[44] Before he turns the conversation to the practical purpose of survival, an unkind thought crosses Prendick's mind, a condemnation that must be kin to his upbringing or descent: "It was hard to deal with such ravings."[45] This voice rejecting spontaneity as excess that is hard to bear brings back what it brought about: Prendick's deprivation in early childhood.

But when early memory was first triggered by the contact with Dr. Moreau, what had come back extended only to adolescence. Ten years ago, before science scandal caused him to withdraw from the public sphere, Dr. Moreau offered his know-how as latter-day Baroque play. Prendick remembers a screen word that then fills with a horror that has trouble finding its name: " 'The Moreau—Hollows' was it? 'The Moreau—?' Ah! it sent my memories back ten years. 'The Moreau Horrors'."[46] Mourning means, in bottom line, that a place can be found in psychic reality for absence. But in another psychic constitution the bottom line that has been reached is

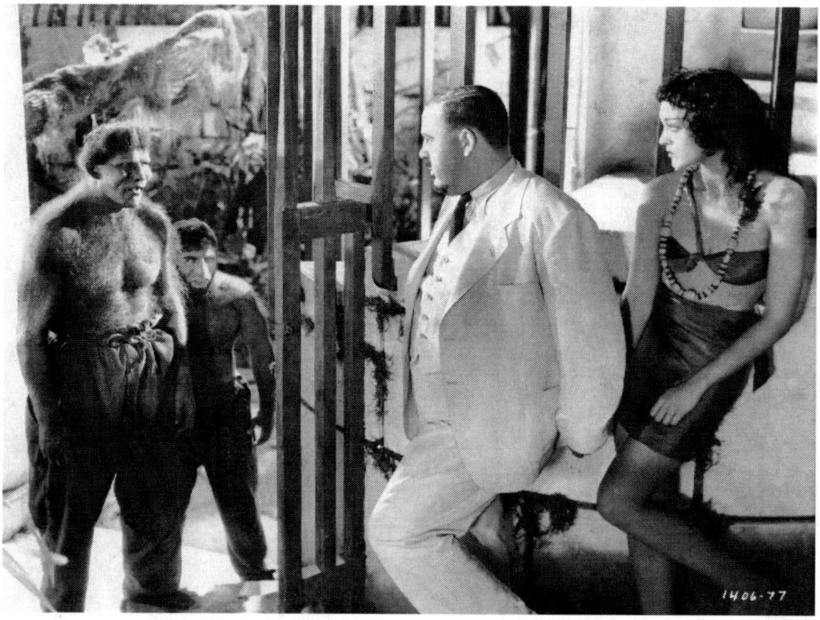

Figure 19.1 Dr. Moreau (Charles Laughton) confronts Ouran (Hans Steinke) in *Island of Lost Souls* (1932). (Courtesy of Paramount Pictures).

a "hollow," the vacuum of meaninglessness as nothingness that can contain itself only through multiplication as more and more fragments and voids. Dr. Moreau's menagerie fulfils this gap.

The border between human and animal is where the psychopath as older child or teen rehearses a certain lack of concern about the suffering of the other (as nuanced in Figure 19.1). When swaying and saying the precepts of the Law with the creatures around the bend or blend between animal and human Prendick can only imagine that he "was already dead and in another world."[47] It's an image that is supposed to call to mind derangement, though in the Christian frame it is also the image of release obtained through neglect of mourning: Let the dead bury the dead.

Since Prendick, who has been "an abstainer from . . . birth,"[48] will not join in mourning carousal following Dr. Moreau's demise, Montgomery turns to the Beast People to comfort him by partaking of drink and dirge with him. When Prendick nevertheless rushes to Montgomery's aid, though the gunshots that summon him also signal that he's too late, he knocks over a lamp that lights the displaced pyre and destroys the inheritance of Dr. Moreau. Now he survives under the protection of the dog hybrid alone, while at best tolerated by the rest of the Beast People, who are devolving. The canine–human protection restores a breach and brings Prendick back to the border that could not withstand the deprivation.

If canine companionship as the delegation of our first contact with animal trainability represents a prosthetic missing link, then the monkey hybrid is the missing link proper, simulated as monstrosity of language. But the devolution that packs relationality inside the person of the dog travels the same transference tracks as the sliding scale of the man/animal distinction overheard in the language of aping. Prendick's disdain for the Monkey Man's accomplishments is that of a first-generation academic for his student body transmitting loss in generation.

> He had a fantastic trick of coining new words. He had an idea, I believe, that to gabble about names that meant nothing was the proper use of speech. He called it "big thinks," to distinguish it from "little thinks"—the sane everyday interests of life. If ever I made a remark

he did not understand, he would praise it very much, ask me to say it again, learn it by heart, and go off repeating it, with a word wrong here or there, to all the milder of the Beast People. He thought nothing of what was plain and comprehensible. I invented some very curious "big thinks" for his especial use.[49]

Prendick is able to join the Monkey Man's network by a double mimicry of and in the medium of "big thinks" that, after all, subsumes their efforts. Countertransference says that there is nothing to the teen idiom of wordplay and acronym. And yet it is the regenerative power of language the teen comes into as metabolization of the pressures upon him of technologization and massification. Not restricted to second-generation adolescence, the initial personalization of language continues as jargon in scientific and theoretical work or as the idiom of news-speak.

"Big thinks" attains recognition value in the retrospect of devolution that afflicts language at the same time as it erodes the Law, the totemic system organized around the control release of the double issue of food and death:

My Ape Man's jabber multiplied in volume, but grew less and less comprehensible, more and more simian. Some of the others seemed altogether slipping their hold upon speech, though they still understood what I said to them at that time. Can you imagine language, once clear-cut and exact, softening and guttering, losing shape and import, becoming mere lumps of sound again?[50]

As the anthropomorphism slips away there remains to Dr. Moreau's creatures a monstrosity sustained as blending or fragmenting of traits into "the animal," the single term that "big thinks" reserves for an otherwise highly differentiated nonhuman world or word:

Of course these creatures did not decline into such beasts as the reader has seen in zoological gardens—into ordinary bears, wolves, tigers, oxen, swine, and apes. There was still something strange about each; in each Moreau had blended this animal with that; one perhaps was ursine chiefly, another feline chiefly, another bovine chiefly, but each was tainted with other creatures—a kind of generalised animalism appeared throughout the specific dispositions.[51]

Monstrosity emerges then out of a doodling visualization of the taxonomies of zoology as they recombine into "the animal" of the philosophical distinction between animal and man.

The distinction between human and animal remains on the verge of coming across as long as the change of devolution is gradual. "For them and for me it came without any definite shock. I still sent among them in safety, because no jolt in the downward glide had released the increasing charge of explosive animalism that ousted the human day by day. But I began to fear that soon now that shock must come."[52] The shock that comes with the murder of Prendick's canine protector is carried forward into his post-rescue existence. He is "haunted" by memories of Dr. Moreau's island. In time the "terror" becomes his "disease."

My trouble took the strangest form. I could not persuade myself that the men and women I met were not also another, still passably human, Beast People, animals half-wrought into the outward image of human souls; and that they would presently begin to revert, to show first this bestial mark and then that. But I have confided my case to a strangely able man, a man who had known Moreau, and seemed half to credit my story, a mental specialist—and he has helped me mightily.[53]

That the psychiatrist who treats Prendick credits the story and even knows Moreau is transferential by-product of the talking cure. Nevertheless, Prendick has to leave London where his horror of the shock of devolution was so hard to contain. Somewhere away from the mad-making crowds, he remains stable between his books and chemistry experiments. But it is in the contemplation of the night sky that he obtains a sense of "infinite peace and protection": "There it must be, I think, in the vast and eternal laws of matter, and not in the daily cares and sins and troubles of men, that whatever is more than animal within us must find its solace and its hope."[54] We're at the end of the narrative, though first "hope" is mentioned two more times: "I hope, or I could not live. And so, in hope and solitude, my story ends."[55]

The night sky in which Prendick finds hope restored is an external image of his relationship to the inner world of his good objects, which remains up in the air, uninherited, and up for grabs. As Klein writes with regard to a similar scene of contemplation,[56] "I would also interpret his intent gazing at the stars as an attempt to regain his good objects which he feels are lost or far away."[57] Later on, she links this literary figure to the experience of patients: "such phantasies have far-reaching consequences and vitally influence the structure of the ego. They have the effect that those parts of his self from which he feels estranged, often including his emotions, are not at the time accessible either to the analyst or to the patient."[58]

TRANS-PARENT

What subsumes all of the above is the literary figure of Prendick's autoanalysis dependent upon a hope that is taken from animals. In Wells's next liminal science fiction, *The Invisible Man,* the protagonist is lost to mad science and psychopathic violence, while those who witness his rise and demise must build upon the assumption that the protagonist engaged in animal vivisection as containment of the violence preliminary to the onset of the capacity for mourning. The protagonist's inability to take responsibility for his dead father, which precedes the successful experimentation, is carried forward as the charge of vivisection his neighbors make against him, which first breaches the confidentiality of his experiments with the stolen inheritance.

When "after three years of secrecy and exasperation" the man who would be invisible found that owing to shortage of funds, the completion of his experiments with omnipotence would be "impossible—impossible," he robbed his old man, who then killed himself because the money taken wasn't his.[59] The thought Winnicott wagered that the unconscious significance of stealing was to get back what was one's own, namely the maternal relation, completes itself as the father killing himself over a loss that was not his own. The thieving or reclaiming son completes this significance by splitting the scene of the dead father's commemoration. Though the "current cant required . . . attendance at his funeral," the man in search of his own invisibility found it an "unmeaning tragedy."[60] He continues, "I appreciated my loss of sympathy, but I put it down to the general inanity of things. Reentering my room seemed like the recovery of reality. There were the things I knew and loved. There stood the apparatus, the experiments arranged and waiting."[61] We're now on the same page with his history: "In all my great moments I have been alone."

He is alone with the missing object relation, the object of which he was deprived but which he hopefully reasserts claim to by his antisocial acting out. His psychopathic industry keeps him moving along the lines of reality testing, however displaced from the maternal objective that remains buried in the past. What is hard to recombine is the environment the psychopath tests for its capacity to endure him—complete with his feeling or feelings unattractive—and its origin in or as the mother, in whom, at the time of deprivation, he couldn't find fault.

What follows his first crime, then, was his first successful experiment with a bit of white wool: he saw it "fade" like a "wreath of smoke," like the respect he paid his father, "and vanish." When he tested invisibility on a cat, however, the animal didn't vanish: "there remained two little ghosts of her eyes."[62] He lets the virtually invisible cat go when the animal's crying in his abode threatens to belie his rejection of the charge that he is a vivisectionist. The failure of the animal experiment leads to thoughts of his father's funeral.[63]

In his experiments with invisibility, he discovers not only that man is better suited than glass or diamonds—"*he's more transparent*!"[64]—but even that an albino like himself is the perfect vehicle since the pigments were next to impossible to make disappear. Now he could only imagine "what it meant to be an albino with such knowledge."[65] Invisibility thus confers on him the doubling of the sense or direction of oversight: overlooked as albino outcast he overlooks the environment as mastermind once he completes his albino condition as the new and improved status of invisibility or, more specifically, transparency. While he can steal upon objects in the environment, the objects remain visible, on the outside as well as inside the transparent man. Here, we see clearly the illumination of the importance of the environment that Winnicott underscores as basic to the hopeful significance of delinquent acts.

The ease with which he will be able to steal once invisible is his most available omnipotent thought. When criminality appears as the logical consequence of being able to operate invisibly, he is disappointed to discover that everything he can indeed obtain unseen he can never enjoy unseen. Since the loot is visible, stealing it is as difficult as it looks. If someone gets in his way during a covert operation, then he simply knocks him out, ties him up, and leaves him there. To become recognizable in the field of his stealth, whether to obtain basic services or to enjoy the objects of theft, he must become a mummy: "And for this I had become a wrapped-up mystery, a swathed and bandaged caricature of a man!"[66] The melancholic ingredient that's under wraps can be read off the back of this incarnation not only in name but also in the alternation this occult figure undergoes, like the werewolf, with exhibitionism.

In following out his discovery and invention, the invisible man repeats his undercover status in the psychopathic milieu of academe:

> I had to do my work under frightful disadvantages. Oliver, my professor, was a scientific bounder, a journalist by instinct, a thief of ideas.... I simply would not publish, and let him share my credit. I went on working, I got nearer and nearer making my formula into an experiment, a reality. I told no living soul, because I meant to flash my work upon the world with crushing effect—to become famous at a blow.[67]

Following the lead of his albino status, he "took up the question of pigments to fill up certain gaps"[68] and by accident, coincidence, or merger discovered that blood can be rendered colorless while leaving its functions intact.[69] It is this great step forward—toward incorporation of the original blood bond—that coincided with the exhaustion of funds and the recourse to stealing backing from his father.

For the overlooked academic, there's the mad science of invisibility or there's the allotment of life as "a shabby, poverty-struck, hemmed-in demonstrator, teaching fools in a provincial college."[70] It is also, then, responsibility to and for the transferential relationship that the invisible man abandons for his new existence as stealth actor-out. But it is the transference he threw away that now must come around for the narrative of his case. Only when the invisible man fortuitously encounters in his flight someone from his own pre-invisibility milieu at the university, Dr. Kemp, who knew him well enough to overlook him, does he tell his story: "Practically, I thought I had impunity to do whatever I chose, everything—save to give away my secret."[71] Thus it is up to Dr. Kemp to respond, like a therapist, in lieu of the invisible man's missing response:

> "Knocked him on the head!" exclaimed Kemp.
>
> "Yes—stunned him—as he was going downstairs.... He went downstairs like a bag of old boots."

"But—I say! The common conventions of humanity—"

"Are all very well for common people."[72]

That the invisible man finds no respite from the scrutiny of "common people" and thus becomes, in response, increasingly violent, beginning with the cat experiment that miscarries while carrying forward his dead father. Invisibility elevated his outcast status as albino to ultimate precondition for this experiment: of all test subjects, the albino is the most "transparent" or, in other words, the one least fettered by parental guidance. And yet any intake of the environment—the point of maternal contact—annuls his transparency.

In the course of his invisibility he staggers the crime against his father, of which his animal experiment is the souvenir, as stealing first, then murder. "This invisibility, in fact, is only good in two cases: It's useful in getting away, it's useful in approaching. It's particularly useful, therefore, in killing."[73]

Kemp is to serve as the invisible man's "goal-keeper," "helper," and "hiding-place," a place of rest and transition that will allow him to go beyond the small-time antisocial behavior of his solo acting out. Thus the invisible man proposes not "wanton killing, but a judicious slaying."[74] What he now proposes is a "Reign of Terror." But the host of his last resort or respite was, while actively listening to the invisible man, waiting for the authorities to descend upon him. When the invisible man escapes, Kemp reduces the man's discourse of exchange and support to criminality beyond the pale: "He is mad," said Kemp; "inhuman. He is pure selfishness. He thinks of nothing but his own advantage, his own safety. I have listened to such a story this morning of brutal self-seeking!"[75] Kemp promptly comes up with the strategy of strewing powdered glass on all the roads to let invisibility bleed and read.[76] When the police chief issues the understatement that the strategy is "unsportsmanlike,"[77] Kemp reassures the posse, once again, that the man hiding out in invisibility has become "inhuman."

In no time the invisible man's first fatal act of violence takes place. The motivation is "impossible to imagine"—"save in a murderous frenzy."[78] "Indeed, the theory of madness is almost unavoidable." But a "voice heard about sunset . . . wailing and laughing, sobbing and groaning"[79] confirms reservations held on behalf of the invisible man:

> He was certainly an intensely egotistical and unfeeling man, but the sight of his victim, his first victim, bloody and pitiful at his feet, may have released some long pent fountain of remorse which for a time may have flooded whatever scheme of action he had contrived.[80]

But then he loses all empathy upon issuing his first proclamation as "Invisible Man the First"[81]: he will execute Kemp to establish his power as "Death, the unseen Death."[82]

And yet the reservation is held by Kemp for us, the readership. When Kemp tries to stay the mob execution, it's too late. Like the transparent man of anatomy lessons, the dead man begins putting on invisibility from the inside out. "And so, slowly, beginning at his hands and feet and creeping along his limbs to the vital centres of his body, that strange change continued. It was like the slow spreading of a poison."[83] The relationship to the body—to the mother's body—returns as discard, as toxic waste. His "crushed" body, the "drawn and battered features" of his face, the expression of "anger and dismay," come into focus, whereupon they cover him with a sheet.

THE SCHIZOID

At the close of "Transitional Objects and Transitional Phenomena," Winnicott places psychopathy on one side of the parting of ways at the end of the transitional phase.[84] On the one side we find the development of so-called cultural interests. But if it's not that way, the other way is the path of addiction (fixation on the unchallenged transitional phenomenon), fetishism (persistence of a specific object or type of object dating from infancy and linked to the "delusion of a maternal phallus"), and pseudologia fantastica and thieving (which follow out the "unconscious urge to bridge a gap in continuity of experience in respect of a transitional object"[85]).

The underside of the urge to bridge the gap, which drives the delinquent activity of stealing, is the insistence that only the gap exists, as in the case of a schizoid patient Winnicott includes in his remix of the original transitional article for *Playing and Reality*.[86] Underexposed to the graduated experience of the mother's failure, which is the other meaning of the requirement that the mother be "good-enough," this patient just can't deal with what Winnicott regularly terms, between valuation and photographic development, the negative side of relationships. Over time the patient "reached the position . . . that the only real thing is the gap; that is to say, the death or the absence or the amnesia."[87]

And yet the urge to deny this absence as the only positive or real element is also still in attendance: as in the chain through which in her dream she is tied to an eagle. Another client, who used strings to deny his separation anxiety, was similarly in a "tie-up" on the range where the transitional phenomena of interweaving are at home. While the string can be viewed as another technique of communication (like the telephone[88]), once its function changes from communication into denial of separation (which can also happen with the use of the phone)—once strings are attached—it "becomes a thing in itself, something that has dangerous properties and needs must be mastered."[89] Used as a communications device, the string still contains hope. But when the hope is gone with the transformation, "a much more complex state of affairs has arisen—one that becomes difficult to cure, because of the secondary gains that arise out of the skill that develops whenever an object has to be handled in order to be mastered."

In "The Absence of a Sense of Guilt,"[90] Winnicott elevates the schizoid to join the company of teens and psychotics, with the difference that, as verso of the psychopath, the schizoid also struggles with the developmental norm to which he stands in the relationship of near miss:

> And now finally let me introduce you to some of the things that our schizoid patients teach us, or require us to know. These patients are in some ways more moral than we are, but they are of course terribly uncomfortable. They perhaps prefer to remain uncomfortable and not to be "cured." Sanity spells compromise. That is what they feel to be wicked. Extra-marital intercourse is of no consequence to them as compared with betrayal of the self. And it is true (I think I could show you) that sane people relate to the world by what I call cheating.[91]

If the child can early on amp up the basic experience of the object given as the object the infant found and then created to include his sense of creation of the world—thereby allowing a surfeit of experience of omnipotence preliminary to giving it over to external reality or to God—then, and only then, can an "ethically respectable" sanity be obtained before "cheating" becomes of consequence. What the schizoid teaches Winnicott is this deep sense of cheating between the norm and the other norm.[92] As in the case of the psychopath, then, the schizoid is in a failing relationship to his omnipotence. More specifically, however, Winnicott lodges the schizoid plaint against the sense of guilt.[93]

When the infant becomes aware that he has impulses and entertains ideas (as entertaining) which are destructive—I love you, I eat you—"there is a clear and natural beginning of a personal sense of guilt," as Freud says. He continues, "the sense of guilt enables the individual to *be* wicked."[94] Being wicked means to feel just awful after the thought of eating mother crosses your mind. The urge to be constructive or reparative springs from this awfulness. "If the child's sense of guilt is absent in the pattern," Freud says, "then the child does not get so far as allowing the impulse. Fear is there instead, and the child is inhibited in respect of the whole of the feeling that naturally builds round this impulse."[95] But if the sense of guilt proves overwhelming, babies die of it or, if they cannot, they organize a compliant or false self—or, in the case of the schizoid-to-be, a holy war against the false self. The false self is seen to betray the true or core self in so far as it seems to succeed in terms of what the onlookers believe to have value. The schizoid is wrecked by this success (the success of cheating).

In the case Winnicott presents episodically in "Withdrawal and Regression,"[96] that of a "schizoid-depressive patient,"[97] it was his interpretation of this patient's initial absences in session as regressions that called attention to the existence of a "medium,"[98] or the need for one, between patient and analyst. This interpretation, which he marks as only possible after his 20 years of work largely with nonclassical, non-neurotic patients, culminates in the patient's being able to hold, finally, the headache he brings to session as the placeholder for his otherwise missing mourning for his dead father.[99] This headache, which seems "as if it were situated just outside the head," and which doesn't cause him to stay home from analysis because his wife didn't provide sympathy, signifies, Winnicott interprets, his wish to have his head held.[100] Then the patient again experiences a momentary withdrawal during which he had the "feeling" that Winnicott had a machine in the office "which would supply the trappings of sympathetic management."[101] In other words, if, rather than interpret, Winnicott had in fact held the patient's head, the gesture would have been mechanical. What emerges from these experiences of a desire to have his head held, via the patient's sudden recollection in session that he (a medical doctor) recently held the head of a child who was undergoing a minor operation and, despite the local anesthesia, was uncomfortable, is the more abiding recollection: the patient feels that he has come up against the fact "that he had never accepted his father's death."[102] It was his father who would have held his child's head: "In other words, after his father's death there was no one to hold his head should he break down into experiencing grief."[103] From a Freudian and Kleinian perspective, it is clear that the father's death signifies the capacity for mourning: he had never been able to mourn.

Winnicott can't get around his sense that for too many patients regression happens, though it may go unrecognized and unused in the session. To this end, he demonstrates here how a patient's withdrawal from the session can be reclaimed for the process by identifying it as regression in the transference. When the patient tells Winnicott about his "withdrawn moment,"[104] he adds that he at the same time had the idea of being curled up precariously positioned to fall. Winnicott recognizes in the withdrawal as regression the first "direct evidence . . . of a spontaneous self."[105] Winnicott already mentioned the loss of the father at age 18 in introducing the case subject. But we weren't ready yet for its communication through the "medium."[106] Winnicott spells out the baby steps of interpretation to follow: "In speaking of yourself as curled up and moving round, you are at the same time implying something which naturally you are not describing since you are not aware of it; you imply the *existence of a medium*."[107] That seems a mouthful for someone who strives to withhold interpretations, and the conclusion as formulation seems abstract and obscure. But the patient is a professional whose own diction may have been, since he was schizoid, constitutively abstract and full of the makeshift syntax of distance. What's more, "the existence of a medium" underscores a séance quality to this medium as to their session which from his own conceivable dabbling in occult news topics he might well have been prepared to follow. The patient immediately understood, though, shifting from the occult to the technical register (which also means, however, that one can shift back again): "Like the oil in which wheels move."[108] Winnicott continues,

> Following this the patient had a very important dream, and the analysis of this showed that he had been able to discard a shield which was now no longer necessary since I had proved

> myself capable of supplying a suitable medium at the moment of his withdrawal. It appears that *through my immediately putting a medium around his withdrawn self I had converted his withdrawal into a regression,* and so had enabled him to use this experience constructively.[109]

Weeks later "the patient (unexpectedly from his point of view) came up against the fact that he had never accepted his father's death."[110] The therapeutic use of regression—the viscous medium in question—is theoretically compatible with Freud's lodging of regression inside hallucinations and dreams as their momentum or motor. But therapeutically applied, Winnicott's understanding of regression replaces the throwaway quality of withdrawal of attention, for example, while keeping its ability to travel back in time—or move reality in the past as past reality into the place of the present setting—up and running.

Winnicott discovers this medium via the schizoid, the double of the psychopath on the new frontier of psychoanalysis. The schizoid was as close as Winnicott could get to the mourning. Winnicott, who tended to abandon his own difficulties with mourning to the melancholic legacy of his mentors, Freud and Klein, theorizes and performs the introduction of the prospect of mourning into psychopathic industry and nonrelationality via specialized doubling or regression.

For H. G. Wells, the medium first took off or returned as time machine (which also reclaimed withdrawal of narcissism as regression within the transference), which then, in becoming capable of space travel after four more years, opened up the sci-fi externalization that got him out from under his maternal legacy. The medium took him back in the tracks of animal identification to the original environmental provision. From there he transferred out of the impasse of stealing and hiding into science fiction proper, the hub for rewiring psychopathic preconditions to the productivity of mourning.

NOTES

1. H. G. Wells, *The War of the Worlds, Seven Famous Novels by H. G. Wells* (New York: Alfred A. Knopf, 1979), 334.
2. Wells, *The War of the Worlds,* 334.
3. Wells, *The War of the Worlds,* 380.
4. H. G. Wells, *Experiment in Autobiography: Discoveries and Conclusions of a Very Ordinary Brain (Since 1866)* (New York: The Macmillan Company, 1934), 274–275.
5. Wells, *Experiment in Autobiography,* 310, 354, 364.
6. Wells, *Experiment in Autobiography,* 233.
7. For a more complete reading of *The Time Machine* in terms of the lost objective of mourning, see volume 3 of my *Nazi Psychoanalysis* (Minneapolis, MN: University of Minnesota Press, 2002), 172–178.
8. Wells, *The War of the Worlds,* 385.
9. D. W. Winnicott, "The Psychology of Separation," *Deprivation and Delinquency,* ed. Claire Winnicott, Ray Shepherd, and Madeleine Davis (London and New York: Routledge, 1990), 132.
10. D. W. Winnicott, "The Anti-Social Tendency," in *Collected Papers: Through Paediatrics to Psycho-Analysis* (New York and London: Brunner-Mazel, 1958/1992), 306–315.
11. Friedrich Kluge, "hoffen," in *Etymologisches Wörterbuch der Deutschen Sprache* (Berlin and New York: Walter de Gruyter, 1975), 313.
12. D. W. Winnicott, *Human Nature,* ed. Christopher Bollas, Madeleine Davis, and Ray Shepherd (London: Free Association Books, 1988), 105.
13. See Melanie Klein, "Infantile Anxiety Situations Reflected in a Work of Art and in the Creative Impulse" (1929), in *Love, Guilt and Reparation and Other Works 1921–1945* (New York: The Free Press, 1975), 210–218.

14. See Melanie Klein, "Mourning and Its Relation to Manic-Depressive States" (1940), in *Love, Guilt and Reparation and Other Works 1921–1945* (New York: The Free Press, 1975), 344–369.
15. See Klein, "Infantile Anxiety Situations Reflected in a Work of Art and in the Creative Impulse."
16. Klein, "Infantile Anxiety Situations Reflected in a Work of Art and in the Creative Impulse," 210.
17. Klein, "Infantile Anxiety Situations Reflected in a Work of Art and in the Creative Impulse," 211–212.
18. Melanie Klein, "The Role of the School in the Libidinal Development of the Child (1923)," in *Love, Guilt and Reparation and Other Works 1921–1945* (New York: The Free Press, 1975), 69.
19. H. G. Wells, *The Island of Dr. Moreau* (New York: Dover Publications, 1896/1996), 26.
20. Wells, *The Island of Dr. Moreau,* 51.
21. Wells, *The Island of Dr. Moreau,* 53.
22. Wells, *The Island of Dr. Moreau,* 104.
23. Wells, *The Island of Dr. Moreau,* 54.
24. Wells, *The Island of Dr. Moreau,* 55.
25. Wells, *The Island of Dr. Moreau,* 58.
26. Wells, *The Island of Dr. Moreau,* 59.
27. Wells, *The Island of Dr. Moreau,* 61.
28. Wells, *The Island of Dr. Moreau,* 61.
29. Wells, *The Island of Dr. Moreau,* 61.
30. Wells, *The Island of Dr. Moreau,* 62.
31. Wells, *The Island of Dr. Moreau,* 66.
32. Wells, *The Island of Dr. Moreau,* 71.
33. See Henri Bergson, *Laughter*, trans. Cloudesley Breretson and Fred Rothwell (New York: The Macmillan Company, 1921).
34. See Theodor Adorno, *Minima Moralia: Reflections From Damaged Life*, trans. E. F. N. Jephcott (London: Verson, 1989).
35. For an annotated discussion of this relay of readings that begins with Ella Freeman-Sharpe's identification of the problem of food and death, see my *Ulrike Ottinger. The Autobiography of Art Cinema* (Minneapolis, MN: University of Minnesota Press, 2008), 187–190, 194–195.
36. Wells, *The Island of Dr. Moreau,* 72.
37. Wells, *The Island of Dr. Moreau,* 69.
38. Wells, *The Island of Dr. Moreau,* 74.
39. Wells, *The Island of Dr. Moreau,* 74.
40. Wells, *The Island of Dr. Moreau,* 74.
41. Wells, *The Island of Dr. Moreau,* 73–74.
42. Wells, *The Island of Dr. Moreau,* 73.
43. Wells, *The Island of Dr. Moreau,* 45.
44. Wells, *The Island of Dr. Moreau,* 82.
45. Wells, *The Island of Dr. Moreau,* 82.
46. Wells, *The Island of Dr. Moreau,* 22.
47. Wells, *The Island of Dr. Moreau,* 43.
48. Wells, *The Island of Dr. Moreau,* 20.
49. Wells, *The Island of Dr. Moreau,* 96.
50. Wells, *The Island of Dr. Moreau,* 96.
51. Wells, *The Island of Dr. Moreau,* 97.
52. Wells, *The Island of Dr. Moreau,* 97.
53. Wells, *The Island of Dr. Moreau,* 102.
54. Wells, *The Island of Dr. Moreau,* 104.
55. Wells, *The Island of Dr. Moreau,* 104.
56. Melanie Klein, "On Identification," *Envy and Gratitude and Other Works 1946–1963* (New York: The Free Press, 1975), 141–175.
57. Klein, "On Identification," 152.
58. Klein, "On Identification," 166.

59. H. G. Wells, *The Invisible Man* (New York: Dover Publications, 1897/1992), 66.
60. Wells, *The Invisible Man,* 67.
61. Wells, *The Invisible Man,* 67.
62. Wells, *The Invisible Man,* 68.
63. Wells, *The Invisible Man,* 69.
64. Wells, *The Invisible Man,* 65.
65. Wells, *The Invisible Man,* 66.
66. Wells, *The Invisible Man,* 88.
67. Wells, *The Invisible Man,* 65.
68. Wells, *The Invisible Man,* 65.
69. Wells, *The Invisible Man,* 66.
70. Wells, *The Invisible Man,* 66.
71. Wells, *The Invisible Man,* 87.
72. Wells, *The Invisible Man,* 85.
73. Wells, *The Invisible Man,* 90.
74. Wells, *The Invisible Man,* 91.
75. Wells, *The Invisible Man,* 92.
76. Wells, *The Invisible Man,* 93.
77. Wells, *The Invisible Man,* 94.
78. Wells, *The Invisible Man,* 95.
79. Wells, *The Invisible Man,* 97.
80. Wells, *The Invisible Man,* 96.
81. Wells, *The Invisible Man,* 97.
82. Wells, *The Invisible Man,* 98.
83. Wells, *The Invisible Man,* 108.
84. D. W. Winnicott, "Transitional Objects and Transitional Phenomena," in *Collected Papers: Through Paediatrics to Psychoanalysis* (New York: Brunner-Mazel, 1958/1992), 229–242.
85. Winnicott, "Transitional Objects and Transitional Phenomena," 242.
86. D. W. Winnicott, "Transitional Objects and Transitional Phenomena," in *Playing and Reality* (London and New York: Routledge, 1970/2002), 1–25. Subsequent references are given in the text.
87. Winnicott, "Transitional Objects and Transitional Phenomena," 22.
88. Winnicott, "Transitional Objects and Transitional Phenomena," 17.
89. Winnicott, "Transitional Objects and Transitional Phenomena," 19.
90. D. W. Winnicott, "The Absence of a Sense of Guilt," *Deprivation and Delinquency,* ed. Claire Winnicott, Ray Shepherd, and Madeleine Davis (London and New York: Routledge, 1990), 106–112.
91. Winnicott, "The Absence of a Sense of Guilt," 111.
92. Winnicott, "The Absence of a Sense of Guilt," 111.
93. Winnicott, "The Absence of a Sense of Guilt," 109.
94. Winnicott, "The Absence of a Sense of Guilt," 109.
95. Winnicott, "The Absence of a Sense of Guilt," 109.
96. D. W. Winnicott, "Withdrawal and Regression," in *Collected Papers: Through Paediatrics to Psychoanalysis* (New York and London: Brunner-Mazel, 1958/1992), 255–261.
97. Winnicott, "Withdrawal and Regression," 255.
98. Winnicott, "Withdrawal and Regression," 260.
99. Winnicott, "Withdrawal and Regression," 260.
100. Winnicott, "Withdrawal and Regression," 260.
101. Winnicott, "Withdrawal and Regression," 260.
102. Winnicott, "Withdrawal and Regression," 260.
103. Winnicott, "Withdrawal and Regression," 260.
104. Winnicott, "Withdrawal and Regression," 256.
105. Winnicott, "Withdrawal and Regression," 256.

106. Winnicott, "Withdrawal and Regression," 260.
107. Winnicott, "Withdrawal and Regression," 260.
108. Winnicott, "Withdrawal and Regression," 257.
109. Winnicott, "Withdrawal and Regression," 257.
110. Winnicott, "Withdrawal and Regression," 260.

CHAPTER 20

WHY IS THE *TENSION* SO *HIGH*? THE MONSTROUS FEMININE IN (POST)MODERN SLASHER FILMS

DEJAN OGNJANOVIĆ

THIS CHAPTER DEALS WITH THE MONSTROSITY CONTAINED IN THE INSTABILITY of the killer's gender in horror films. Its purpose is to question the gender politics of slasher (and of horror film in general) by investigating: (1) the connection of the monstrous with sexual difference, especially homosexuality; (2) the role of "The Final Girl" in slasher films; and (3) the connection between The Final Girl and the "Monster" (i.e., the Slasher).

A relatively recent horror film, *High Tension* (*Haute Tension*, a.k.a. *Switchblade Romance*, Alexandre Aja, 2003), provides a telling case study. My analysis answers the questions set forth earlier and creates a better appreciation not only of this rather misunderstood genre masterpiece but also of developments in horror film since the late 1970s, when slasher subgenre was fully shaped. I chose this film because it represents a conscious homage *and* a clever, postmodern critique of the slasher tradition and its concept of the monstrous.

(UN)ORIGINAL BONES OF A QUEER SKELETON

Few horror films in the first decade of the millennium have caused as much dispute among fans and misunderstandings among critics as it is the case with *High Tension*. Divided reactions were largely caused by the film's infamous twist in which the heroine (The Final Girl) is eventually revealed to have been the one and the same as the Monster, that is, the brutish male slasher. As it turns out, *he* has been just a figment of *her* deranged mind, an alter ego along the lines of Tyler Durden in *Fight Club* (David Fincher, 1999).

This twist was more than many could take. The reception of the film was characterized largely by two dominant feelings: (1) *exasperation* with slasher subgenre itself, in the eyes of those who saw it as inherently inferior, and (2) *frustration* with the twist, which allegedly spoiled the otherwise well-made genre film for the horror fans.

Among the loudest critics was Roger Ebert, who, in 2005, could not see the logic of the twist and claimed that "clever viewers will be able to see for themselves that the movie's plot has a hole that is not only large enough to drive a truck through, but in fact does have a truck driven right through it."[1] Ebert's "clever" viewing deserves to be singled out because he has a history of misunderstanding slasher films: Carol J. Clover's influential *Men, Women and Chain Saws*[2] was in part written as an answer to his essay "Why Movie Audiences Aren't Safe Anymore,"[3] which explicitly accused slasher films of inviting (male) audience's identification with the killer through the first person camera's view. The carelessness of his viewing of *High Tension* is evident in the erroneous account of its plot in his one-star review.[4]

Other respectable publications were equally mystified by the logic and purpose of the twist. The pattern in their criticism is clear: the mainstream point of view claims that *High Tension* would have been a superior film had it been content merely to provide a variation on the well-known clichés, without straying into the gender-twisting territory. The twist is "perceived" as a mere gimmick in an otherwise generic, unoriginal film, as summed up by *Beyond Hollywood*'s "Nix": "*Haute Tension* has no real original bone in its body (unless you consider the surprise twist at the end)."[5]

However, I disagree with the majority opinion. *High Tension*'s originality lies in the way in which it deconstructs and reassembles the well-known ingredients of slasher, especially the figures of The Final Girl and the Monster, and what it does with the minutiae of their particular interplay. The movie seems to follow the genre rules, which lull viewers—only to have those rules ultimately turned upside down.

Alexandre Aja's film may not have an original bone in its body, but it dares to reassemble slasher's bones into a rather novel skeleton. And then, in the shocking twist, it takes it out of the closet.

Bad Reception

Many reviewers have been puzzled by *High Tension*'s alternate title, *Switchblade Romance*. The nature of the love story at the center of this film is key to its understanding, and yet, it is both sad and worrisome that so many professional movie-watchers failed to read the film's rather obvious signs. Roger Ebert is curious: "The film's British title is *Switchblade Romance,* which, if you see the film, will seem curiouser and curiouser."[6] Along those lines, *The Times* could not see anything past splatter: "More gore, this time from France, in the strangely titled *Switchblade Romance*."[7]

Some reviewers had problems setting straight the film's basic facts. So, before analyzing the romance aspect, perhaps it is helpful to provide a brief account of what really happens, as opposed to what is shown in the film. Some critics were dumbfounded because they noticed the switchblade,[8] the axe, the barbed wire, and the power saw, but they could not see the romance. They seem to have trusted the obviously unreliable narrator a bit too much, because this is what really happens in the film.

High Tension's central plot is a framed narrative, a flashback recounted by Marie (Cecile de France), seen in the present only in a few brief shots at the very beginning and end. She narrates it from a vaguely shown institution. This mysteriously unspecified environment (hospital? insane asylum? prison?) is the first sign which makes its inmate at least *suspicious* as a *narrator*. In the flashback, Marie and Alex (Maiwenn) go to a country house belonging to Alex's family. Marie has a one-sided (possibly erotic) attachment to her friend. All she gets from Alex are jealousy-inspiring flirts with boys, taunts about Marie's shyness with men, cold shoulders, and insensitive pranks. Seeing her friend taking a shower, attractive but forever distant, Marie goes into a psychotic episode. While masturbating alone in her room, she "summons" a brutish psycho killer (Philippe Nahon), actually an alter ego from her subconscious. Marie kills Alex's family, ties and silences Alex, places her in the back of her car and goes on the road, imagining that she's pursuing "the killer" (in his nonexistent truck). She alternates between moments in which she is Marie and those in which she is completely the sadistic slasher. When she notices a gas pump attendant acting suspiciously, she kills him. She drives to the woods where she hallucinates or simply invents her struggle with the killer. However, when she releases Alex and imagines herself as a savior, the girl tries to run away, so Marie has to kill the driver who stops to pick her up. Alex refuses Marie's advances and stabs her in the shoulder. Marie is sent to an asylum, where she recounts *her* version, that of a romance-like, heroic rescue of her friend from the psycho killer. She still believes that the two of them can be together forever, with no one between them.[9]

There are several problems this story poses for the American audience and critics. First, American genre film has spoilt its viewers into spelling everything explicitly for them. *High Tension* takes a more European stance of leaving certain things unspoken, unspecified, or downright irrational. It is typical of European film, including Euro-horror, to supplant the pragmatic Protestant American logic with a surreal, dream logic. That is why even distinguished critics could not comprehend that a lot of the things shown in the film either did not happen at all or did not happen the way they were presented. There has never been any old truck to drive through the plot's holes: it is the product of Marie's delusion. She was driving Alex, neatly tied up, in the back of her car, imagining a truck in front of her. She was not bumped off the road by the truck, but by her own disturbed mind.

What makes *High Tension* especially hard to take is the fact that for most of its running time it pretends to follow the American model of slasher subgenre, only to overturn this model in its final 20 minutes. Thus, lovers of the (sub)genre felt frustrated and angered by the film's "betrayal" in its climax. It seemed to tell one kind of story, but in the end revealed to have been telling something completely different. But did not *Psycho* do exactly the same thing 50 years ago?

The other problem is its attitude to sexuality and romance, which is different from that usually found in American film. "In the American horror film, women are usually murdered because of their having had sex, or desiring sex. In the Euro-horror film, women murder because of their carnality!"[10] This situation Totaro lucidly connects to the fact that "American horror, like its popular culture in general, is generally prudish and too deeply entrenched in a Puritan past to really engage in sexuality, which is so important to the horror film."[11] It is too often forgotten that *High Tension* is actually a European reinterpretation of American genre tradition, with a far more liberated and complex stance toward eroticism. Also, the timeless trope of horror—that things are not what they seem—is taken to such extremes that in this instance it applies not only to the content but also to the form itself.

Nothing here is what it seems: the friendship is not friendship, The Final Girl *is* the Monster, the savior is the torturer, male is female is male, love is murder. *High Tension* deals with notions of appearance and essence, but the point of it all is largely lost on the viewers. Even the film's defenders didn't seem to grasp the film's essence, relegating it to a playful, but superficial and ultimately pointless fooling around with generic clichés. This is exactly how Peter Hutchings "defends" the film's inclusion among 100 best European horror films:

> It is clearly not meant to be taken too seriously. The idea that the psychological double of the youthful France is a fat, middle-aged man is particularly ludicrous, and while the lesbianism of her character—and the association of this with her violence—might well raise the hackles of a politically sensitive audience, one suspects that for the film-makers this too is just part of the game, a game that is by turns amusing, inventive and cheerfully irresponsible.[12]

A child's play, almost. Gory, funny, suspenseful, well-made, but ultimately illogical, pointless, and irresponsible. This attitude is especially damning when it comes from those who actually liked the film. The above quote points to a major misunderstanding of the film's two central issues. One has to do with Marie's doubling, while another is related to her "lesbianism." These should be the key questions:

1. Why is Marie doubled at all, that is, why is her alter ego played by a different actor?
2. Why is Marie's alter ego male?
3. Why doesn't this male correspond to her age and appearance? In other words, why isn't "the killer" played by a young, slim, good-looking man? Why is "he" a fat, middle-aged, unpleasant brute?

In the process of answering these questions, another significant question will also become clearer: is Marie a lesbian, and if she is, does her murderous rampage present a reactionary, negative, homophobic slant that identifies homosexuality with monstrosity, as some have claimed—or is there a more complicated explanation than that?

What follows is an attempt to answer these questions.

The Romance That Dares Not Speak Its Name

Why Is Marie doubled at all?

This story could have been presented as a typical Jekyll and Hyde scenario, with a single actor: the audience could see Marie transform into her monstrous alter ego from the very beginning. But that would be a completely different film. In the Jekyll and Hyde plot, these two "characters" exist alternately, not simultaneously. Jekyll is only Jekyll, Hyde is only Hyde. The whole point of Marie's peculiar monstrosity is that she can be *both things at once:* both The Final Girl (the hero) and the Monster (antihero). Crucial for this particular story is to see the *schizophrenia of her position,* the internal split that cannot easily be divided into rather simplistic, black–white, good–evil, Jekyll–Hyde binaries.

Marie is a postmodern monster that sheds the old dichotomies and their attendant morality. As Judith Halberstam wrote, "What I want to argue is that The Final Girl, particularly as embodied by Stretch, represents not boyishness or girlishness but monstrous gender, a gender that splatters, rips at the seams, and then is sutured together again as something much messier than male or female."[13] Marie is a perfect embodiment of this kind of monster that refuses to be placed into a limited range of categories (male, female, homosexual). It is a messy gender—"monstrous" precisely because it collapses the usual boundaries.

Also, only through the personified polarities is the twist possible. It is important for the audience to believe that Marie is the archetypal Final Girl, and that the Monster is someone else. Crucial for the film's impact and meaning is for the audience to sympathize with the Girl, to root for her, to invest their undivided interest and emotions in her plight. In *High Tension,* we are made to sympathize with a Monster in Final Girl's clothing: this is not mere playfulness. The Final Girl is used to tell the Monster's point of view.

In classic horror, sympathy for the monster (if any) usually is induced by presenting its plight explicitly, by showing how misunderstood, essentially how tender and kind it can be, if only it were given a chance. An archetypal episode is the episode with a blind hermit in *The Bride of Frankenstein* (James Whale, 1935). However, Frankenstein's creature is a monster in appearance only. In essence, it is "just like us": it likes music, wine, cigars and friends, just like everybody else. While essentially well-meaning, this kind of attitude diminishes the difference in an artificial manner and begs for acceptance on the grounds of "we (monsters) are the same as you (normals)."

Under its surface, this depiction of monstrosity can be labeled reactionary, because it *accepts* the dominant standard and basically craves to be measured in accordance with it. It is similar to the stance of another monstrous feminine, Carrie, anxious for acceptance. In spite of all the evidence to the contrary, she just wants her own piece of "normality." This is reactionary because the story implies that any female monster, deep down, just wants to be a prom queen, with roles of a good mother and housewife as close second and third choices. This standpoint wants to reduce the monstrous to a *surface,* beneath which lies a perfectly good conformist bourgeois. A monster, viewed in this way, is just a creature unfortunate enough to look and behave in a "freaky" and eccentric manner, but if given half a chance, such a creature would bend over backwards to become *one of us.*

The cleverness of *High Tension* lies in the fact that it refuses to present its "monster" as a pathetic, misunderstood creature—until the very end. The filmmakers are aware that inherent homophobia would prevent a majority of viewers from sympathizing with a queer monster from the start, even if she were presented as misunderstood and well-meaning. Thus, they slyly hide her real nature *from her* as well as from the audience, in order to make us sympathize with the lengths she's willing to go to reach her goal. In her paralleling the films with a similar twist (*The Fight Club, Identity* and *High Tension*), Iva Radat pointed to an alienating effect of such a twist for more conventional viewers:

> An important element of all these films is that all three protagonists turn out to be bad guys/gals; the reason behind some viewers' feelings of manipulation could read as a result of having been made to identify with the villain/ness without consent. This might also explain why all three killers manage to stay alive, two of them moreover on the loose. In a marked departure from Clover's psychopaths, these movies do not punish their audience for the shared sadistic gaze, but instead leave them with the knowledge of having participated in the events that took place.[14]

Crucially, the audience's participation is the key here. In my view, once the goal is revealed together with the meaning of the alternate title, *Switchblade Romance,* it is hard to stop liking Marie after the road we have traveled with her. She just wants to love and be loved, despite the circumstances—how monstrous is that?

At the moment we realize that Marie *is* the Monster, we also realize who and what made her monstrous, and this realization purifies her from guilt. She is a victim of impulses fostered by her surrounding. Her fragility, incomprehension, and confusion almost inevitably invoke compassion. She is a martyr for love, reminiscent of Jeanne d'Arc, that famous French martyr and hero, immortalized in Carl T. Dreyer's masterpiece.[15] "I won't let anyone come between us anymore, I won't let anyone come between us anymore," she keeps repeating to her beloved. The sadness lies in her inability to accept that everyone and everything is between them.

WHY IS MARIE'S ALTER EGO MALE?

Her other self is male because, in a world defined by clear-cut binaries, to desire a woman is a masculine property. The beauty of the film is that it does not attempt to confine Marie into any of the recognizable categories that have graced slasher cinema so far: she is not a man trapped in female body (the opposite of the transsexual psychiatrist in *Dressed to Kill*); she is not a girl brought up as a boy (the opposite of the killer in *Sleepaway Camp*); and it is debatable whether she is homosexual, that is, lesbian. The latter option seems the likeliest, and numerous reviewers jumped at that label, but the case as presented in the film seems more complicated.

Superficially, Marie does possess certain traits that position her into the recognizable stereotype of a lesbian, most notably her very short hair, androgynous features, jeans, and incessant smoking. But, since those same "boyish" qualities characterize The Final Girl, a heterosexual audience can accept her as a familiar generic type from slasher film, while a homosexual audience may take pleasure in recognizing in her one of their own. Reading Marie as a (closeted?) lesbian is almost inevitable, although one could argue that she is no more a lesbian than Norman Bates is a transvestite. Alexandre Aja points toward a more complex possibility in his audio commentary on the British DVD edition of his film:

> I think it's more about love, it's about relationship between two persons. We can imagine the same film with a boy and a girl, or two boys. It's the same. I didn't stop to say "I'm gonna write a lesbian story," that was not the purpose of the film. It was just a friendship that was a little bit too strong. And maybe she is not as lesbian as that, because she just wants to be her best friend. Maybe she wants to *be her,* and not with her.[16]

First of all, one cannot imagine the same film with a boy and a girl. With a boy and a girl there would be no need for schizophrenic split personalities or alter egos, especially not of the opposite sex. *High Tension* makes sense only with a homosexual (or some other "un-natural" "monstrous") subtext. Only then is the tension between the surface appearance and the (closeted) essence so high such that it can produce such a grotesque monster and such dramatic results. To imagine this same plot with two boys, however, a similar film could be envisioned: Mark, the passive and shy boy, develops a female alter ego as a result of the tension between him and his (unresponding) friend Alex. In such a hypothetical, "his" female "self" would probably look like a sluttish, male-devouring, witchy monstrous feminine, like those found in Italian *giallo* films, like *Suspiria* (1977).

One could ask why Aja has not made a film with two boys instead of two girls, but the question within this culture is rhetorical, since the answer is too obvious for contemplation. Cinema has always been about "boys photographing girls," as Godard famously said, and the French should know. Besides, the main target audience for slasher horror (adolescent boys) would never accept the film with a romance between two boys at its heart, even a switchblade romance. Many were troubled by the lesbian subtext already; two boys would have been too much and would limit the film's appeal only to the narrow fringe of gay film festivals. By deciding to use the plot with two girls, Aja was able to keep a generic appearance while still instilling the film with an uncommon, subversive subtext.

In any case, it is of lesser importance whether Aja's decision was a result of pragmatic, commercial thinking or of a planned strategy. In my view, Aja intuitively felt that in American culture, a story of two boys who travel to the countryside to "study together" would be far more suspicious for mainstream audiences, and thus would spoil the final twist. Whether he was a male chauvinist who preferred to "photograph girls" or a true filmmaker who knew his tools and trade, or both, Aja has certainly made the best and most effective decision, that is, the only one that could really work. So, he decided the high tension should exist between two girls.

What is more inspiring about Aja's commentary is his suggestion that this relation may not necessarily be sexual, or at least not be entirely reducible to the sexual component. Perhaps Marie just wants to be Alex's best friend. Maybe she wants to *be her,* and not *with* her. These possibilities bring us back to Halberstam's notion of the "monstrous gender," one which is above and beyond the usual polarities. It certainly complicates things for those able to think only in either–or binary options. And it is even more complicated for those who have not openly embraced any recognizable lifestyle, whose sexuality is still not liberated enough to be actualized. Marie's psyche and her orientation may be repressed, closeted, or undecided, but in the world that classifies using binaries, her sexuality still has to be reduced to a recognizable shape, even if it is misshapen in the process. In this instance, her desire for a woman renders that shape as inevitably male.

Why Doesn't Marie's Male Alter Ego Correspond to Her Age and Appearance?

A gender that is forcibly pressed into the preexisting mold will inevitably come out distorted and misshapen. Violence involved in such a process must produce a grotesque distortion. The killer, embodied by Philippe Nahon, is a fitting Mr. Hyde to Marie's Dr. Jekyll. In my view, she is not so much a repressed lesbian as she is someone trying to avoid any categorizing, any mold whatsoever. The film does not provide the slightest hint that she cares for the lesbian lifestyle, values, ideology. All she wants is to be with Alex, as someone "more than just a friend." Whether that someone should be a lover, or a best friend, or a body-double remains unclear. But whatever it is, it belongs to the realm of the unacceptable, of excess. It is "too much." It is, therefore, "wrong." The established concept of wrongness creates a monster.

Thus, Marie's alter ego *cannot* be a young, slim, good-looking man. It is a *distorted* mirror image, and its distortion is twofold.

First, "he" reflects a grotesque parody of slasher subgenre's inherently puritan, antisensual attitude. He is a caricature of the silent, faceless killer of old who comes as punishment to those who indulge in excessive carnality. He is the imprint of the "sex is bad" ideology, as foreshadowed by the two girls' discussion in the car at the very beginning of the film. Marie refers to a recent party during which Alex left her alone, pursuing a male admirer ("Running out on me with God knows who"). When Alex replies that it was worth it, Marie responds, "What a slut," and continues calling her a "bimbo" and a "skank." If Michael Myers and Jason Vorhees talked at all, they would use those same terms to describe Alex's one-night stand. In their dead, puritan eyes, she is a whore. When Alex says, "You're gonna end up an old maid," Marie responds, "I'm not a slut like you." The puritan worldview is defined by such ready-made and unchangeable dichotomies: one can only be either "an old maid" or a "slut;" the age-old Christian duality of Madonna and Whore Viewed in that light, perhaps Marie's alter ego does not abduct Alex in order to rape her, but instead wants to *reform* her, to convert her to the virtues of virginity, or at least monogamy?

Second, the killer in *High Tension* also reflects the denigrating and demonizing urban perception of the rural, which Clover called "urbanoia": "The demonizing impulse that underwrites these films depends on the fiction that country folk always pose an immediate threat of brute force, and for that threat to be sufficiently credible to justify their annihilation, it must be male."[17] There are several Marie's statements telling of her haughty attitude toward the countryside. "Are there any cool places to go out here in the country?" she asks. When Alex says that the town hall is about the only place, Marie says, "Wow, if I had to live here all year round, I think I'd shoot myself." Later on, Alex jokes, "The only real excitement around here is when a train runs through." It is therefore inevitable that a killer roaming this wild, God-forsaken terrain would be a sturdy redneck father-figure with harsh features, dressed in blue-collar attire.

The killer embodies all the major qualities of vintage slashers and their backward ideology—but with a twist. Instead of supporting this repressive ideology, *High Tension* criticizes it by showing the negative, monstrous, schizophrenic effect this ideology can have on those who do not fit into the preexisting molds, yet still incorporate this ideology as a part of their psychological makeup. The film makes us hate the killer, but not Marie, because it clearly shows the reasons for her becoming monstrous. As Halberstam argues,

> Within postmodern Gothic we no longer attempt to identify the monster and fix the terms of his/her deformity, rather postmodern Gothic warns us to be suspicious of monster hunters, monster makers, and above all, discourses invested in purity and innocence. The monster always represents the disruption of categories, the destruction of boundaries, and the presence of impurities and so we need monsters and we need to recognize and celebrate our own monstrosities.[18]

Discourses invested in purity and innocence are shown as schizophrenia-inducing: always eager to label one a slut, a bimbo, a bitch, and a skank, these puritans are the real monster-makers. The most dangerous is the puritan within.

The killing brute that Marie's schizophrenia creates is a caricature of a rural womanizer, an archetypal "male chauvinist pig" whose misogyny is an almost inevitable, or at least logical product of a discourse based on purity, according to which most women are "bitches" and "sluts." This is manifested throughout the film: his sexuality is essentially necrophiliac, as evidenced by the first scene in which he is pleasuring himself with a decapitated female head. Women for him are just notches in his endless line of conquests, as symbolized by the small photographs he keeps as a record of his previous victims. Of course, this character is fictional: there is no killing brute roaming the countryside, there have been no previous conquests; there is no vintage truck to keep the record of his victim count. It is all in Marie's mind. It is her projection, her concept of what it means to be a male (in the countryside).

This is seen nowhere better than in "the killer's" talk with a gas station attendant, a parody of how a woman imagines men talk to each other when they are alone. "On your own tonight?" he asks. "So they left you to mind the store . . . This is the ideal place to bring girls. Don't tell me it's never happened." The young man is uncomfortable with such talk, but tries to please the customer: "If I did, my boss would fire me." But the leering brute is insistent: "Come on . . . The old rich ladies that drive through . . . Don't tell me they never ask for your services. Ain't that right, Jimmy?" The premise here is that men are sex-crazed beasts just waiting for their chance to jump at a woman. Since in reality these words are spoken by Marie, the worker is understandably suspicious and she (or rather "he" inside) eventually has to kill him.

The conventional perception of a male homosexual is that of a man tainted by the female traits: "The female here serves as the source of the monstrous taint: the male homosexual or queer is monstrous precisely because he embodies characteristics of the feminine, either in outward displays or in the selection of a sexual object choice traditionally reserved for women."[19] In Marie's case, the opposite is true: here, a woman is tainted by the embodied characteristics of what is perceived as a typical male behavior. If a lesbian is monstrous because of a sexual object choice traditionally reserved for men, then her male "taint" will be exemplified through an unrealistic, exaggerated caricature of "maleness." Just as some gay men assume a body language, way of talking. and entire psychological makeup in accordance with what the society perceives as "feminine" (although few women, if any, actually behave that way), Marie's "male" persona (in constant pursuit of women and booze) is a product of prejudice, stereotyping, and binary reductiveness.

THE MONSTER INSIDE

High Tension is a progressive film because it shows that "the monster is often a figure less of an external threat to an essentially good social order than of exaggeration of the most normal features of that very order."[20] Thus, the film distances itself from the old-fashioned morality of the classical horrors (society = good, monster = evil), and shows the monster as a creation of the societal cultural apparatus that forms individuality. Jeffrey Jerome Cohen agrees because he sees the monster as "an extreme version of marginalization, an abjecting epistemological device basic to the mechanics of deviance construction and identity formation . . . a code or a pattern or a presence or an absence that unsettles what has been constructed to be received as natural, as human."[21] The monster is the shadow cast by the society, and its ugly head speaks volumes.

What makes *High Tension* especially poignant is the tragedy of a monster unable to cast off the scarifying imprint of the monster-making apparatus of society. Marie's main problem is not her "monstrous gender" that drives her toward an "improper" object, that is, her female friend. The main problem is that she lives in a society that still renders such a desire "monstrous." This barely hidden Puritanism engenders cracks in the frail and brutes in the crude; saddest of all are the frail ones who confuse the brute for desire. *High Tension*'s sympathetic depiction of such a condition shows that the film is not homophobic.

If the film's aim were to portray lesbianism as a cause of dangerous psychosis, and lesbians as potential monsters who like Frankenstein's monster, are running rampant across the countryside, claiming innocent victims,[22] it would have little use of the twist and the *doppelgänger* aspect. Its alleged purpose would have been better served with a straightforward portrayal of a lesbian psycho right from the beginning. Instead, Aja provides a consistently sympathetic portrayal of Marie's character (helped by deFrance's nuanced and energetic acting) that is always tinged with melancholy and sadness.[23]

It is true that lesbians have appeared in horror films as monsters, usually vampires. But, the common lesbian-as-bloodsucking-predator figure in this film is supplanted by the melancholy lesbian-as-victim-turned-monstrous. Aja does not present lesbian love as morbid, monstrous, or threatening. It is a sad love because it is doomed and unable to speak its name.

Also, if gimmickry was the director's main intent, he could have placed the twist about the killer's identity much later in the film, such as the last minute or two before the credits. Instead, Aja chooses to unveil Marie's secret a good 20 minutes before the end. This is very important, because it enables the audience to readdress their sympathies and allegiances, only to realize that they have no one else to sympathize with but with "the monster." One cannot hate Marie at the end of *High Tension* any more than one could hate Carrie, Norman Bates, or Helen (from *Candyman,* 1992, Bernard Rose) once their murderous personae have been revealed. And the reason is the same: because the film has, by that time, clearly shown the mechanisms of identificatory monster-making.

The link between homosexuality and murderous rage may exist, but its origin, effect, and overall nature is more complex than the simplistic formula: lesbianism = murder. This is evidenced by the reception of this film from a lesbian perspective:

> If no trauma is referenced to account for the amount of self-hate Marie feels as a result of her lesbian drive (and providing the viewer does not believe the latter is or should be inseparable from the former), then the question that begs an answer is where such fierce hatred comes from. The answer to that question—from the society Marie grew up in—can shed more light on her motivation for the merciless killings she performs on the family unit. This kind of reasoning led me to better understand the exhilaration I felt at the sight of Marie poised with a chainsaw in hand; I came to accept her sadism and her murderous rage, the fantasy of getting even. Marie's outlet for anger and revenge can become the female, feminist, and/or lesbian viewer's outlet as well; and why should we not allow ourselves the fantasy of righteous wrath or even unabashed sadism?[24]

In other words, Marie's murderous rage can have a cathartic effect similar to Carrie's explosion of anger at the end of de Palma's film. The only difference is that de Palma explicitly shows the process of monster-making: the taunts, the jeers, the laughs, the savage punishments, the misunderstandings, and the humiliations. The structure of Aja's film does not allow that much, but he manages to instill a few telling hints for the careful viewers.

The most obvious clue was not obvious enough for Roger Ebert because he completely misrepresents this scene in his review: "Marie is one of those goofy sorts who wanders into a cornfield for no better reason than for Alex to follow her, shouting 'Marie! Marie!' while the wind sighs on the soundtrack."[25] The fact that there is no wind sighing on the soundtrack in this particular scene—only silence, crickets and night birds—is a minor gaffe which shows the critic's contempt for the material. A more grievous error is that it is not Marie, *but Alex* who wanders into the cornfields, while Marie is going after her, shouting "Alex! Alex!" This is not a benign *lapsus memoriae* but a crucial sign of a failure to understand the vital importance of this scene for the characters and plot.

In said scene Alex pretends to see something in the cornfields while Marie goes after her, worried. To an impatient viewer, this may seem an unnecessary scene which has nothing to do with the film except to provide a pointless false alarm, a tired staple of slasher tradition. To an attentive and sympathetic viewer, the film reveals a lot. First, it makes explicit that Alex is a rather *insensitive person,* prone to making cruel jokes at Marie's expense. Second, it exemplifies what was previously hinted through dialogue: that Marie has a strong *fear of being abandoned by Alex*. The cruelty of the joke is twofold: (1) Marie is made to fear, not for herself, but for her (unworthy) friend, who is actually quite safe; and (2) Marie is made to fear that her "friend" (who has already snuck into the car behind her back) would drive away and leave her alone in the cornfield in the middle of the night. Third, the scene hints at Marie's darker side when she yells: "If this is a joke, I'll *make you regret it*!" As it turns out, it *is* a joke, and Marie does *make her regret it* that very same night.

Therefore, the scene is vital to understanding the psychological profiles of these characters: Alex's indifferent cruelty and Marie's fear of abandonment. These help trigger the violent turn the events take later that night, when Marie "snaps," awakening her murderous persona. If the first trigger is this insensitive prank, then the second one is Alex's teasing act of showering in front of the window (knowing that Marie is outside for a smoke).

If reality is against Marie, so much the worse for reality. She has to invent a romance in the original sense of this French word. Marie invents a "dragon," a Monster to slay Alex's family (so that "no one can ever be between them") and to abduct Alex, too, so that she can become a Knight on a white horse to save the damsel in distress and thus earn her eternal gratitude and love.[26] The inherent sadness of this fantasy is that ultimately, she has to save herself from the Monstrous within.

High Tension shows that The Final Girl and the Monster are siblings, twins of opposite sexes but equally queer genders. Both of these character types, as reinterpreted in this film, "call for new sexual vocabularies that acknowledge sexualities and genders as styles rather than life-styles, as fictions rather than facts of life, and as potentialities rather than as fixed identities."[27] As such, the film cleverly builds upon the gender-twisting tradition inaugurated by Hitchcock's *Psycho*:

> For what was really scary about this movie was precisely the fact that we finally couldn't be sure of either the gender or the sexuality of what was scaring either us or the people in the movie. It was precisely these kinds of dislocations of the film—between normal and psychotic; between masculine and feminine; between Eros and fear; even between the familiar Hitchcockian suspense and a new, more frankly gender-based horror—that constituted the historically new terror of *Psycho*.[28]

This new kind of monster, whose instability is gender-based, and who frightens, puzzles, and attracts us precisely because of its in-between-ness, beyond the either–or option, is cleverly reconstructed. Rather than merely recycling generic clichés, *High Tension* brings a long-delayed maturity to a questionable subgenre because of the film's postmodern, progressive attitude toward the gender politics of horror film.

NOTES

1. Roger Ebert, "High Tension," June 9, 2005, *Chicago Sun Times,* accessed August 20, 2009, http://rogerebert.suntimes.com/apps/pbcs.dll/article?AID= /20050609/REVIEWS/50601001/1023
2. See Carol J. Clover, *Men, Women, and Chainsaws: Gender in the Modern Horror Film* (Princeton, NJ: Princeton University Press, 1992).
3. Roger Ebert, "*Why Movie Audiences Aren't Safe Anymore,*" *American Film* 6, no. 5 (March 1981): 54–56.
4. Ebert, "High Tension."
5. Nix, "High Tension (2003) Movie Review," February 16, 2004, *BeyondHollywood.com,* accessed August 20, 2009, http://www.beyondhollywood.com/high-tension-2003-movie-review/
6. Ebert, "High Tension."
7. Wendy Ide, "Switchblade Romance," September 23, 2004, *The Times* [London], accessed August 20, 2009, http://entertainment.timesonline.co.uk/tol/arts_and_entertainment/film/article1076058.ece.
8. Actually, no switchblade is seen in the film, only a razor.
9. For a film with such a big twist, *High Tension* is a straightforward narrative, and a second viewing reveals numerous hints about the real state of things, as opposed to Marie's narrative. In my view, the only "cheat" is a beginning scene in which the killer is fellated by a decapitated female head. It is unnecessary and illogical.
10. Donato Totaro, "The Final Girl: A Few Thoughts on Feminism and Horror," *Offscreen,* January 31, 2002, accessed August 20, 2009, http://www.horschamp.qc.ca/new_offscreen/final_girl.html.
11. Totaro, "The Final Girl."
12. Peter Hutchings, "High Tension," *100 European Horror Films,* ed. Steven Jay Schneider (London: BFI, 2007), 105.
13. Judith Halberstam, *Skin Shows: Gothic Horror and the Technology of Monsters* (Durham, NC: Duke University Press, 1995), 143.
14. Iva Radat, "Haute Tension: Lesbian Audience and the Slasher Film" (presentation, *Transgressing Gender* Conference: Two is not enough for gender (e)quality, Zagreb, Croatia, October 7–9, 2005).
15. One wonders whether the striking physical resemblance between Cecile de France and Maria Falconetti is a coincidence, especially in light of Aja's numerous close-ups of his short-haired, androgynous, teary-eyed, upward-glancing, anguished, gentle, ethereal, not-of-this-world but still faithful heroine.
16. Alexandre Aja, "Audio Commentary by Director," *Switchblade Romance,* DVD (Lions Gate Films Home Entertainment, 2004).
17. Clover, *Men, Women, and Chainsaws,* 161.
18. Halberstam, *Skin Shows,* 27.
19. Harry M. Benshoff, "The Monster and the Homosexual," in *Horror: The Film Reader,* ed. Mark Jancovich (London: Routledge, 2002), 107.
20. Michael Ryan and Douglas Kellner, *Camera Politica: The Politics and Ideology of Contemporary Hollywood Film* (Bloomington, IN: Indiana University Press, 1990), 179.
21. Jeffrey Jerome Cohen, Preface to *Monster Theory,* ed. Jeffrey Jerome Cohen (Minneapolis, MN: University of Minnesota Press, 1996), ix.
22. See Benshoff, "The Monster and the Homosexual," 103.
23. It is strange how few critics noticed that the murder scenes in the film are not accompanied by the conventional suspense-pumping horror score, but by melancholy, elegiac themes by Francois Eudes.
24. Radat, "Haute Tension."
25. Ebert, "High Tension."

26. In his DVD commentary, Aja explicitly compares Marie to a knight on a white horse from medieval romances.
27. Judith Halberstam, "F2M: The Making of Female Masculinity," in *Feminist Theory and the Body: A Reader,* ed. Janet Price and Margrit Shildrick (Edinburgh: Edinburgh University Press, 1999), 125.
28. Linda Williams, "When Women Look: A Sequel," *Senses of Cinema* 15 (2001), accessed August 20, 2009, http://archive.sensesofcinema.com/contents/01/15/horror_women.html.

CHAPTER 21

BLOOD AND BITCHES: SEXUAL POLITICS AND THE TEEN FEMALE LYCANTHROPE IN YOUNG ADULT FICTION

JUNE PULLIAM

THE YOUNG ADULT FEMALE WEREWOLF OFFERS POWERFUL AND VIVID, even visceral versions of the dangers of traditional femininity. Lycanthropy represents our worst fears that we all harbor a primitive, bestial nature that must be tightly controlled lest civilization degenerate into chaos. The werewolf is an apt metaphor for adolescence, a developmental period in which teens are often characterized as hormonally crazed savages who must learn to master their baser impulses before they can mature into productive adults. The teen werewolf, then, can be seen as an atavistic monster incapable of mastering its "primitive" emotions to develop the restraint necessary to become an adult. This aptly describes Tony Rivers, the hapless protagonist of the 1957 film *I Was a Teenage Werewolf.* Tony is immature because he cannot control his anger, so he constantly fights with his peers. Tony's anger becomes monstrous, however, after his therapist's experimental anger-management treatments exaggerate his anger, forcing him to regress to what is described by the film as a primitive human state. This primitive state, when imposed upon a human adolescent, takes the form of a prototypical werewolf.

While the werewolf represents an atavistic human state, it is also a gendered monster that is most typically coded as male. The werewolf's sudden growth of body hair and aggressive behavior link it to the changes associated with *male* adolescence. Although the werewolf's explosive anger and intense desires for food and sex place him outside of the boundaries of civilized humanity, they are also extreme iterations of normative masculinity, a subject position whose single most evident marker is violence.[1] So, for example, Larry Talbot, the werewolf protagonist of *The Wolf Man* (1941) and its remake, *The Wolfman* (2010), is dangerously uncivilized, yet unambiguously masculine.

Because the werewolf is typically coded as male, the female werewolf is especially monstrous. Her lupine body both puts her outside of the boundaries of normative femininity and recalls a "pervasive cultural association of femininity with nature, embodiment and biology."[2] The female lycanthrope's body cannot be permanently groomed into culturally sanctioned boundaries of femininity: it is strong and athletic, and sprouts hair in places where women are supposed to be smooth. Moreover, the female werewolf's "unfeminine" appetites for sex make her incapable of acting like a "good girl" for long. As a werewolf, her connection to blood and the moon link her to pervasive negative cultural associations of women with the natural world, while as a woman, her hormones and the cycles of her body are perceived as keeping her perpetually prisoner to her emotions. But the most threatening aspect of the female werewolf is her capacity for extreme anger, an emotion incompatible with stereotypical femininity. As a consequence, the female werewolf is no lady; rather, she is the embodiment of the inferior and dangerous creature that all women are suspected of being.

Yet, while some accounts of female lycanthropy reproduce sexist concepts of women's essential nature, others challenge these concepts. If horror teaches us anything, it is that repression is dangerous: the repressed always returns, in monstrous form, to wreak havoc on citizens of the society who have necessitated its banishment. Yet the monster is not necessarily a creature that must be destroyed at all costs. In fact, the word "monster" derives from the Latin *monstere,* meaning "to show."[3] This return of the repressed then is more than retribution on the part of the monster; it is a warning about the dangers of disavowing certain knowledge or parts of the self.

The teen female werewolf emphasizes the dangers of repressing one's desires and emotions too thoroughly. As a result, this creature can transform a reader's/viewer's consciousness and permit her to refuse the crippling subordinate feminine role she is being pressured to occupy. Gender is not the "natural" consequence of biological sex, but a type of subjectivity that underpins a culture's hierarchal division of labor.[4] The powerful perpetuate ideas about the naturalness of gender roles in order to facilitate women's domination, so that culturally specific notions of masculinity and femininity seem to be the innate consequence of being male or female, and so resisting these roles seems futile. The werewolf's ability to pass back and forth between the boundaries that supposedly separate animal from human—and male from female—undermines these categories by revealing their permeability. The teen female lycanthrope, whose overt sexual desire and anger are essential facets of her being, can stifle these feelings only at her peril, thereby providing an object lesson to girls about the dangers of repressing emotions and denying the body in order to be normatively feminine.

For example, Annette Curtis Klause's novel *Blood and Chocolate* and the film *Ginger Snaps* offer typical representations of how the teen female werewolf reveals the constructedness of gender in a way that causes the reader/viewer to question the desirability of what is represented as normal and natural. In these texts, the trope of lycanthropy is used to explore how girls resist being cowed into a subordinate feminine subjectivity, which necessitates that they silence their voices and repress their desires for sex, and sometimes even food, and then disavow the resulting anger over being subordinated. *Blood and Chocolate* draws on the genres of gothic and paranormal romance[5] as well as horror to explore cultural prejudices about women. Klause's sympathetic lycanthrope protagonist questions the idea that woman's presumed interrelationship with nature makes her into an irremediable, abject Other. John Fawcett's 2000 film *Ginger Snaps* builds upon stereotypical cinematic representations of the werewolf as a creature born of someone's inability to deny "primitive" emotions. While Ginger, Fawcett's werewolf protagonist, is not a sympathetic character even when she is fully human, the bland and vicious suburban teens that she menaces are equally unsympathetic, and their presence in the film calls into question the desirability of being normal.

Beauty and the Beast: Conventional Femininity and Monstrosity

While the male werewolf is monstrous because he is dangerously uncivilized, the female werewolf is monstrous because she is not conventionally feminine. The female werewolf's hirsutism is the most obvious marker of her deviation from normative femininity. Because biological femaleness is not sufficient to differentiate women from men, it is necessary for women to perform their gender through a stylized repetition of acts that constitute femininity. Susan Brownmiller describes femininity as a performance that "constantly reassures its audience by a willing demonstration of difference, even when one does not exist in nature."[6] The performance of femininity includes grooming the body into culturally specific parameters of feminine beauty. Beauty standards are part of a wider sexual politics that maintain feminine subordination. Women whose bodies are not groomed into the parameters of normative feminine beauty face serious consequences, particularly in the twenty-first century. Naomi Wolf argues that in a post-second-wave-feminist world where men feel threatened by women's increased economic independence, beauty standards have replaced the feminine mystique as a way of controlling women.[7] Wolf terms these ubiquitous standards the "Beauty Myth."[8] Women who deviate from this feminine aesthetic are considered unfeminine, and as a result can be rejected by potential male mates, the eventual power brokers in a patriarchal society, and may even be shunned by their peers. Additionally, a woman who does not conform to cultural standards of beauty might find her employment opportunities limited, a consequence that significantly diminishes her ability to be autonomous.[9]

The contemporary Beauty Myth affects adolescent girls' feelings of self-worth by encouraging them to "make the body into an all-consuming project in ways young women of the past did not."[10] Young women pursue the Beauty Myth, in part, because it is represented to them by mass culture as a way of being empowered. The Beauty Myth promises to empower the girl who has dieted, exercised, and manicured her body into a magical combination of perfection that will supposedly make her irresistible to all men, the power brokers in a patriarchal society. Yet this promise of empowerment is hollow, as the reward for embracing the Beauty Myth is not agency and autonomy, but becoming an object of desire for men. Ultimately, societal expectations that cause women to aspire to be beauties deprive them of agency: if women are kept occupied with a "body project" that necessitates eternal vigilance against hairiness, odor, weight gain, and aging, then they are less likely to notice, let alone challenge, cultural forces that perpetuate their subordination.

Feminine beauty, however, is more than skin deep. The conventionally feminine woman is also lithe and petite, rather than strong and athletic. The teen female werewolf possesses physical strength, which makes her athletic and competitive, traits still reserved for normative masculinity.[11] In fact, her strength, which often makes her stronger than any human male in a lycanthropy narrative, flies in the face of a patriarchal culture where women's participation in sports, particularly competitive sports or those that are not conducive to developing a lithe and petite female form, is still discouraged, in spite of changes ushered in by Title IX to encourage female athleticism.

Finally, even in the twenty-first century, femininity is predicated on sexual passivity. One way that girls are subordinated involves the threat of being labeled a slut. The girl who is designated a "slut" by her peers becomes a sort of untouchable: she marks the outer limits of normative femininity, serving as a warning to other girls to curtail their own behavior lest they share her fate as an outcast.[12]

The figure of the teen female werewolf, with her exaggerated representations of gender, can assist girls in rejecting debilitating characteristics of normative femininity. The teen female werewolf allows a coded exploration of issues of gender, sexuality, and agency. This coded exploration is particularly important for teens, whose relative powerless and inexperience makes them fearful of examining the incongruity between their own feelings and pressures to be "normal" girls in the way represented through contemporary discourses of gender.

Vivian, the werewolf protagonist of *Blood and Chocolate,* and Ginger in *Ginger Snaps,* deconstruct normative femininity. Vivian originally desires to be a "normal" girl, but her lupine body cannot be made conventionally feminine in any lasting way. In Klause's novel, humans cannot be turned into werewolves. Instead, werewolves are a parallel species who appear human when they are not in their pelts. Vivian, who has always lived with other members of her species in an extended family pack, initially is disdainful of her kind because she views werewolf culture as sexist. At the beginning of the novel, Vivian wants nothing to do with the young men of her kind, whose swaggering, vulgar, sex-crazed performance of masculinity leads them to attempt to dominate her.

Vivian believes that she has found an alternative to her species' sexist masculinity in Aiden, a sensitive human boy with long hair and a love for poetry. Aiden's interest in the occult leads Vivian to hope that he would also love the beast within her, a facet of her self that she cherishes, though she is alarmed by her own anger, which she fears could make her lose control. Therefore, Vivian pursues Aiden, believing that a relationship with him would free her of being forced to accept a restrictive sex role in her own culture.

Ironically, Vivian's brief relationship with Aiden causes her to become ensnared within the parameters of stereotypical femininity. Because Aiden is human, Vivian must perform a sort of double drag in his presence, passing as both human and normatively feminine. In Klause's novel, werewolves must always give a convincing performance as human when not among their own kind so that humans will not be alerted to their existence and hunt them to extinction. Therefore, Vivian must be careful not to be near Aiden when the moon is full because her body changes into its wolf form. When Vivian is with Aiden, she must also convincingly perform as normatively feminine so as not to frighten him, even though he is supposedly an enlightened man who does not subscribe to conventional gender roles. Performing in this way means that she cannot overtly express her sexual feelings, at least at first. This is difficult for Vivian, as she and others of her kind openly desire sex, and she longs for the time when she feels that she knows Aiden well enough so that she can "teach him to be less polite."[13]

While being conventionally feminine benefits Vivian in the short run, eventually it sets her up for victimization. Vivian reaps short-term rewards for appearing to be normatively feminine—she momentarily becomes Aiden's love interest. However, when Vivian finally decides to stop performing as conventionally feminine *and* human, the results are disastrous. On the night they are to consummate their relationship, Vivian comes to Aiden in his bedroom and reveals her wolf form, hoping that he will see "something beautiful, and wild, beyond imagining."[14] Instead, Vivian out of "drag" is so beyond Aiden's concept of reality that he trembles and cries, then chases her from the room.[15]

Aiden's reaction to Vivian's lycanthropic body in effect punishes her for expressing her sexuality outside the parameters of stereotypical femininity. Human females find male werewolves attractive, as their lycanthropy is an extension of normative masculinity.[16] However, human males find female werewolves repugnant because they are the antithesis of conventional femininity. Days later, when Vivian corners Aiden to discuss their last encounter, he can only express loathing for her now that he knows her secret: "Every time I think of kissing you I see that other face" and think "what has that mouth done?"[17] Aiden's phrasing is reminiscent of how males have typically described their reactions to their girlfriends after discovering that they had been previously sexually active, and indicates that he is as repulsed by Vivian's sexuality as he is by her lycanthropy, which was revealed to him in a moment of sexual intimacy. Later Aiden is so horrified by Vivian's lycanthropy that he shoots her in order to put her out of the misery he believes she must be suffering. Aiden's actions, however, maintain traditional gender roles rather than help Vivian. Vivian easily survives the attack, but remains a chimera, stuck between forms, because she cannot yet fully accept her lycanthropy, that part of her that is the opposite of the conventionally feminine, as something that makes her strong and beautiful.

Ginger, the protagonist of *Ginger Snaps,* embraces the Beauty Myth as a consequence of being bitten by a werewolf. Ginger's new conformity to the Beauty Myth is a symptom of how she is turning into a hormonally driven, sexually insatiable animal. However, Ginger as werewolf is also not so different from her peers, whom she scorns as part of what she characterizes as the "total hormonal toilet" of high school culture. In her lycanthropic state, Ginger embodies essentialist concepts of women as inherently dangerous, sexually insatiable beasts governed by their hormones.

In the opening of *Ginger Snaps,* we learn that Ginger and her sister Bea already have rejected the Beauty Myth. The teen sisters, with their dark-hued thrift shop finery and teased Goth hair, set themselves apart from their peers. The sisters' sartorial defiance is part of their larger rejection of hegemonic femininity and of the white middle–class values of their community. However, the sisters' rejection of hegemonic femininity is represented as due to their lack of female sex hormones rather than the result of a reasoned intellectual position. Both sisters are not yet "women" according to this logic: 15-year-old Bea and her nearly 16-year-old sister have not yet entered menarche. As a result, neither is interested in heterosexual relationships, and both have disdain for their sexualized peers.

However, everything changes for Ginger after she starts her period and is bitten by a werewolf moments later. Overnight, she suddenly conforms to the Beauty Myth by adhering to a standard of teen female beauty that encourages girls to demonstrate their "maturity" by dressing in sexualized ways. The day after Ginger is attacked, she comes to school sporting a stylish hairdo and form fitting clothing, drawing appreciative glances from the boys and disapproving glares from other girls. Ginger transforms over the next lunar cycle from a human girl with no interest in boys or dating into a sexually insatiable beast for whom desire and anger are inextricably linked. She is particularly sexually active and dangerous when she ovulates and menstruates for the second time in her life, phases in a woman's monthly hormonal cycle that increase libido. Ginger's newfound interest in heterosexual relations makes her normatively feminine, while her hormonally driven emotions link her to patriarchal fears about women's closer relationship with nature. However, while her conventionally feminine peers manage to keep their sexual desires under control, these feelings erupt violently in Ginger, who has been transformed into a teen femme fatale.

The female werewolf's lupine body is also an iteration of patriarchal fears about women's alleged closer relationship to nature. This relationship makes her dangerous and justifies her subordination. *Ginger Snaps* reproduces in monstrous form the Enlightenment nature–culture division, in which women are more closely affiliated with nature, while men are more closely affiliated with culture. Ginger is linked to the natural world both because she is female and because she is a werewolf. Ginger's lupine characteristics are associated with her becoming a young woman. When Ginger enters menarche and is bitten by a werewolf in nearly the same instant, she is transformed into a sexually mature woman *and* a monster, which calls attention to the association between the category of woman and the category of nature. Moreover, Ginger's menstrual cycles and lycanthropy are both governed by the moon, a connection that further links her to nature.

The werewolf's bite has also made Ginger monstrous by making her body resemble what Julia Kristeva terms the abject body, whose manifestation is the feminine/maternal body.[18] The feminine/maternal body is the prototype of the abject body because its lack of corporeal integrity, demonstrated through its secreting of blood, among other fluids, signifies its connection to the natural world.[19] Ginger's menstruation is represented as something as repugnant as her lycanthropy. In two scenes, Ginger cannot staunch her menstrual flow: it courses down her legs in one instance, and visibly drips on the floor in another. The combination of lycanthropy and menarche changes Ginger's body from girlish to maternal, a transformation connecting her to the natural world.

Ginger's menstruation is also tied to her sexual desire, which reaches its peak when she menstruates and ovulates, again, times in a woman's cycle when she often experiences increased libido due to higher levels of estrogen in her blood. Ginger's behaviors are regulated by her menstrual cycle, which is in turn controlled by the phases of the moon. Days after Ginger begins her period, she goes from having no interest in dating to becoming a slave to a biological imperative to mate.

While lycanthropy transforms Ginger into the embodiment of patriarchy's fears about women, it also ironically disqualifies her as conventionally feminine. Instead, lycanthropy makes Ginger more masculine, which is demonstrated in part by her aggressive sexual desire. When Ginger is about to ovulate, she is so eager to lose her virginity that she sexually assaults her boyfriend Jason. In the backseat of Jason's car, Ginger's sexual desire is so fierce that she pushes her boyfriend into the car seat, ignoring his screams of protest. Their coupling infects Jason with lycanthropy, which emasculates him. The next day Jason has a bloody discharge in his urine that stains his pants and causes his male peers to joke that he is "on the rag." As Jason's infected body changes, his voice becomes higher and more feminine, and unlike Ginger, he is incapable of using violence effectively, as evidenced by his inability to victimize a child who is half his size.

Ultimately, Ginger's association with the moon makes her completely monstrous, a connection that underscores her affiliation with nature. Although Ginger is dangerous while she is ovulating, she is even more threatening on the night of the full moon, when she is about to menstruate for the second time in her life. On this night, when Ginger will fully transform into a werewolf, she is also at her most sexually active: she attempts to sequentially seduce several men. Afterwards, Ginger will permanently change into her werewolf form, a metamorphosis that has been occurring over the past 28 days. The relationship between the werewolf and menstruation is nothing new. Walter Evans sees the werewolf, regardless of its sex, as related to the menstrual cycle because its "bloody attacks . . . occur regularly every month."[20] As a female werewolf, Ginger is doubly tied to the phases of the moon. Lunar cycles are generally associated with women's menstrual cycles, which loosely follow the moon's phases. Before Ginger fully metamorphoses into a werewolf, she is a seductive combination of woman and animal, representing what men find bestial in themselves and have projected on to women's bodies.[21] In this context, Ginger's ability to incite desire in all who come her way is as monstrous as her need to tear things apart.

ANGER AND VIOLENCE

While the teen female lycanthrope is threatening because of her overt sexual desire and inability to appear conventionally feminine, her most monstrous aspect is her anger. Anger is that most unfeminine of emotions, and women's expression of it is met with great disapproval and cultural sanctions. This disapproval is not surprising since reasoned anger "is tied to self-respect, a sense of entitlement, and lucid thinking about wrong-doing"[22] that can lead to action. Angry women "take themselves seriously" and "believe that they have the capacity as well as the right to be judges of those around them, even of those who are said to be their 'superiors'."[23] As a result, women's expressions of anger are viewed by those in power as inappropriate, and even insubordinate. For this reason, girls are trained early on that their expression of anger is incompatible with being a "nice" girl who will ostensibly be "listened to, accepted, rewarded, included."[24] The teen female werewolf exposes that this promise is hollow: "nice girls" are not listened to when it counts, but instead, rewarded by being further silenced and subordinated.

Vivian's expression of anger completely disqualifies her as normatively feminine. At the beginning of *Blood and Chocolate,* Vivian is fearful of the expression of all anger, particularly her own. While Vivian belongs to a werewolf culture that views women's anger as healthy, and even allows women to express this emotion through violence, she initially considers anger to be an emotion that is at best undignified and at worst extremely dangerous. In the beginning of the novel, Vivian is mortified to learn that her mother Esmé has been brawling with Astrid, another female werewolf, over the affections of a man, though Vivian too has harbored violent feelings of jealousy. When Kelly, a rival for Aiden's affection, gives Vivian a dirty look, she momentarily contemplates brawling with the girl. But Vivian has seen how anger is also potentially dangerous, regardless of the sex of the person expressing it. In extreme cases, anger is something that can wipe away the human part of a werewolf and permit the "animal to reign supreme,"[25] which endangers the entire pack. A year previously, Vivian's father was killed and the pack forced to relocate after one of their members could not control his anger. As a result, he murdered a human girl, an action that revealed the pack's existence to local humans, who burned the pack's compound. Vivian's father, the pack's leader at the time, died trying to save the others.

Vivian will eventually come to reconsider her feelings about anger when her expression of it comes about as a consequence of her emerging feelings of self-respect, which prompt her to fight injustice. This emotion causes Vivian to take the swift action required to save her mother's life. In Klause's werewolf culture, both males and females fight in their wolf skins to settle differences, and pack leaders are chosen through physical contests rather than through acclimation. For example, all adult women can fight in the Bitches' Match in their wolf skins to determine who has the right to become the leader's mate and the female head of the pack. When Vivian's mother and her rival, Astrid, fight in the Bitches' Match, Astrid badly injures Esmé during the fray. Vivian jumps in without thinking and saves her mother's life by savaging her opponent.

Still, because Vivian has been influenced by a human culture that views women's anger as toxic, she continues to fear this emotion in herself. Vivian's anger over Aiden's rejection of her causes her to believe that "the animal in her has reigned supreme" and prompts her to get drunk, break into Kelly's house, and vandalize her room. Vivian awakens the next morning with the taste of blood in her mouth and little recollection of the previous night, fearing that she has done more than damage property after the mauled body of a biker is found behind a local bar.

Astrid takes advantage of Vivian's fear of her own anger, setting her up to appear guilty of the recent string of maulings of humans, including the one found on the night that Vivian blacked out. While humans have attributed the maulings to a wild animal, the werewolf community is on edge because they realize the deaths were caused by one of their own. Gabriel, the pack's new leader, is obligated to find and execute the perpetrator whose actions threaten to reveal the pack's existence to humans.

Vivian can only accept her anger as a natural and desirable after Gabriel reveals to her that she was not responsible for the killings. Only then can Vivian can appreciate her anger as something positive that leads her to protect those she loves instead of an emotion that permits "the animal to reign supreme." However, Vivian's acceptance of her anger at the end of the novel does not constitute a complete repudiation of conventional femininity. Gabriel, Vivian's eventual romantic partner, is charmed by her anger, which he sees as evidence of her fierce ability "to care" for those she loves. In this way, Vivian's anger makes her *more* feminine in that it is linked to that stereotypical feminine affinity for caring and connection, rather than to self-respect.

Ginger's anger also disqualifies her as conventionally feminine. However, anger is not merely confined to female lycanthropes in the film. *Ginger Snaps* accurately represents how contemporary teen girls labor to suppress open expressions of anger in the interests of being "nice." This repressed anger does not disappear, but seethes beneath the surface, erupting into girlfighting,

Lyn Mikel Brown's term for the bitchy, backbiting relational aggression that frequently characterizes girls' relationships with one another, and that is viewed as the "natural" consequence of being female.[26] Dominant girls police the borders of femininity through girlfighting, ostracizing from their groups any girl who is different and so does not exhibit prevailing notions of girlness. Girls who are too outspoken, or who don't meet other, generally white, middle-class notions of femininity, are branded as sluts, a designation that configures their sexualities as marking the outer limits of conventional femininity. Girlfighting perpetuates a "climate of division and distrust among girls [that] eventually undermines women's psychological strengths and their political potential."[27] In this way, girlfighting maintains the status quo—girls grow into women who see one another as rivals for the attention of men, the power brokers in a patriarchal society, rather than become women who question the value of this attention in the first place.

Ginger and her sister Bea have always been the victims of girlfighting. The sisters' running feud with other female peers is established in an early scene in gym class. Ginger and Bea make nasty comments about Trina St. Claire, one of the school's more popular girls, characterizing her as the school slut. (Trina will later make the same accusation against Ginger.) Trina overhears the sisters' remarks, and the violence of her retaliation demonstrates the long-standing nature of their grudge. During a game of field hockey, Trina knocks Bea to the ground in a way that appears accidental from the gym teacher's distant perspective. But this move is also characteristic of girlfighting. Girl-on-girl relational aggression is often hidden so that it will fly under the radar of adults who could intervene in what they might see as bullying behavior: "In a culture so deeply infused with white middle-class values" girls must appear to be "nice" in order to be acceptably feminine.[28] Thus, "girls who buy into prevailing views of femininity are likely to hide the 'bad' or 'shameful' parts of their relationships."[29] This type of "accidentally on purpose" violence is one way that girls hide from adults their aggression toward one another.

When Ginger becomes a werewolf, the power dynamic shifts between her and the girls who excluded her: while Ginger is still the target of girlfighting, she can now defend herself. But from her new, stronger position, Ginger still perpetuates these persistent divisions between women rather than attempting to overcome them. When Ginger becomes a beauty whose appearance gets her attention from boys, she becomes Trina's rival. Ginger begins dating Jason McCardle, one of the more popular boys in school, and the relationship makes her an even more powerful rival as Jason's popularity makes him one of the school's power brokers.

Ginger's changed status also alters her relationship with Bea: fights erupt because Ginger's new interest in boys causes her to privilege her relationship with Jason over her relationship with Bea. Now that Ginger is more like a "normal" girl, she is even less likely to benefit from the sisterhood resulting from female friendship. As a consequence, Ginger's anger is not a political emotion that frees her from a crippling subordinate feminine subjectivity. Instead, it further isolates her from others and causes her to revert to what is stereotypically represented as both women's and adolescents' essential nature as atavistic creatures in thrall to "primitive" emotions such as anger.

As Ginger becomes more isolated from other girls, she becomes more angry and violent. Though Ginger has always seen herself as a "lone wolf," even before becoming a werewolf, she has depended on her close relationship with Bea. However, this relationship is threatened by Ginger's lycanthropy. As Ginger transforms into a werewolf over the next 28 days, she becomes increasingly jealous of anyone who pays attention to Bea and kills those she perceives as intruding on that relationship. In one of the film's more bloody scenes, Ginger savages the elderly school janitor who is kind to her sister, justifying her actions with a weak claim that her victim was looking at Bea's breasts. Ginger later kills Sam, an older teen marijuana dealer who uses his knowledge of plants to try and help Bea cure Ginger. Ginger makes a similar weak claim about Sam's alleged predatory sexual feelings toward Bea.

What Monsters Can Teach Us

So, if the monster is a creature meant to show us something, then what can the teen female werewolf teach us about the terrible cost to young women of being conventionally feminine? Barbara Creed explains that "the concept of a border is central to the construction of the monstrous."[30] Anything crossing this border, or attempting to cross it, is menacing because it brings about "an encounter between the symbolic order and that which threatens its stability."[31] The threat to that border, however, is educational: it reveals that the boarders that define us are not stable and absolute, but permeable, and so they can be modified or even obliterated.

Ultimately Ginger can only fit into the category of monstrous Other. However, her ability to pass through boundaries shows the viewer that these categories are constructed rather than the immutable result of a biological imperative. Ginger's metamorphosis from human to werewolf is a sort of drag performance: her transforming body is both more masculine and more animal, requiring her to labor to successfully pass as female *and* human. Judith Butler sees drag as a performance that can destabilize the category of gender by mocking "the notion of a true gender identity."[32] Ginger's lupine body threatens the symbolic order because it is a perversion of the notion of a stable gender identity. As Ginger becomes more of a femme fatale, she is also more normatively masculine in some aspects of her appearance. She sprouts hair on her chest and her coccyx elongates into a budding tail, which is alarmingly erect, like a tiny penis. As the tail grows, Ginger must tape it to her leg in order to continue passing for human and female. Strapping down her new appendage in this way is similar to how drag queens tape down their penises to more convincingly create the illusion of femininity. Like the body of the drag queen, Ginger's body also cannot be neatly categorized as male or female, human or animal. Instead, her body crosses borders and calls into question the stability of these boundaries.

But finally, Ginger will have passed through so many borders that cannot be anything else but monstrous Other. As a werewolf, Ginger is neither male nor female, but an animal that does not resemble any sort of creature found in the natural world. She is now a hairless, hideous gray beast who walks on all fours and is intent on destroying everyone she meets, so she must be "put to sleep" for her own good and for the good of those threatened by creatures who cross borders. Dead, Ginger is now wholly a monstrous Other.

Yet the film's conclusion is not an unproblematic affirmation of the normal. Rather, Ginger is damned by her culture even before the werewolf's bite. As a young woman, her choices were to either embrace a conventional femininity that would make her into a vapid "pleasure model" like her rival Trina St. Claire or be perpetually scorned as an outsider. The film's adult women characters hint at Ginger's destiny were she to opt to become normatively feminine. She could become like her mother or the school nurse, both intelligent women in traditional roles whose words are discounted as a result, and whose visible aging marginalizes them in a culture that values youth and beauty in women.

While Ginger offers a fairly normative representation of woman as monstrous Other, Vivian in *Blood and Chocolate* hints at possibilities for a liberated feminine subjectivity. *Blood and Chocolate* emphasizes the pressure that teen girls feel to embody a normative femininity that necessitates they disavow their desires for sex—and sometimes even food—while swallowing the justifiable anger they experience as a result. Unlike Ginger, Vivian has successfully deconstructed this subject position, while Ginger loses her ability to deconstruct it.

Blood and Chocolate is a paranormal romance, a hybrid genre that gives Klause multiple strategies for exposing gender as constructed, rather than natural. "Paranormal romance" is defined as a narrative with supernatural elements where the love relationship between main characters is the focus of the plot.[33] *Ginger Snaps* is not a paranormal romance; though Ginger has a male love interest, the relationship is secondary to the story. In *Blood and Chocolate,* however, Vivian's romantic relationship is crucial to the development of her emerging sense of self as an adult woman. Moreover, her romantic relationship is altered because she is a werewolf. In the romance narrative, the heroine must successfully reinterpret the hero's surliness as evidence of his affection, rather than behavior that should drive her away. This semantic sleight of hand is not difficult for the heroine to perform (or for the typical romance reader to accept) since contemporary discourses of masculinity have already predisposed her to view his gruff, dismissive behavior as compatible with his gender.[34] The presence of a werewolf figure, however, transforms the typical relationship between the heroine and hero of the romance. Because the female werewolf is the embodiment of all that women are compelled to repress in the interest of being stereotypically feminine, the lycanthropic Vivian can deconstruct normative masculinity. As a consequence, she can avoid becoming entangled with someone who would deprive her of autonomy.

Harriet Margolis argues that romance fiction can be read as a type of female *bildungsroman* in that "it considers questions of female identity, with a particular interest in the female protagonist's subjectivity."[35] Unfortunately, in the romance genre, these questions are usually answered in a way that represents the female protagonist as subordinated and effectively silenced. In the conclusion of most romance novels, the heroine's development is achieved after she finds her true love, with whom she will retreat into the domestic sphere and live a fairly conventionally feminine existence.[36] Paranormal romance, on the other hand, depicts alternatives for women to the typical marriage plot. Lee Tobin-McClain describes paranormal romance as a genre whose fantastic elements allow "for the exploration of unspeakable elements of contemporary gender identity and relationships,"[37] such as women's anger and empowerment and feelings of desire. The fantastic elements of *Blood and Chocolate* allow Vivian's anger and sexual desire and sense of herself as powerful to be represented as natural facets of her personality rather than abject qualities that must be disavowed. Lycanthropy enables Vivian to accept these parts of herself rather than attempt to eradicate them, permitting her to develop beyond the narrow confines of the typical romance novel protagonist. *Blood and Chocolate* ends with Vivian's developing into a strong and relatively autonomous woman who will never quietly and completely retreat into the domestic sphere.

The paranormal elements of *Blood and Chocolate* enable Vivian to deconstruct the romance genre's discourses of normative femininity that set women up for victimization. Vivian initially attempts to emulate the typical romance heroine's behavior, a behavior that typifies what it means to be a "good" and "normal" woman in our culture.[38] However, eventually Vivian realizes that this behavior is self-destructive, in part because it is antithetical to her nature as a werewolf. As a result, she comes to understand how normative femininity is a confining subject position, rather than a "natural" facet of adult womanhood.

The basic framework of *Blood and Chocolate* follows the trajectory of the Harlequin romance: a young, inexperienced woman becomes involved with an older man who is "mocking, cynical, contemptuous, often hostile,"[39] and his behavior confuses her—since the man is obviously interested in her romantically. Vivian too is young and inexperienced in the ways of adult relationships (though it is implied that she has been sexually active). Gabriel, the man who will become her partner at the end of the novel, is older than Vivian by about a decade, strong, and more experienced than she. Although Vivian is initially attracted to Gabriel, she dismisses her feelings because of what she sees as his mocking, cynical, and contemptuous behavior, especially toward her.

The supernatural elements of horror denaturalize the repressed, thereby making accessible the terrors of daily life,[40] as well as deconstruct and redraw the boundaries that perpetuate subjectivity.[41] In this way, *Blood and Chocolate* uses supernatural elements to critique the sexist representations of erotic love that inform the romance. Though Klause frames her heroine's life through the conventions of romance, she also manipulates these conventions of the genre in order to challenge its sexist assumptions. She does this in part through the use of paranormal elements more commonly found in horror.

Vivian is more than an animal in drag in human skin or a normatively feminine werewolf. Unlike Ginger, Vivian is a true hybrid: she can *continuously* pass between the boundaries separating human and animal, male and female, and even adult and child, thereby revealing the permeability of these borders. Judith Butler writes of how the drag queen's parodic performance exposes "the phantasmic effect of abiding identity as a politically tenuous construction" because the audience always understands that there is in this performance "the possibility of a failure to repeat, a de-formity."[42] The female werewolf's hybridity similarly undermines "an illusion of the unity of gender," which "is maintained through the constant repetition of stylized acts."[43] Ultimately, this hybridity endows Vivian with agency that Ginger and her normatively human sisters lack.

Klause's female werewolf invites readers to consider a subjectivity that transcends boundaries between male and female, human and animal, nature and culture. For the teen female lycanthrope, overt sexual desire and anger are natural facets of herself that give her autonomy, rather than feelings that must be repressed because they have the potential to unsex her. These feelings are so greatly a part of who she is that they can be disavowed only at her peril. In this way, the teen female werewolf provides an object lesson to girls about the dangers of truncating the self in the interest of normative femininity.

Klause's werewolves derive their power not from their animalistic natures, but due the flexibility afforded to them by lycanthropy. Like Ginger, Vivian crosses boundaries. However, this mutability gives Vivian more agency than she would have if she were a human girl. At the end of the novel, when Aiden shoots Vivian, she momentarily becomes stuck between forms. Her resulting body is a chimera that deprives her of agency in that her mismatched parts do not permit her to live comfortably as either a wolf or a human. Vivian can only regain her autonomy after Gabriel helps her understand that her hybridity is empowering. Humans too have "a beast within," Gabriel tells her, yet they are weaker than werewolves because this beast will "break out in evil ways"[44] if it suppressed too fiercely. Werewolves, with their ability to pass between boundaries separating human and animal, can give this beast a voice, and make use of the strengths it affords them, without necessarily losing touch with their own humanity. After remembering the strength inherent in her changeable body, Vivian regains her ability to transform along with the agency that this ability gives her. The fluidity of Vivian's form finally means that she cannot be relegated to the position of object.

The teen female werewolf implies that normative femininity is not the natural consequence of being female, but is a fragile construction that can be maintained only at a terrible cost to young women. Ginger demonstrates how threatening a girl is to the dominant culture when she will not, or cannot, perform as normatively feminine. Ultimately Ginger is locked into a type of stereotypical femininity where she is ensnared in the body of a beast that embodies patriarchy's worst fears about the supposed essential nature of women. Yet her "normal" female peers are similarly trapped: they too are locked into a type of stereotypical femininity that sets them up for an adulthood where they will be deprived of agency. In 20 years, Ginger's rival, the popular Trina St. Claire, can become like Ginger's mother, rewarded with a life of middle-class privilege where her husband, her children, and her culture in general silence her by ignoring her words. As a hybrid of human and animal, Vivian is uniquely able to reject normative femininity. Vivian's hybridity gives her the resources to develop strategies that permit her to express these supposedly unacceptable parts of herself without provoking the wrath of members of the dominant culture. In both instances, however, the figure of the teen female werewolf causes us to question what we have believed to be "natural" and "true" about women and adolescents.

NOTES

1. Michael S. Kimmel, "Masculinity as Homophobia: Fear, Shame, Silence in the Construction of Gender Identity," in *Theorizing Masculinities,* ed. Harry Brod and Michael Kaufman (Thousand Oaks, CA: Sage Publications, 1994), 132.
2. Chantal Bourgault du Coudray, *The Curse of the Werewolf: Fantasy, Horror and the Beast Within* (London: I. B. Tauris, 2006), 112.
3. Anthony Fonseca and June Michele Pulliam, *Hooked on Horror III: A Guide to Reading Interests* (Westport, CT: Libraries Unlimited, 2009), 155.
4. In *Paradoxes of Gender* (New Haven, CT: Yale University Press, 1994), Judith Lorber examines how gender roles perpetuate women's subordination by keeping them economically dependent on men.
5. "Paranormal romance" is a term describing romance fiction with the addition of supernatural creatures such as vampires, ghosts, or werewolves. Romance fiction itself is, according to Kristin Ramsdell in *Romance Fiction: A Guide to the Genre* (Englewood, CO: Libraries Unlimited, 1999), defined as "a love story in which the central focus is on the development and satisfactory resolution of the love relationship between the two main characters, written in such a way as to provide the reader with some degree of vicarious emotional participation in the courtship process."
6. Susan Brownmiller, *Femininity* (New York: Ballantine, 1984), 15.
7. Naomi Wolf, *The Beauty Myth: How Images of Beauty Are Used Against Women* (New York: Harper Perennial, 2002), Naomi Wolf situates the Beauty Myth as part of the present antipathy toward feminism documented by Susan Faludi in her book *Backlash:* "The ideology of beauty is the last one remaining of the old feminine ideologies that still has the power to control those women whom second wave feminism would have otherwise made relatively uncontrollable. It has grown stronger to take over the work of social coercion that myths about motherhood, domesticity, chastity, and passivity, no longer can manage" (pp. 10–11).
8. Wolf draws here from Betty Friedan's earlier work *The Feminine Mystique* (Harmondsworth, UK: Penguin, 1963).
9. Wolf, *The Beauty Myth,* 220–257.
10. Joan Brumberg, *The Body Project: An Intimate History of American Girls* (New York: Random, 1997), xvii.
11. For a more thorough discussion of how women's athleticism is undermined by cultural ideas about their alleged innate frailty, see Colette Dowling's *The Frailty Myth: Redefining the Physical Potential of Women and Girls* (New York: Random House, 2000).
12. The most salient aspect of the figure of the slut is how her abjection is connected to her perceived sexual excesses, which are rooted in a sexual double standard in which overt sexual desire is antithetical to normative femininity. Emily White (*Fast Girls*), Lyn Mikel Brown (*Girlfighting*), and Leora Tannenbaum (*Slut!*) deconstruct the figure of the slut, noting that girls are put in this category by peers not due to their sexual practices, but because they do not fit within the boundaries of stereotypical femininity. While the slut can be the girl who is sexually active, she is more likely to be the girl who came to the school in the middle of the year and so is not protected by a coterie of friends, the girl who ran afoul of the reigning "mean girl," or a member of a racial or class minority within her school's population.
13. Annette Curtis Klause, *Blood and Chocolate* (New York: Delacourt Press, 1997), 52.
14. Klause, *Blood and Chocolate,* 166.
15. Klause, *Blood and Chocolate,* 168–169.
16. This is particularly true in paranormal romances with werewolves such as Stephenie Meyer's *Twilight Saga* and Kelley Armstrong's *Women of the Otherworld* Series.
17. Klause, *Blood and Chocolate,* 194.
18. Julia Kristeva, *The Powers of Horror: An Essay on Abjection,* trans. Leon S. Roudiez (New York: Columbia University Press, 1980), 102.
19. Barbara Creed, "Dark Desires: Male Masochism in the Horror Film," in *Screening the Male: Exploring Masculinities in Hollywood Cinema,* ed. Steven Cohan and Ina Rae Hark (London: Routledge, 1993), 122.

20. Walter Evans, "Monster Movies: A Sexual Theory," *Journal of Popular Film* 2 (1973): 357.
21. Susan Griffin, *Pornography and Silence: Culture's Revenge Against Nature* (New York: Harper and Row, 1981), 12–14.
22. Lyn Mikel Brown, *Raising Their Voices: The Politics of Girls Anger* (Cambridge, MA: Harvard University Press, 1998), 10.
23. Brown, *Raising Their Voices,* 11.
24. Brown, *Raising Their Voices,* 12.
25. Klause, *Blood and Chocolate,* 171.
26. See Lyn Mikel Brown, *Girlfighting: Betrayal and Rejection among Girls* (New York: New York University Press, 2003).
27. Brown, *Girlfighting,* 33.
28. Brown, *Girlfighting,* 6.
29. Brown, *Girlfighting,* 6.
30. Barbara Creed, "Horror and the Monstrous-Feminine: An Imaginary Abjection," in *The Dread of Difference: Gender and the Horror Film,* ed. Barry Keith Grant (Austin, TX: University of Texas Press, 1996), 40–41.
31. Creed, "Horror and the Monstrous-Feminine," 40–41.
32. Judith Butler, *Gender Trouble: Feminism and the Subversion of Identity* (New York: Routledge, 1990), 137.
33. Kristin Ramsdell, *Romance Fiction: A Guide to the Genre* (Englewood, CO: Libraries Unlimited, 1999), 4, 221.
34. In *Flirting with Danger: Young Women's Reflections on Sexuality and Domination* (New York: New York University Press, 2000), Lynn M. Phillips identifies what she terms "The Male Sexual Drive" discourse, a description of "normal" masculinity depicted in popular culture that represents men as in possession of a sexual drive "that is inherently compelling and aggressive in its quest for fulfillment." This discourse normalizes much masculine misbehavior, assuring "women (and men) that sexualized male aggression, from street harassment to gang rape, is neither a crime nor an act of violation, but just another case in which 'boys will be boys.' It is what tells us that 'working out a yes' from a nonconsenting woman is not rape, but merely what any 'red-blooded American male' would do when aroused. It is what allows defense lawyers to 'justify' such behaviors as fraternity gang rape on college campuses and acquaintance rape of women who are drunk or unconscious" (pp. 57–58). Furthermore, "The Male Sexual Drive" discourse eroticizes these behaviors.

    So pervasive is the privileging of male entitlement that aggressions moves well beyond merely being naturalized as inevitable; indeed, male domination is often posed as something positive—erotic, flattering to women, indication of the powers of desire. Such messages are communicated clearly—to women as well as to men—in the eroticizing of women's powerlessness and objectification in pornography [as well as in romance fiction] (p. 59).
35. Harriet Margolis, "A Childe in Love, or Is It Just Fantasy? The Values of Women's Genres," *Paradoxa: Studies in World Literary Genres* 3, nos. 1–2 (1997): 124.
36. Margolis, "A Childe in Love," 125.
37. Lee Tobin-McClain, "Paranormal Romance," *Journal of the Fantastic in the Arts* 11 (2000): 300.
38. Lynn Phillips discusses how discourses of normative masculinity and femininity are perpetuated by romance fiction, as well as in other forms of mass media such as women's magazines.
39. Tania Modleski, *Loving with a Vengeance: Mass-Produced Fantasies for Women* (New York: Methuen, 1982), 36.
40. Isabel Cristina Pinedo, *Recreational Terror: Women and the Pleasures of Horror Film Viewing* (Albany, NY: State University of New York Press, 1997), 39.
41. Creed, "Horror and the Monstrous-Feminine," 46.
42. Butler, *Gender Trouble,* 141.
43. Butler, *Gender Trouble,* 141.
44. Klause, *Blood and Chocolate,* 261.

Section VII

Teratologies and Ethics

Chapter 22

The Queer Ethics of Monstrosity

Patricia MacCormack

Teratology is most importantly informing theories of alterity, such as feminism, post-structuralism, anti-species-ism, and queer theory. Monstrosity, initially an act of taxonomical and ontological naming of certain subjects as aberrant—both fetishized and maligned—can be thought as an imperative in forming relations which enter subjects into becomings. In continental philosophy, self is constituted not by subject and object but as an event of relation, particularly desire. The ambiguous state of wonder which defines monstrosity demands that political, cultural, and aesthetic relations are themselves monstrous. Relations shift from dialectic to monstrous, so each entity's elements and qualities metamorphose into a mobile negotiation premised on fabulation of extraordinary singularity. Each element is changed and future potentialities of relation go from knowledge to creation. In continental philosophy, these relations are premised on desire, not for an object or toward satisfaction, but as flow which occupies, exceeds, and transforms. Queer theory emerged as a response to the persistence of polarity in sexual identity, suggesting that sexuality is mobile, metamorphic, and ambiguous. Monstrous relations, in their fluid invocation of desire as wonder and horror, where the other collapses in on the self because it is neither same nor opposite, are queer and queer theory itself could similarly be described as monstrous. Teratological relations in this chapter are evinced in many examples: Deleuze and Guattari's demonological,[1] werewolf and vampire philosophy, extreme body modification read through Lyotard,[2] Serres's Venusian contract,[3] Irigaray's mucosal encounters[4], and Braidotti's transpositional pleasures.[5]

Affective Ethics

> The unity of a world is not one: It is made of a diversity and even disparity and opposition. It is in fact, which is to say that it does not add or subtract anything. The unity of a world is nothing other than its diversity, and this, in turn, is a diversity of worlds. A world is a multiplicity of worlds; the world is a multiplicity of worlds, and its unity is the mutual sharing and exposition of all its worlds—within this world.[6]

In his book on Spinoza, Deleuze explicates ethics through the concept of common notions: "In short a common notion is the representation of a composition between two or more bodies, and a unity of this composition .... For when we encounter a body that agrees with ours we experience an affect or feeling of joy-passion, although we do not adequately know what it has in common with us ....”[7] Crucial to Spinoza and Deleuze's definition of ethics borne of common notions is that each element or entity does not come to the relation already fixed in its qualities, which will therefore either be or not be clearly commensurable with the other. Deleuze emphasizes that a defining element of the experiencing of affects of joy comes from an encounter even when we do not (or cannot) know the commonality from which the affects arise.[8] This requires we think carefully about what is meant by “commonality.” Refining this ethic, we can interpret commonality not as resemblance but by the openness of each element to experiencing the other as self and thus the self as other.

> “Now rejecting this way of defining by kind and specific difference,” explains Deleuze, Spinoza suggests a completely different way, linked to common notions; being will be defined by their *capacity for being affected,* by the affections of which they are capable, the excitations to which they react, those by which they are unaffected, and those which exceed their capacity and make them ill or cause them to die. In this way one will obtain a classification of beings by their power.[9]

Defining, signifying, classifying, and placing certain kinds of subjects into a hierarchy is an act, which is based not on the quality or essence of an entity but by the powers that constitute the capacity to define. The history of teratology has been a history of powers of expression in mechanizing and controlling taxonomical structures. Monster ontology manifests the truth of the aberrant in order to affirm the shift of the “normal” from a cultural, arbitrary category to an idealized natural phenomenon. Enriching ethical encounters are also expressions of power. “A manifest truth,” writes Foucault,

> disappearing not when it is replaced by another one that is fresher or sharper but when one begins to detect the very conditions that made it seem manifest; the familiarities that served as its support, the darknesses that bought about its clarity, and all those far away things that secretly sustained it and made it ‘go without saying’.[10]

Affective expressions that elicit joy and novel passions emerge through each entity's capacity to act and be affective not as *what* it is but *that* it is. By virtue of openness to the alterity of the other, commonality is reduced to the majestic but simple notion of openness itself. Encounters are not conditional based on preconceived definitions of the other to which one comes. This would mean the other is experienced before the event of experience and thus the other as a singularity is denied its specificity. This encounter with the preconceived is no encounter, but a reification of self through confirmation of opposition or commonality based on structures that by their very definition cannot locate two entities without one subsuming the other through exertions of the power to define. Ethical encounters are encounters of both affectivity and liberty. Alterity and openness, relinquishing reliance on preexistent signifiers to become lost in the flows of affectivity, are essential to ethical encounters. Alterity of other catalyses alterity of self. Similarly, commonality is not recognized through identical resemblance but by a common intensity that is present but not necessarily transparent in its meaning or capacity for apprehension. Difference is commonality, that is, commonality is a way of differing (from other groups based on their own commonalities), and sameness is imperceptible. If we include desire as an integral part of the ethical configuration, alterity is seductive because it is not complementary in its opposition. This would affirm sameness of self to self. Difference is desirable because it is difference that cannot be subsumed, because it is mobile as a protean experience rather than a position occupied and defined by the other. Desire is neither dialectic nor reiterative of self and other. It is an event upon which we can only reflect fleetingly and that can neither be repeated nor predicted. Ethical desire cannot operate in the positioning of two entities aware of themselves as closed subjects.

Heterosexuality/heterosociality (commonality as complementarity) and homosexuality/homosociality (sameness as repetition) privilege position over affect. Ethical desire cannot be maintained in a relation that privileges the being of each entity rather than the space between. Clearly, an ontology of "sexuality" does not work in this context. Ethical desire cannot be framed as a particular form of sexuality. Fluid, formless sexuality is queer sexuality. Claire Colebrook adds, "Our theory would not be queer, for we might well be in agreement with the general structure of subjects being constituted through social norms and structures; the queerness would lie in the attention we paid to those supposedly failed or extrinsic modes of subjectivity, to which we may accord a privileged transgressive value."[11] The occupation of space *as* something is resistant to the mobile affectivity of forces that interact as a mediation of desire and where passion and joy come from the not-knowable of self or other. Yet it is problematic to offer this constitution of ethics as an exploratory future without a social contextualization of the effects of powers of discourse on others in history. Just as "good" ethics seeks to enhance joy and passion, so "bad" ethics emphasizes those affects that exhaust or enclose the other, exacerbating their capacity to express. In terms of reflections on specific entities whose capacity to effect have been oppressed through signifying systems, the monster stands as iconic. The monster describes many things while not itself being specifically defined as anything that has been consistent in history. The monster is alterity as both wonder and horror, as the limit of humanity and proof that the human always exceeds the parameters of what we think it is capable of. The monster crosses species and boundaries; it is hybrid, metamorphic, but it is not properly something that *is* so much as something that fails to be something else—the traditional dominant human subject. Certain subjects, such as embodiment, have been privileged in their proclivity toward monstrosity.

The body has traditionally been maligned as a monstrous necessity of human subjectivity. Bodies are the medium through which we access pleasure and horror beneath and beyond signifying and cleansing rituals that repress the knowledge that we all are vulnerable and volatile bodies. Where fantasies of volition, self-authorization, stability, and identity itself are perceived as residing in the mind, the persistence of Cartesian proclivities has redeemed the body's excesses and frailties by subsuming it into the social "mind"—science, epistemology, and discourses seeking and claiming absolute knowledge. Bodies are not in opposition to minds but stand at and as threshold between mind and anatomically signified body/neurophysiologically or psychiatrically signified brain (as flesh not self). Bodies are already more than we can bear in their treason against our subjectivity—we feel we occupy them but we are occupied by their irrefutable ownership of us. Theories of corporeality have underpinned many post-structural philosophies of alterity precisely because the other has been relegated to a purely corporeal expression. The other thus fails to pass as subject defined by mind over body or embodied mind. Rather the subject is territorialized by color, sex, age, and other trajectories of signifying difference. Monstrosity is at its most spectacular when it is visible deformity in form or action. Monstrous bodies are also those that have certain qualities—sticky, not demarcated, compelling in spite of their repugnance, interspecies, multiple, or generally resistant to both signification and subjectification. The following section will offer deliberately brief sketches of monstrosity that emerge through these qualities, always initially premised on the body. Taxonomically, women reside beneath men and animals beneath humans. Further hybridity coalesces all three.

WILLFUL MONSTROSITY? BODY MODIFICATION

As an introduction to the organizing of the body through the flesh/text will/body inflection, the heavily modified body is a *despositif* which, we imagine, shows selection of creating signifying punctums on the flesh, forcing the flesh to be read differently. A persistent reinscriber of the body, one that makes the body illegible by demanding a new mode of perception as encounter, is the extreme body modifier. The sociological enunciation is silenced in an aesthetic-ethical relation of joy at wonder and desire as jubilant confounding. An entire occupation of surface by ink, swirling skin, punctuating piercings with no sentences to organize, hybrid making horns, scars as enigmatic coveted wounds, and other examples of body modification deny the skin its function as the inscribed surface, where subjectivity is identified through encounter with flesh as text. I deliberately use the word "extreme" to include modifications which the fashion assimilation of tattooing would still find unpalatable or monstrous. The face as the primary plane of subjectivity recognition is rarely tattooed as it is perceived to be the residence of self. Tattooing a face operates a new production of facial recognition via finite binary options—black/white, male/female—"faces are not basically individual, they define zones of frequency or probability, delimit a field that neutralises in advance any expressions or connections unamenable to the appropriate significations."[12] Assimilating such a face into the binary of tattooed/not tattooed cures the monstrous tattooed face through being explained by the nontattooed interpreting voice. Scarification through branding expresses the "primitive" civilized subject, cutting scarification/patterning the nonmedical subject with a scalpel operating external to appropriate medical operations. The "becoming animal through full tattoos of cheetah spots, zebra stripes or semi-mythic goat-satyr" modifier who inserts and grows coral horns is the new humanimal monster. Lyotard says of the body organism that exceeds the letter (description, taxonomy):

> The letter is not directed to the body; the line however exists only through the echo that it will encounter in the bodies where it will generate itself as danceable volume, polyphony, scene, texture at palpitating fingertips. It will suspend speech. It will be the other side of words, the order of silence, of the scream, hushing all emitters and receivers.[13]

Line as trajectory launches the self encountering the body modified (whether modified or not—this is operation not coalition or fetishism) upon an adventure in desire as ambivalent and ambiguous. Lyotard's syntax of flesh[14] offers echoes—lost, ghostly, stuttering repetition which loses original meaning, dance—the body in movement without meaning, polyphony—many voices in one, one voice as many, scene—movement through space as context rather than occupation of space by subject, texture—apprehension through touch rather than sight, but here sight is another form of touch, not excluded, and the many excesses inherent in the letter as enclosing speech—the silence that is not lack but where words are not enough, the scream, the horror of the thrill of silence. The emitter who describes the other, the receiver told who they are and what they mean, do not figure in this inflection between planes of flesh. Sociological systems presume certain volition in the deliberate "monstrization" of the body, seeing their function as decoding these willful acts. They demand the other speak in the language of the dominant so they may be interpreted. This presumes that body modification is always done for a reason, that each inscription or modification has a symbolic meaning which is commensurable with established symbols, and that the modifier wants to speak in order for their language to be interpreted and spoken back to them to give them some kind of liberation through being told why they really modify—a kind of psychoanalysis of the transgressive who modifies a secret code awaiting translation. To ask the modifier "why" both imagines logical, causal, and necessary volition and fails transparent reflection from the questioner. "But to ask someone a question," Lyotard adds, "is to presuppose that the person understands it and wants to reply . . . do we ask ourselves this question about ourselves."[15] The sociological compulsion to ask "why" annexes this body to the Cartesian privileging of will over flesh, where the heavily body modified is not a subject with reasons so much as an encounter between the interrogator and object, but an encounter or question itself. All monstrous bodies come as questions. Seeking an answer dams up the liberatory pleasures and terrors of monstrosity, converting the question to an event of encounter that creates a queer relation with monstrosity.

MUCOSAL MONSTERS

> A great deal of these physical and morphological mutations are expressed in the language of monstrosity, abjection and horror... what horror has to do with is the lifting of categorical boundaries between human and their others; racialised or ethnic others, animals, insects or inorganic and technological others. The main function of horror, consequently is to blur fundamental distinctions and to introduce a sense of panic and chaos. The monstrous body fulfils the magical or symptomatic function of indicator of the register of difference, which is why the monster has never been able to avoid a blind date with women.[16]

What kind of queer relation could a monstrous configuration lead us to through monstrosity? Irigaray offers the concept of mucosity to explore relations of difference which meld flesh as liquid, sticky, inflecting materiality. She states,

> In order to bring about [sexual difference's] ethics, however, we must constitute a space that could be inhabited by each sex, body or flesh... that threshold which has never been examined in itself: the female sex. It is a threshold unto *mucosity*. Beyond the classic opposites of love and hate, liquid and ice lies this perpetual *half open* threshold.[17]

The monstrosity of female difference is culturally lucid in fictional and historical discourses on monsters: the sticky, oozing materiality of the collapse between monsters and women in film, and, paradigmatically, the horror of relation as viscous connectivity rather than clean, closed dichotomy. Irigaray's refusal of the binarization of love and hate resonates with the doubling of fear and wonder the monster elicits, as well as queer theory's seeking the beyond of hetero and homo. What is vital in Irigaray's idea is her affirmation that the elements which mediate in mucous still nonetheless have their own place and history. Monstrous femininity and female monstrosity offer a threshold in reference to relation and to opening up infinite new configurations of desire, making each entity itself a threshold. However, we cannot deny the other a space of its own as not assimilated or subsumed. Additionally, an ethics of monstrosity will celebrate the potentialities of future experiments in flesh and subject but will not forget or ignore the history of oppression that has constituted the category at all. This is why historical studies and memories of monsters are always part of thresholds, not to anchor monstrosity as a site of oppression but to acknowledge the transgression that the monster offers is the transgression for which it was maligned. A feminine monstrous discourse is a mucosal discourse, challenging the petrifaction and reification that phallologocentric discourse exerts on the monster.

MONSTROUS ANIMALITY

A lower level still than woman in the taxonomical failure to be human comes as those whose flesh or psyche congenitally or behaviourally resonate with the arbitrary homogenizing concept of the animal. Arguably the animal is both the most horrifying and ubiquitous point of coalescence of other and subject. It is the moment of discourse and no discourse; although animals have unique forms of communication, because animals become "animal" in teratology, the specifics of these animal forms of communication are denied. It is the point of nature's threat to subsume culture, evincing that all culture is, is dependent on nature's foundation to create and support bare life. Mary Douglas analyzes the patterns of oppression and subsumation culture uses to dam the fluidity of monstrosity that shows the slippages inherent in any categorization. In reference to teratology, she states, "when a monstrous birth occurs, the defining line between humans and animals may be threatened. If a monstrous birth can be labeled an event of a particular kind, the categories can be restored."[18] Mythical Minotaurs and Sirens become the Elephant man (protean syndrome) and congenital sirenomelia (mermaid syndrome) which, both named after Greek monsters, show mythical monsters inform modern teratology rather than being disproved and rationalized by it. Animal, mythical monster, and syndrome "sufferer" all solicit a "cure." Hermaphroditism, the queer body in and for itself, is almost always "corrected" and the myth transforms from the mystical Hermaphridite to the occult (often converted to Satanic) Baphomet who, in addition to intersex features, has hooves and horns. Pig hearts in baboons aspiring to human transplant are our new Frankensteinian monsters, but while these animals are good enough to stand in for the human, they are denied basic ethical address as not being good enough to be treated at the same level. Like the hero slaying the mythic hybrid, animals are tortured because they are considered aberrant, bodies as commodities, while becoming the zenith of medical sciences' capacity for creation. The ethical issues raised here, clearly antagonistic to Spinozan ethics,[19] show myth has constituted scientific reality rather than being deposed by it, and, while claims to transcendental *a priori* truth in bodies and subjects through their prehuman "nature," concentrate on objects of study rather than self-reflective tendencies of desire for knowledge—what Adams calls the "arrogant eye."[20] What is most crucial for such unethical situation is the distance between the subject and object, while queer ethics and monstrosity both collapse and refuse the possibility of this distance.

MONSTERS WITHOUT METAPHOR

If myth informs science, rather than the converse, then the power of social imaginings of "impossible" fictional fabulations exerts as much power on our constitution of irreducible "nature" as does the idea of distant objective scientific discourse. Monsters emerge in science, medicine, criminology, and psychology as predetermined by genes, chromosomes, congenital destiny, and other reasons authenticated by a fantasy of phenomena that precedes the discourses that describe them. This has seen real bodies deemed monsters and addressed as those who must be either cured or ostracized, those who deserve sympathy or extraction from the "healthy" social *corpus*. For historical studies, as with all minoritarians, this actual system of teratology must be remembered; however, a queer ethics shifts science's claim to truth in monsters as something that needs to be studied and described to abstract monsters, who demand imagination and renegotiation of self precisely because they cannot be studied or known. Braidotti points out a tendency in modern relation with monsters "the contemporary trend for borderline or liminal figures of sexuality, especially replicants, zombies and vampires, including lesbian vampires and other queer mutants."[21] There are two reasons we can see this turn occurring, but neither entirely extricable. The first is the fear of a residually superstitious fantasy that comes directly from a concept of the fictional in order to act as a catharsis to rectify anxieties about the elements of fantasy that operate in reality. For example, lesbians create anxiety because they show that nonphallic desire is possible without being exhausted by description or need of gender opposition. The vampire is the seducer which takes the victim away from the grounding performed by the phallus in sexuality, offering a scenario of fear and ambiguity as its own sexuality without epistemology. The lesbian-vampire coalesce these two figures of mystery. Zombies unite food and sex, death and the idea that the death of the human gives birth to a living nongendered, nonintegrated, oozing, suppurating, perhaps mucosal, "something else." This is especially true for representations of metamorphic zombies rather than those belonging to voodoo or mindless consumerist lore.

Deleuze and Guattari see fictional monsters as neither metaphor nor fantasy but as invoked for a politics of virtuality which can actualize material, political, ethical, creative becomings, always founded on desire.[22] Where science that nomenclatures monstrosity sees nature as having produced mistakes, Deleuze and Guattari see ethics as coming from relations that are "combinations neither genetic nor structural; they are interkingdoms, unnatural participations. That is the only way Nature operates—against itself."[23] This theory performs an elliptical, infinite function. Entering into relations with the monstrous other—woman, animal, body modifier, fictive creature of horror—creates an unnatural participation, an interbreeding, a truth created from incommensurability. Hybridity and mobility, inherent elements in monstrosity, describe these relations. Nature is always already against itself, folded into a multifaceted chaotic elegant creativity; nothing is normal or aberrant, nothing a mistake as by virtue of nature creating it; it cannot be unnatural. Only participations that majoritarian discursive systems see as unnatural, via the cultural interpretation of nature, are observed as incorrect phenomena and mistakes. Unnatural structures exploit and develop their becomings through inconceivable but nonetheless possible infections of unlike intensities, and for this reason becoming-woman and animal are not bifurcated from fictional becomings, such as participations with werewolves, demons, and vampires. The intensities, not the biological givens, constitute these monsters, nonfictional and fictional alike so that this categorization itself is moot. "Becomings," Deleuze and Guattari infer, "produce nothing by filiation: all filiation is imaginary."[24] That the monster is not the "brother of man," outside of the family tree of the evolutionary zenith of the human, means there is no family for the monster so the only relations possible are unnatural. The monster can neither reproduce itself nor its subjective discourse because every relation is a singularity. In this sense, Deleuze and Guattari emphasize that ontology is fiction, becoming actualizations of nature. Werewolves, demons, vampires, and other post-teratological monsters multiply the multiple of the assemblage as they are already more than one—packs of wolves, contagions of vampires and zombies, demons as legion or pandemonium. Within their own emergence they are hybrid—the werewolf half-animal half-man thus neither and both; the vampire transforming undead to wolf, bat, and always sexually ambiguous; the demon seducing as it damns, reflecting the self of the one who makes the pact while showing infinite potentialities of self as otherwise. Deleuze and Guattari state, "we are not interested in characteristics, what interests us are modes of propagation, occupation, contagion, peopling. I am legion . . . ."[25]

MONSTROUS ETHICS

Monsters no longer contain characteristics; they cannot be described, signified, or inserted into a hierarchy or nosological system. A queer ethics of monstering becomes a *practice,* an activity to evoke affects and open up to affects unthought of. Michel Serres writes,

> Fear, hideousness, vampires, dragons, the multiple at first, inspire fear. What terrifies is not the meaning of the noise—the thing spoken, forspoken—but the increasing multiplicity that says it . . . . But these demons are nothing but the calls of the world or the moans of the others who are crying for help. Would you be frightened by this wailing?[26]

Love for monsters acknowledges their suffering within a certain regime of signification. Just as fear and wonder emerge when relating with monstrosity, opening to this fear bears witness to a suffering based on the incapacity to speak within a certain discourse, described but not heard. When we succumb to the wondrous desire of unnatural participation, this wail is also a seductive call to hear without interpretation or epistemology, to encounter with the self become otherwise.

A monstrous language, sonority frightens only the human, the refusing, the dividuated, and the integrated. The multiple shifts, the band twists as a moebian strip and the self is lost to the many within one, the one within many, the community of the unlike.

> "Everything flows," writes Serres, and, Objects are springs . . . . thus perception is an encounter, a collision or an obstacle, one of many intersections along the way. The perceptive subject is an object of the world, plunged into the objective fluencies. Receiver, in its place, transmitter from every point of view. Beaten, struck, wounded, sometimes ravaged, burned, painful.[27]

Proximity with monsters here constitutes the monster only as its own object or object in the world which itself as space does not perceive as the world is not constituted as its own object per se. The monster, as all perceivers, is object as receiver. It cannot be objectified for or by the other. It is one among many proliferative objects within a teeming world where the only demarcation of objects comes through proximity and vibration or turbulence. Why in this argument I maintain the monster as monstrous object is twofold. First, the monster is frequently that which is most likely demarcated as object for the other due to its particularly emphatic modes of collision affected by its extreme difference. Constituted as aberration, this collision makes likely the monster as receiver more likely to receive in Serres's[28] warning way—beaten, struck, and so forth. The ethical turn of the perceiving other will be a part of this sensation of diminishing affect toward the other. But from a queer creative perspective, the emphasis on turbulence of familiar and stabilizing vibrations, waves and flows that the monster catalyses, means perception is most likely to form new, unthought-of relations that encounter the monster as molecular synthesis rather than obstructive traumatic collision.

Love for Monsters

Serres describes two systems of knowledge or, more correctly, modes of perception, one of which opens out through perception as creation, the other which slaughters through signifying practices, the Order of Mars:

> The atomist, a friend to Venus, does not feel the hatred by which a subject is invented, or the detestation of the body that makes it other to the world; these are vices of Mars and his philosophical followers. The senses are faithful, like all other receivers. They are under contract to Venus, as are the objects among themselves. This natural pact is something like an equivalent of harmony, and functions like it. Established by an immanent Venus. The fluctuating network is stable for itself. The so called errors of the senses can be reduced to the canon.[29]

The Order of Venus is an order of desire for fluctuating self without lack or opposition. Constituted by the Order of Mars, the subject in proximity with the monster cannot sense because sense is blocked by knowledge, just as harmony is destroyed by collision. Errors are of sensation as perception, so an object cannot be an erroneous subject, the monster not an erroneous human. Monstrosity is experienced as a viscous seduction of perturbation. We can only name monstrosity under these conditions as mucosal, inextricable molecular alteration of both objects as they are perceived by their conditions of singularly expressed collusion. Serres's call to sense is both a sensuousness and sensation as asemiotic relation.[30] Sensuous relations are ones of corporeal desire, where the flesh comes before the constitution of its form as subject by science, religion, capitalism, and so forth. Sensation similarly refuses the hardness, surface, or outline of bodies as being objects independent of the world in which they arise. Those who name monsters imagine they stand outside of the world, where the world is defined as the conditions which produce our capacity to know through naming and name through knowing. In this context, knowledge belongs to the Order of Mars, to finality and to absolutes of qualities nomenclatured by definitions of forms. Two singulars stand in opposition in the Order of Mars, the aggressor and the invaded. But the aggressor does not define itself, masquerading as the distant voice of reason, logic, or any other mode of elocution independent of subjective investment in power. The aggressor defers speech and operations of naming the monster to external, higher order unities—Law, "nature" as preceding culture, God. The monster represents two vulnerabilities in the system of the singular—the abject as the collapse between subject and object, I and other, demarcated and integrated. It also shows to the I that it is always and already part of this collapse. Discourse is both a description and an activity of separation. Two elements in space standing against each other are also a continuing practice in time of maintenance and assurance through repetition. The beings, those who are the "to be"—to be the monster and to be the not-monstrous—is always a consistency of being as durational separative practice. Monstrous ethical desire is movement without cessation or destination. "The place and law of the One," Julia Kristeva writes, "does not exist without a series of separations."[31] Elaborating the work of Douglas[32] on the clean and the unclean, the holy and the unholy, and the sacred and the taboo, Kristeva[33] relates the structure of abjection as a strategy of taxonomical demarcation. The tendency to make the monster sacred, to fetishize it, to elevate it to an equal or superior position as mystical savior or esoteric portal to world, where knowledge means enlightenment more than observable truth, continues series of separation, inverting the arboreal taxonomy without relinquishing the patterns of objects in space to be studied and placed within a hierarchy. This fails to address that "every body is a well and every body is a fountain."[34] Fluidity is not of one body but can only be between bodies, and each body is a volume which is empty and full, creative and created. Attraction as interdependence is an act of both love and grace—love in Venusian seeking of sensation and grace in forsaking the human inclination to exert and maintain power through the Order of Mars. Desire is found in both, but fluid, nonoppositional Venusian desire aligns itself with queer desire in their shared qualities. While queer has been understood as coming after heterosexual and homosexual differentiation, as a kind of post-post modern sexuality, Venusian desire occurs before the separation of forms, "desire is constituted *before* the crystallization of the body and the organs, *before* the division of the sexes, *before* the separation between the familiarized self and the social field."[35]

At this final stage of thinking, queer monstrosity comes as perplexing questions. Through the many phases and explications of monstrosity—the female, the animal, the modified, the fictive—what, in the Order of Venus does it mean to be a monster? The troubling but somewhat necessary persistence of syntaxes of "we" and "they" have become confounded. "We" speak of "those" who name, while speaking of "those" who are named. I have deliberately used this oscillating and sometimes frustrating pronoun use for two reasons. The first acknowledges "we," as in all subjects, are complicit in naming and exerting power through practices of knowledge. This is most evident in historical genealogies of monstrosity, taxonomy, and teratology. But it continues in any space where extrication from another is activated for purposes of preserving dominance or simply demarcation. The second conversely welcomes and addresses the monstrosity that all subjects contain and the risks certain subjects take through political activities that enhance monstrosity through occupying spaces and performing actions that resist, disrupt, and make the concept of the normal transparent. We are all monsters and all not monsters depending on our relation with signifying systems. Power is its own act of desire. Imagination through encounters with alterity that catalyze loss of self is a form of desire that is, like the spectacle or encounter with the monster itself, both frightening and compelling, seductive and dangerous. Thus monstrosity, in its final definition as the simple turbulence that collides or harmonizes with the fluidity of our own selves, is nothing more than a wondrousness possible in all things which requires not the monster as entity, but monstrous encounter. The monster in this (de)structure is independent of all objects as it is a state of relation. It is the in-between, the threshold, and we are left with our selves as constituted as part of and through this relation. Without a relation of desire we can no longer speak of monstrosity, just as without human configurations based on polarity we cannot speak of "the" monster. Taking the monster lover in the way Deleuze and Guattari configure the friend, "the friend who appears in philosophy no longer stands for an extrinsic persona, an example or empirical circumstance, but rather for a presence that is intrinsic to thought, a condition of possibility of thought itself, a living category, a transcendental lived reality."[36] Without desire there can be no ethics, as ethics is a power of affective and porous force. Monsters have stood as symbols of a need for ethical address in the face of an entity that refuses the modes through which we have come to be used to addressing otherness and self. The shift from the symbolic to asemiosis, from form to relation, and from atrophy to metamorphosis—all monstrous intensities—transforms the monster from that position of symbolism, denied specificity, to an imperative for action. Monstrous queer ethics is a form of activism as well as an experiment and expression of desire.

NOTES

1. See, for example, Gilles Deleuze and Fèlix Guattari, *A Thousand Plateaus,* trans. Brian Massumi (Minneapolis, MN: University of Minnesota Press, 1987).
2. See, for example, Jean-Françoise Lyotard, *The Inhuman,* trans. Geoffrey Bennington and Rachel Bowlby (Palo Alto, CA: Stanford University Press, 1988); *Driftworks,* trans. Richard Lockwood (New York: Semiotext[e], 1984); and *Libidinal Economy,* trans. Iain Hamilton Grant (Bloomington, IN: Indiana University Press, 1993).
3. See, for example, Michel Serres, *The Birth of Physics,* trans. Jack Hawkes (Manchester: Clinamen Press, 2000).
4. See, for example, Luce Irigaray, *An Ethics of Sexual Difference,* trans. Carolyn Burke and Gillian C. Gill (Ithaca, NY: Cornell University Press, 1993).
5. See, for example, Rosi Braidotti, *Transpositions* (Cambridge: Polity, 2006).
6. Jean-Luc Nancy, *Being Singular Plural,* trans. Robert D. Richardson and Anne E. O'Byrne (Palo Alto, CA: Stanford University Press, 2000), 185.
7. Gilles Deleuze, *Spinoza: Practical Philosophy,* trans. Robert Hurley (San Francisco: City Lights Books, 1988), 55–56.
8. Deleuze, *Spinoza.*
9. Deleuze, *Spinoza,* 45.
10. Michel Foucault, "For an Ethics of Discomfort," in *Power,* ed. James D. Faubion, trans. Robert Hurley (London: Penguin, 1994), 447.
11. Claire Colebrook, "How Queer Can You Go?," in *Queering the Non-Human,* ed. Noreen Giffney and Myra J. Hird (Surrey, England: Ashgate, 2008), 21.
12. Deleuze and Guattari, *A Thousand Plateaus,* 168.
13. Lyotard, *Driftworks,* 85–86.
14. This concept is found throughout both in *The Inhuman* and in *Libidinal Economy.*
15. Lyotard, *The Inhuman,* 128.
16. Rosi Braidotti, *Metamorphoses* (Cambridge: Polity, 2006), 191.
17. Luce Irigaray, "Sexual Difference," in *The Irigaray Reader,* ed. Margaret Whitford, trans. Sèan Hand (London: Blackwell, 1992), 175.
18. Mary Douglas, *Purity and Danger* (London: Routledge, 2007), 49.
19. Ubiquitous in all Spinoza's work and in Deleuze's *Spinoza.*
20. Carol Adams, *Neither Man nor Beast* (New York: Continuum, 1995), especially Part 1.
21. Braidotti, *Metamorphoses,* 179.

22. This is their project catalyzed especially in *Anti-Oedipus: Capitalism and Schizophrenia,* trans. Robert Hurley (Minneapolis: University of Minnesota Press, 1996).
23. Deleuze and Guattari, *A Thousand Plateaus,* 242.
24. Deleuze and Guattari, *A Thousand Plateaus,* 238.
25. Deleuze and Guattari, *A Thousand Plateaus,* 239, 241.
26. Michel Serres, *Genesis,* trans. Genevieve James and James Nielson (Ann Arbor, MI: University of Michigan Press, 1995), 67.
27. Serres, *The Birth of Physics,* 49.
28. Primarily throughout *Genesis.*
29. Serres, *The Birth of Physics,* 49.
30. My interpretation here comes from *The Five Senses: A Philosophy of Mingled Bodies,* trans. Margaret Sankey and Peter Cowley (London: Athlone, 2008).
31. Julia Kristeva, *Powers of Horror: An Essay on Abjection,* trans. Leon Roudiez (New York: Columbia University Press, 1982), 94.
32. Mary Douglas, *Purity and Danger* (London: Routledge, 2007).
33. Kristeva, *Powers of Horror.*
34. Serres, *The Birth of Physics,* 89.
35. Fèlix Guattari, *Soft Subversions,* trans. David L. Sweet (New York: Semiotext[e], 1996), 153.
36. Gilles Deleuze and Fèlix Guattari, *What Is Philosophy?,* trans. Hugh Tomlinson and Graham Burchill (London: Verso, 1994), 3.

Chapter 23

Reopening the Question of the Human and the Animal (Extract)

Dominick LaCapra

Striking in its insistence and durability is the quest or desire for a decisive criterion with which to differentiate humans from other animals as well as the human from the animal in human beings. At issue in this quest is both the nature of a judgment that distinguishes between the human and the animal, along with humans and other animals, and the consequences or implications it may have for interactions both among humans and between humans and other species. I would like to reinforce and contribute to the argument (which, despite indications to the contrary, I hope is becoming increasingly prevalent) in favor of judgment that is differential in complex, qualified ways, does not assume a decisive binary opposition or caesura between human and animal, is attentive to complex differences within what is classified as human or animal, and does not have self-serving, anthropocentric, oppressive or exploitative functions or consequences.

The point of my inquiry is not to deny all differences or distinctions between humans and other animals. But it is to question both the adequacy of the concept of exclusively human rights and the motivation as well as the functions of the misguided quest for a kind of holy grail—a decisive criterion or conceptual Grand Canyon that divides into two the deceptively massive categories of human and animal. I would also ask whether differences that may be adduced are sufficient to serve as a criterion or divider that justifies the human practices and attitudes in the treatment of animals that presumably follow from such a criterion. In the absence of such a decisive, differentiating criterion, any attempted justification of a given treatment of animals (for example, killing and eating or experimenting on them) has to be based on considerations that are typically controversial and debatable, involving problematic normative judgments, that do not have the logical, ethical, or religious force—and conscience-calming function—of a decisive criterion or clear-cut divide in which much of importance is obviously invested.[1]

Humanism itself has often been defended or attacked for dubious reasons: defended as the most enlightened philosophy in the history of "mankind" or attacked as a departure either from true religion or from what is taken to be an even more enlightened or perhaps suitably disabused, nihilistically accomplished theoretical perspective. Without entering into the complexities and functions of various defenses and attacks, one may recognize the basic inadequacies of humanistic idealism and argue that the most valid and ethicopolitically pertinent dimension of the critique of humanism is that which points to humanism's possible role in an anthropocentric perspective that, at least surreptitiously or unintentionally, validates whatever serves human interests and, as a consequence, projectively situates other animals, or animality in general (including the animal in the human being), in the position of bare life, raw material, or scapegoated victim. In fact the human/animal divide is often premised on a dubious comparison between an idealized, rights-bearing, "normal" human—usually a healthy adult in full possession of his or her faculties—and an excessively homogeneous category of the animal.[2] The obvious question is whether these mutually reinforcing frames of reference provide a sufficient basis for the understanding of problems or the elaboration of viable alternatives.[3] A related issue is whether the concept of human rights should be replaced, or at least supplemented, by that of claims that are so basic or fundamental that they are situated beyond sovereignty and should not be infringed by supposedly sovereign states (or other entities). Indeed legitimate claims that limit human assertiveness would place the concept of sovereignty in doubt and apply in important respects to other animals or even ecological systems. [. . .]

A question concerning humanism is whether it has always required a radical other, perhaps even a quasi-sacrificial victim and scapegoat, in the form of some excluded or denigrated category of beings, often other animals or animality itself. As categories of humans (such as women or nonwhite "races") have been critically disclosed as the encrypted other of humanism, however universalistic in its pretensions, the other-than-human animal in its animality has been left as the residual repository of projective alienation or radical otherness. Indeed forms of posthumanism may still divorce the human from the animal and anthropocentrically seek the differential criterion (or essence) identifying the human, even when that criterion paradoxically points to an enigma or indistinction: a traumatic split, signifying stress, or anxiety-ridden form of self-questioning that serves to set apart the human or its "post" avatars such as *Dasein* or creaturely life.[4]

One especially dubious function or consequence of a decisive divide between humans and other animals is to situate the latter in a separate sphere that makes them available for narrowly anthropocentric uses and even exposes them to victimization as if they were simply beyond the pale of ethical and political concerns. At best, actions, including violent actions, against other animals are subject to much lesser legal sanctions than comparable actions performed against humans.[5] Paradoxically, the projection of other animals into a separate sphere may take two seemingly contradictory but at times conjoined forms: the reduction of the other to infra-ethical status, for example, as raw material, purely instrumental being, or mere life, and the elevation of the other to a supra-ethical status as sacrificial or quasi-sacrificial victim as well as utterly opaque or enigmatic other (whether within or outside the self). One may also foreclose the issue of denigration or victimization of other animals as an ethical and political problem by restricting one's concern to humans and leaving other animals out of the equation or at best referring to them only or predominantly in anthropocentric ways, including their reduction to a form of radical alterity. Here anthropocentrism may serve invidious functions insofar as it ascribes certain abilities or considerations only to humans and induces an excessive generalization of the category of anthropomorphism, typically on the unexamined assumption that one has an unproblematic, clear-cut idea of what is distinctively human and that there is indeed a decisive criterion that divides the human from other animals or perhaps the human from animality in the human being. (The charge of anthropomorphism may even serve as a screen for anthropocentrism.[6])

A decisive difference between humans and other animals may, in certain contexts, also be linked to the postulation of decisive differences between categories of humans based on gender, sexual orientation, race, and class. Traditionally women were seen as closer to nature and to other animals, for example, with respect to menstrual cycles. They have also been seen as dominated by sensation, passion, and emotion, indeed hysteria and suggestibility, and, by that token, less open to reason and self-control. Their putative affinity for suffering, compassion, melancholy, and endless mourning has functioned to make them seem peculiarly suited for abjection. At times same-sex acts have been classified as animalistic. People of color and entire societies have been presented as *Naturvölker*, in the tell-tale German term, ahistorically caught or captivated in more or less compulsive cycles of repetition, mired in a magical, mythical, or ritualistic "mentality," and marked by subhuman, animalistic practices such as sexual license and cannibalism.

[. . .]

The paradoxical, complex relations between figuration of the other as raw material (or bare life) and as scapegoated, quasi-sacrificial victim demand sustained attention, for they are often objects of neglect, disavowal, or confusion. They share the crucial function of placing the other-than-human animal, or animality itself, in a separate sphere or category of otherness to which ethical and political considerations do not apply, or at best apply in very reduced form, because the other is either sub- or supra-ethical in status. But they perform this operation in significantly different and seemingly contradictory ways . . . . [W]ithin the very same sentence, the animal may be presented as sacrificed, utilized, or eliminated as a pest for the good of humans. Similarly, a discriminated-against or persecuted group of humans may be figured as other-than-human animals of an infra- or supra-ethical sort, and responses may oscillate between different linguistic, representational, evaluative, and affective registers. (*Pace* Giorgio Agamben, Nazi discourse about Jews pushes prevalent equivocal tendencies to contradictory extremes, with the Jew figured as a powerful, world-historical, subversive force, a phobic, ritual contaminant, a pest or vermin, and even a rag, piece of refuse, excrement, or, in Agamben's sense, mere life.) [. . .]

[. . .]

NOTES

1. For a statement of opposed positions on the question of animal rights, see Carl Cohen and Tom Regan, *The Animal Rights Debate* (Lanham, MD and Oxford: Rowman & Littlefield, 2001). Cohen assertively argues that humans are fundamentally different from animals. This fundamental difference has far-reaching consequences, including the denial of rights to animals and the justification of their use by humans for food and experimentation, with very limited restrictions on human practices (for example, the prohibition of ill-defined unnecessary cruelty) . . . . For a discussion of empathy and morality, including a sense of fairness, in primates, see Frans de Waal, *Primates and Philosophers: How Morality Evolved* (Princeton, NJ: Princeton University Press, 2006). Moreover, as Richard Sorabji notes (*Animal Minds and Human Morals: The Origins of the Western Debate* [Ithaca, NY: Cornell University Press, 1995], 216) with reference to Regan's book, *The Case for Animal Rights* (Berkeley, CA: University of California Press, 1983), Regan believes that inherent value is equal and admits of no degrees, and he relies on a unifying principle (or theory) in terms of inherent value. See also Peter Singer's groundbreaking *Animal Liberation: A New Ethics for Our Treatment of Animals* (New York: Avon Books, 1975) as well as the book he edits, *In Defense of Animals* (Oxford: Blackwell, 1985). My argument has implications for the question of animal rights but does not directly engage that complex debate.
2. As a result, any proximity between human and animal may well be seen as paradoxical and derive from a questionable comparison between an excessively generalized notion of human extremity if not pathology and of abused animals deranged by extreme stress or trauma . . . . See Eric L. Santner, *On Creaturely Life: Rilke, Benjamin, Sebald* (Chicago: University of Chicago Press, 2006) and Slavoj Žižek, Eric L. Santner, and Kenneth Reinhard, *The Neighbor: Three Inquiries in Political Theology* (Chicago: University of Chicago Press, 2005).

3. The widespread but not universal public outcry in the summer of 2007 against the role of the star football player, Michael Vick, in a dog-fighting enterprise, involving the brutal killing (electrocution and drowning) of dogs that did not perform with the desired brutality, is a welcome indication that the issues I discuss are entering the "public sphere" in more than marginal ways....
4. See, for example, Santner, *On Creaturely Life*. See also Žižek, Santner, and Reinhard, *The Neighbor*....
5. In New York State, for example, it is not mandatory for veterinarians to report cruelty to animals. New York State Agriculture & Markets Law section 353A stipulates that cruelty to any animal is a class A misdemeanor making a person subject to up to one year in prison, having the animal removed, and up to three years' probation and a court order barring animal ownership for up to three years. "Lawful" hunting, fishing, trapping, and animal testing are not defined as acts of cruelty.... Agriculture & Markets Law section 351 section B makes it a misdemeanor to own, possess, or keep any animal for fighting. These regulations obviously leave much room for interpretation in both judging that an infraction has taken place and in determining a penalty. And it is debatable whether penalties could be termed prohibitive....
6. For a critique of anthropomorphism, which is self-confidently anthropocentric and follows the prevalent "us-and-them" format, see Clive D. L. Wynne, *Do Animals Think?* (Princeton, NJ: Princeton University Press, 2004). See also the excellent, generally nonanthropocentric exploration of the abilities of various other animals (including language acquisition, inventing, planning, episodic memory, and even deceptiveness) in Virginia Morell, with photographs by Vincent J. Musi, "Minds of Their Own: Animals Are Smarter Than You Think," *National Geographic* 213, no. 3 (March 2008), 37–61.

CHAPTER 24

Where Reality and Fantasy Meet and Bifurcate: Holocaust Themes in *Pan's Labyrinth* (2006), *X-Men* (2000), and *V* (1983)

Caroline Joan (Kay) S. Picart, John Edgar Browning, and Carla María Thomas

Introduction: Classic and Conflicted Frames

The theoretical framework of this chapter begins with Picart and Frank's *Frames of Evil: The Holocaust as Horror in American Film.*[1] In this book, Picart and Frank discuss the cross-fertilizations that have evolved, binding Holocaust films, usually shot in a documentary or docudramatic mode, and horror films, usually visually coded as drawing from the Gothic fictional tradition. An auxiliary part of the argument is that there is a "Gothic criminological" element that enables this cross-fertilization across the realms of fact and fiction: "Gothic criminology gestures toward an account that moves in between the realms of Gothic fiction and film, which entertains its horrified and fascinated readers with unreal horrors attended upon a realistically/cogently imagined fictional world and factual cases (e.g., of stalkers, serial murderers, terrorists, rogue cops) framed in Gothic terms, which are essential to plotting the social construction of where evil resides in modernity."[2] Yet the point of *Holocaust as Horror* is not to show that there is no such thing as "fact" or "fiction" but that there is a mode of narrativizing that clearly privileges the *look* of the "real," even in the use of horror-derived cinematic techniques (such as in *Schindler's List* (1993), where the Nazi Goeth's [Ralph Fiennes] roving and penetrating gaze upon Helena [Embeth Davidtz], his maid, in the basement scene, is reminiscent of shots seen from the point of view of Hannibal Lechter [Anthony Hopkins] in *Silence of the Lambs* [1991]) or motifs (as in *Schindler's List's* visualization of the Schindler women's descent into the "showers" is reminiscent of *Psycho's* (1960) shower scene, with a reverse ending: the Schindler women are saved, rather than killed).[3] Part of the book's conclusion is that "realistic" documentary modes actually draw from "fictional" Gothic modes, which themselves have a complex relationship with the real: all fictional cinematic serial killers, beginning with the iconic Norman Bates from *Psycho,* in some way draw their heritage from the historically real Ed Gein. Yet the appropriation of fictional Gothic modes into factual documentary or docudramatic modes are acceptable or convincing as "true" only if these cinematic footnotes masquerade as partaking of the look of the "real."

But how does one analyze cinematic genres that reference the Holocaust, but defy the privileging of the documentary mode, for more fantastic modes of narrativizing? What do the cinematic modes of fantasy and science fiction, for example, tell us about how the legacy of the Holocaust has seeped into the way that we collectively imagine and tell stories about heroes and monsters, and "good" and "evil"? From whose perspective do we tell these stories? Is there an ethics of spectatorship that can be glimpsed through science fiction and fantasy referents to the trauma of the Holocaust? What do, for example, *Pan's Labyrinth,* the *X-Men* trilogy, and *V: The Original Miniseries* (hereafter *V*) tell us about how we cope with the trauma of the Holocaust through more fantastic, rather than documentary films?

A crucial tool in tackling this set of questions is again derived from Picart and Frank's *Frames of Evil,*[4] partially derived from Isabel Christina Pinedo.[5] This tool lies in the distinctions drawn between a "classic horror frame" and a "conflicted horror frame."[6] The classic horror frame, more characteristic of Hollywood horror films of the 1930s and 1940s, demands the creation of a monster so utterly Other that only his or her killing/sacrifice can render closure, and with that, the restoration of normalcy, to the story. As Pinedo writes, "the boundary between good and evil, normal and abnormal, human and alien is as firmly drawn as the imperative that good must conquer evil, thus producing a secure Manichean worldview in which the threats to the social order are largely external and (hu)man agency prevails, largely in the figure of the masterful male subject."[7] In contrast to the classic horror frame, the conflicted horror frame views evil as residing within the "normal." Whereas classic horror monsters "breach the norms of ontological propriety,"[8] such as the classic Hollywood Frankenstein monsters, monsters of the conflicted horror frame seem "ordinary" at a first glance, much like Norman Bates. While the classic horror frame breaches the ontology of "normal time," the conflicted horror frame, as Steffen Hantke observes, "violates the integrity and separateness of the two spheres"—the normal and the fantastic.[9]

Whereas the focus in *Holocaust as Horror* was in showing the differences between the two frames, the focus of this chapter is in mapping how the classic and conflicted frames, in fantasy and science fiction modes, are less diametrically opposed, than paired, in mirror-imaging ways, like Siamese twins. The resulting narratives, because they are not as constrained by "documentary" or "moral" binaries, are much more complex, and have much to tell us about the teratological reimagination of the Holocaust and its iconic monster, the Nazi.

PAN'S LABYRINTH

Marketed as a fairy tale for adults, *Pan's Labyrinth (El Laberinto del Fauno)* juxtaposes the horrors of two worlds: the horrors of fantasy in an archetypal world of fairies and fauns and the horrors cemented by a fascist regime, of psychopathic military men and their minions. Its story can be simply sketched, as a starting point. Nearing the end of the bloody Spanish Civil War, 10-year-old Ofelia (Ivana Baquero) is ordered to go to an isolated mansion along with her extremely pregnant mother, Carmen (Ariadna Gil). Lonely and alienated from her new stepfather, Captain Vidal (Sergi López), Ofelia, summoned by a grasshopper-fairy, discovers an ancient labyrinth where she meets the Faun, who recognizes her as the long-missing "Princess Moanna" and regales her with stories of the fairy world. The plot takes an unexpected twist when Ofelia's mother suddenly becomes ill because of what seems like a pregnancy worthy of Mary Shelley's

Frankensteinian nightmares. Devoted to her mother, Ofelia makes an agreement with the Faun, to save her mother. Yet to prove that Ofelia/Princess Moanna's spirit has remained "whole," and uncontaminated by her mortal flesh, Ofelia/Princess Moanna also has to perform three tasks. Much like all mythical quests, these challenges transport her on an Odyssean quest, where she must use her guile and wit, and trust her own instincts to overcome all monsters who stand in the way of her reclaiming her royal status in the fairy world.

The plot of the film meanders across these two worlds: one rooted in fairy tales and the other in Franco-ite Spain. The two worlds initially seem completely separate, but then slowly begin to infiltrate and influence each other, as evidenced, for example, by the filters used to shoot the two worlds. Despite the hypersaturated color of the daytime world of Franco-ite Spain, its night scenes have a cold, bluish-gray tint. In addition, the camera work in the world of the diegetic real, likewise, has a linear, less active perspective. By contrast, the nocturnal underworld or labyrinth scenes predominantly have a light green sheen that lights up the moss that seems to populate not only the background but also the trees and the figure of the Faun himself. In general, the color palette of the Faun's world is more vibrant: its reds and golds are particularly luminous, and the camera work in this fantasy world, initially as well, seems more active and meanders about imaginatively.

Later, as the film develops to arrive at a climactic conclusion, the two worlds begin to bleed into each other, with the turning point being Ofelia's mother's near-miscarriage and descent into a fever that induces delirium. Interestingly, it is the fantasy world that influences the real world first, as Ofelia, following the Faun's instruction, immerses a mandrake root, shaped like a boy, in a bowl of milk and feeds it two drops of blood, and slips it underneath her ailing mother's bed. Increasingly, the reds and golds of the fantasy world seep into the real world as her mother begins to recover.

Yet when Ofelia's stepfather, Vidal, finds what appears, to his eyes, to be a decaying root soaked in putrefying milk, another turning point ensues. Choosing her second husband over her daughter, Carmen rejects her daughter's impassioned pleas and disciplines her by throwing the mandrake into the fire. As the mandrake transitions, through Ofelia's gaze, from being simply a root to becoming a human-like creature that writhes in pain and lets off a shrill cry, Carmen's fate, which she has chosen by rejecting the fantasy world in favor of the real, becomes clear. Carmen dies as she gives birth to Vidal's son, and the color palette of the film again begins to shift. The golden color undertone is replaced by an ash gray that predominantly marks Captain Vidal's harsh universe and seems reminiscent of the color tones of Picasso's *Guernica*.[10] The colors of the diegetically real become more dominant as Ofelia is forced to report to the Faun that she failed to heed his advice in the accomplishment of her second task, and experiences utter despair.

On one hand, *Pan's Labyrinth* seems to have a clear, practically literal reference to the nightmare of the Holocaust through the figure of Captain Vidal, who is clearly a sadist in military uniform. He has set up camp in an isolated farmhouse in northern Spain to stamp out the pestilence of leftover anti-Fascist rebels from the Civil War. Vidal's only other obsession, all too reminiscent of the Nazis, is to produce a pure-blooded son.

One of the most violent scenes, shown very early, and one of the very few sequences visibly referencing horror methods of narration in relation to the Holocaust, illustrates how the captain indifferently tortures one of two captured "rebels" who turn out to be innocent peasants hunting rabbits. Shot in Gothic low-key lighting, and seen from a high-angle shot, from the point of view of Vidal, we see an extreme close-up of the prisoner's face, systematically mashed into a pulp by a bottle, which, unlike the prisoner's face, does not break.[11] Then, with the same degree of aloofness, the captain simply shoots the protesting father of the man he just killed. When an examination of the now-deceased prisoners' belongings reveals two dead rabbits (and thus verifies the alleged rebels' story to be true), Vidal simply shrugs, and walks away, expressing irritation that his staff had even bothered him with such an inconsequential matter.

Yet it is less the captain, a clear appropriation of the Nazi-as-monster type, who is of interest to us. Rather, it is the second of the monsters, the "Pale Man," who bears closer scrutiny, precisely because his connection to the monstrosities of the Holocaust is more oblique, and therefore, given the vividness of Del Toro's imaginative universe, more revelatory. The original design of the "Pale Man," according to the director's notes, was an obese man who suddenly lost a lot of weight, leaving the excess flesh hanging over an extremely tall, skeletal frame.[12] Del Toro changed the face, such that only the nostrils and bloody mouth remained, as the character's eyes became bloodshot eyeballs that could be inserted into slits in the palms of the hands of the creature. To see, the monster would then hold his hands, fan-like, against his head.

The result was a character both mythic and historical. The Pale Man was a creature, akin to one of the many wondrous beasts encountered by Odysseus during his journey back home, who is forever hungry, surrounded by luxuriant supplies of food, and yet consumes only the flesh of innocents (as evidenced by the pile of children's shoes—a historical reference to the Holocaust), and ironically, is never full. Del Toro, in the director's commentary,[13] was clear that he wanted the *mise en scene* of the Pale Man to resemble both a "church" (meaning Something that commands dread and reverence, much like Otto's notion of the M*ysterium* T*remendum*[14]) and "the Holocaust" (principally through the pile of shoes—now an iconic synechdoche for the millions killed during the Holocaust). Del Toro's interpretation of Ofelia's catabasis into the Pale Man's lair therefore parallels some Holocaust historians' description of the descent into the gas chambers as a "negative sublime."[15]

Nevertheless, Del Toro was also at pains to make the diegetic real world (Franco-ite Spain) and the fantasy world within *Pan's Labyrinth,* increasingly mime each other. In one pivotal scene, Captain Vidal sits at a long, rectangular table, where, as a show of wealth and power, he superciliously feeds the town officials with luxuriant supplies of food during wartime—condition when food is scarce and heavily rationed. In a mirror-imaging way, the Pale Man also sits at a long, rectangular table decked with appetizing displays of food, essentially as alone as the captain is, despite the small crowd gathered around Vidal, engaging in self-serving political small talk. Del Toro takes pains to explain that the predominant visual lines of the camera, in both table scenes, were long and linear, in contrast to the usually circular lines that animate the fantasy world.[16] The lighting, in both, had a yellow, harsh glare, quite unlike the soothing, golden color of Ofelia's story of the rose, which she narrates to her brother, sleeping in her mother's womb.

Del Toro was meticulous in emphasizing that all of his artistic designs had an allusion to fine art rather than "comic book" references. Thus, he embedded a visual footnote to one of Francisco Goya's horrifying Black paintings: that of Saturn devouring one of his sons.[17] In *Pan's Labyrinth,* the Pale Man devours two fairies: a grotesque form of justice, as Ofelia had willfully devoured two juicy grapes from the Pale Man's table despite the fairies' and the Pale Man's warnings. But this is a form of excessive "justice" the Nazis would have well understood, in their attempt to stamp out all rebellion or resistance, much as, interestingly, the Faun later attempts to extract blind obedience from Ofelia for her third task.

Del Toro emphasizes that it is not so much whether Ofelia "succeeds" at her tasks that matters, but her coming to trust her judgment enough to rebel, that is important.[18] It is as much a "coming of age" as it is a paean of praise for those who dared to be disobedient to the Nazis. Del Toro, at the end of his commentary on the film, reveals that he deliberately chose the same actor, for both the Pale Man and the Faun because in his mind, the Pale Man, the Faun, and the Giant Toad were all the same character.[19] In other words, even the sacrifice of the blue and red fairies to the Pale Man's ravenous revenge were simply a ruse to test Ofelia's/Princess Moanna's spirit. As proof, Del Toro states that in the final scene, when Princess Moanna has entered into her kingdom, not only is her mother restored as Queen, beautiful in full regalia beside her king, but also all three fairies are present, vibrantly alive.[20]

What emerges, upon a deeper analysis, are the complex interrelationships binding a classic and conflicted frame, particularly in the figures of the Faun and Ofelia, the two characters who cross most easily across the two diegetic realms of the real and the fantastic. Del Toro was careful to emphasize that "Pan" was referenced in the title only of the U.S. English release. To him, the Faun was a creature more ambiguous—a "neutral" character, neither "good" nor "bad."[21] In the diegetic "real world," the Faun seems a monster both "classic" and "conflicted." With his imposing appearance and agelessness (the reference to Cronos pops up again, when the Faun states that he has so many names, some so old that only the trees can pronounce them), the Faun appears completely "other." Yet because the Faun initially seems so bent in helping Princess Moanna regain her rightful place, he seems wise and good, and therefore, sympathetic enough to understand Ofelia's mortal plight (and therefore, in spirit, passing as humane). It is important to see that the Faun ages backwards, such that he seems oldest (practically blind with cataracts and bent over, perhaps in mimicry of an archetype like the Greek figure of Tiresias, the blind seer) when he is most benevolent. Later, as he gets more tyrannical (and demands that Ofelia sacrifice her younger brother—the brother whose birth has caused her mother's painful pregnancy and eventual death), he becomes younger and more attractive, much like Lucifer. When Ofelia resists the Faun's final command/offer, he surrenders the girl-woman to his diegetic real-life counterpart in this scene. Captain Vidal, who seems an extension of the Faun, in this darkest of moments, shoots Ofelia, and claims his son—only to be assassinated by the triumphant rebels. Much like the Nazis, who prized a severe Aryan form of beauty, the Faun, during the final temptation/challenge in the diegetic real world, appears most attractive and tyrannical. It is in this scene that the Faun appears to the monster of the conflicted frame: someone more akin to the Nazi psychopathic human beasts, who delight in the suffering of innocents.

Yet the story does not end there. In an *en medias res* that returns to the beginning, where the blood dripping from Ofelia's nose and hand had flowed backwards, the blood now drips in a slow but steady stream, forming rivulets that fill the lacunae of the labyrinth, resembling a Mayan sacrifice. As the diegetically "real" Ofelia dies, a hero mourned, the Princess Moanna returns to her kingdom, hailed by her magical royal parents and all the strange and wondrous creatures of the fantastic realm, including, of course, the Faun, who bows to her, much as a devoted courtier does. The Faun, in the fantastic realm, ultimately ends up not a monster, but his counterpart, a citizen-emissary: a catalyst whose function was to help reawaken Ofelia/Moanna's true self.

As Del Toro acknowledges in his commentary on the film,[22] it is important that Ofelia is a girl-woman: someone who has not yet crossed completely over into sexual maturity and motherhood. As such, there is no contradiction, for her, between being a true princess (as opposed to the apparent "princess" in the green dress and shiny black shoes her mother wanted her to be, in order to display her, as an obedient spectacle of femininity, at the captain's long table) and going on these masculine adventures of battling monsters. While Ofelia/Moanna within the diegetic fantastic world, initially appears as the unambiguous heroine of a classic frame (human/Good versus Other/Evil), especially in her battle against the giant Toad, in her battle against the Pale Man, her "goodness" becomes questionable. She appears to have a perverse streak for disobedience, as she does not heed the Faun's earlier warning of not being distracted, and refuses to follow the directives of the fairies, in choosing which door to open, to claim an ancient dagger, and eventually, in stealing two luscious grapes, from the forbidden table of the apparently sleeping Pale Man. Her punishment: the bloody devouring of the two fairies, and her apparent banishment by the Faun. Thus, Ofelia, during her second test or challenge appears more akin to characters who populate narratives of the conflicted frame: she knows evil can lurk within, and she knows the despair of the Fall, with its curse of mortality.

Nevertheless, during the third and final test, Ofelia, though she swears total and absolute obedience to the Faun, defies him, refusing to spill the blood of an innocent (her brother, who inadvertently caused her mother much pain during pregnancy, and eventually kills Carmen, when he is born). Ofelia's "perverse streak" for disobedience thus becomes revaluated, within this context, as a rebellion against Evil, and as a finding of her true self: a "coming home." Indeed, Del Toro, in his commentary, praises the value of learning to become disobedient, and to trust one's own sense of inner decency, in contrast with, in his view, the codified "fairy tales" of politics and organized religion.[23]

To close this analysis of *Pan's Labyrinth,* it is important to see that Mercedes, the maid/militia spy (Maribel Verdú), survives Ofelia in the diegetic real world. As Del Toro in his commentary notes, Mercedes and Ofelia, in some crucial ways, "are the same" (in contrast to the compliant Carmen, Ofelia's mother).[24] Both Ofelia and Mercedes have secret lives and engage in dangerous adventures; both have a propensity to disobey outer directives and honor their inner selves. Mercedes, in some ways, is the grown-up version of Ofelia.

But there are two crucial differences between Mercedes and Ofelia: (1) Mercedes no longer believes in fauns and magic, as Ofelia does; (2) Mercedes is capable of a great deal of violence, as revealed in the scene in which she stabs Captain Vidal, and guts his cheek, calling him a "pig," thus momentarily turning the tables on her would-be torturer to escape.

By contrast, Ofelia not only believes in Fauns and magic: to her, they are the more compelling reality. Unlike Mercedes, Ofelia is incapable of any violence, even against the brother who has caused her beloved mother's suffering and death, or against Captain Vidal, who seems the very embodiment of Evil. Like a Christ-like figure, she absorbs violence unto herself, rather than choosing to direct it outwards, to save herself, or gain entry into the fantastic world, through the sacrifice of another, however justifiable it may seem. Ofelia/Moanna is a character who can only survive within a classic frame as she is, in the final choice, incapable of making compromises with evil and violence. Mercedes, because she has been willing to make such compromises, can survive the diegetic real world, and thus become a "hero," of the conflicted frame. And it is ultimately through her eyes that we survive Del Toro's fantastic and mythic deformation of the nightmare of Spanish Nazism, to look forward, with something resembling hope.

From the fantastic world of *Pan's Labyrinth,* we next move into the science fiction and fantasy world of the X-Men, to see view how traces of the Holocaust have been imaginatively transmitted and transformed to comprise part of the narrative landscape of this futuristic universe, and how we situate ourselves, as spectator-participants, to/in this brave new world.

THE *X-MEN* TRILOGY

Bryan Singer, the director of *X-Men* and *X2: X-Men United,*[25] poignantly explains in a DVD special feature that the story of the X-Men is a commentary on overcoming prejudice, because of one's innate difference (human evolution via mutation), a theme which is threaded throughout the *X-Men* trilogy.[26] The emotive first scene in *X-Men* focuses on young Eric Lensherr (Brett Morris), who later becomes Magneto (Ian McKellen). Lensherr/Magneto is violently separated from his parents (Rhona Shekter and Kenneth McGregor) at the Auschwitz concentration camp in Poland in 1944. The *X-Men* cinematic trilogy utilizes the horror of hatred and persecution of World War II as the underlying metaphor for mutant equality while the overarching theme woven throughout the films is the fight for control. Although the use of imagery from 1944 Auschwitz juxtaposed with the not-too-distant-future United States—a world in which Senator

Robert Kelly (Bruce Davison) urges his colleagues to pass the Mutant Registration Act—does not reoccur in the trilogy, the films do contain scenes in which scientists engage in immoral experiments, evocative of Nazi Germany's infamous Dr. Josef Mengele, and the tyrannical behavior of megalomaniacs, reminiscent of Adolf Hitler himself.[27] Moreover, each film within the trilogy concentrates on individuals' fight for control, either over themselves or over others. After all, this wider theme of control, through domination and elimination, was Hitler's ultimate goal in his Nazi regime. The ways in which the Holocaust and the image of the Nazi-as-monster are portrayed in the *X-Men* trilogy, however, are much more complex than ordinary horror films, either classic or conflicted frames. The science-fiction-action genre forces the parallel to be more discreet and at once more complicated.

Throughout the *X-Men* trilogy, characters are constantly battling for control, which leads to oppression or liberation. In the first installment, *X-Men,* Rogue (Anna Paquin) and Wolverine (Hugh Jackman) lack control of themselves. Rogue's power of borrowing mutants' abilities (and humans' life force) is beyond her control, which renders her a danger to others. Wolverine, on the other hand, lacks the knowledge of his past, and his amnesia wields a kind of internal control over him similar to Rogue's powerlessness. Jean Grey (Famke Janssen) emerges as a third character that loses autonomy over herself in *X-Men: The Last Stand.* Rather than an indiscernible past or uncontrollable power paralyzing her, Jean's problem lies in her other persona, the Phoenix, which is the wildly powerful side of her psyche. Magneto and Professor Charles Xavier (Patrick Stewart), however, are two characters who, while they demonstrate perfect control over themselves, consistently fight one another over the fate of humanity. Perhaps the best way to understand the importance of control in the *X-Men* trilogy is through the Jungian shadow.

The Jungian shadow, according to Rushing and Frentz, is "that which we hate, fear, and disown, and therefore repress into the personal/cultural unconscious."[28] The inferior, or first, shadow rejects anything that is Other or not-ego. Since the white heterosexual male supplies the form of ego in Western culture, the ego rejects the feminine, body, people of color, and "anything else that is clearly the rational negation of ego-consciousness."[29] The overdeveloped, or second, shadow is the ego's attempt at perfection through the control, rather than the blatant rejection, of the Other. In this attempt, the ego "separates from the unconscious and develops itself to an extreme so as to combat increasing threats to its autonomy."[30] Through separation and fragmentation, the overdeveloped shadow creates tools to combat the Other, and these tools may be integrated with the Self only when the inferior shadow is acknowledged through dreams or waking experiences.[31] Through Rushing and Frentz's framework, Picart finds a natural development of the third shadow, the "feminine-as-monstrous" or the female monster. When the third shadow manifests in the "feminine-as-monstrous," the woman's "beauty, intelligence, and ambition" make her dangerous.[32] The third shadow as the female monster is a hybrid construction that is "powerful and vulnerable; compelling and repulsive" at the same time.[33] Ultimately, however, the third shadow must be eliminated even in the conflicted frame; she is "either (justifiably) murdered" or "given no narrative alternative than to choose death."[34]

The theoretical framework of shadows is necessary in understanding the way in which the theme of control unravels for certain characters in the *X-Men* trilogy and links to the overarching metaphor of the Holocaust. Rogue assumes the role of the "good woman," who is horrified at the unmanageable harm that she causes others, and finally she exercises power over herself in *The Last Stand* by willingly taking the vaccine. Jean seems like the good woman in *X-Men* and *X2,* particularly when she faithfully chooses Cyclops (James Marsden) over Wolverine, but the third shadow emerges when the Phoenix rips apart Jean's control in *The Last Stand.* Wolverine's struggle with his victimized past allows him to become the hero required to defeat Magneto's army and to eliminate the threat of the third shadow at the end of the trilogy. Magneto, on the other hand, evolves into the Nazi-as-monster of the conflicted frame, which is socially determined by his victimization at Auschwitz. Professor Xavier remains the steadfast and benevolent guide for the X-Men, which leads to his eventual death in *The Last Stand.*

What follows is a discussion of the representation of the Holocaust-as-horror motif within a cinematic trilogy of the science-fiction-action genre that draws upon the Jungian framework of cinematic "shadows" delineated by Rushing, Frentz, and Picart. In each film, the Holocaust is omnipresent through the underlying metaphor of control and persecution (demonstrated through the application of the shadows) and through the imagery evocative of Nazi science laboratories and tyrannical leaders.

X-Men

Before proceeding, an overview of the first film, *X-Men,* is helpful. Briefly sketched, the film revolves around Wolverine and Rogue whose chance meeting is disrupted by Sabretooth's (Tyler Mane) ambush. Storm (Halle Berry) and Cyclops rescue Wolverine and Rogue and take them to Professor Xavier's school for "gifted youngsters," or the "X-Mansion." As the film progresses, Magneto's distrust in a peaceful mutant–human coexistence pushes him to kidnap Rogue so that he may use her as a conduit for his radiation device. Situated atop the Statue of Liberty, he employs his device in an attempt to mutate every major world leader, all of whom are gathered for a U.N. Summit on Ellis Island. Aware that the forced mutation will result in millions of terrible deaths (as shown from Senator Kelly's earlier demise as a result of complications from the radiation), the X-Men fight and ultimately defeat Magneto, albeit temporarily.

The film begins as Nazi soldiers herd Jewish prisoners through the gates of Auschwitz—although the film only mentions "Poland 1944," it is clear which concentration camp Singer is suggesting. The camera work in this scene is dark, almost black and white, with highlights of color most notably found in the vibrant yellow Stars of David, historically worn by the Jews for identification purposes—a cinematic technique akin to that used in Spielberg's *Schindler's List* in pivotal scenes, such as those of a little girl in red in a ghetto liquidation scene. (Similarly, Senator Kelly's bill would require mutant identification two scenes later.) The darkness of this critical first scene, which is accentuated by the rain, mud, and dark clothing, not only adds to its sinister tone but also makes for a more "realistic" viewing of the past. Similar to scenes found in *Schindler's List,* which was filmed in a docudramatic style, this technique is meant to evoke a sense of horror from a past based on our own reality. In fact, one of Singer's primary goals in the creation of *X-Men,* as well as *X2,* was to make the film seem less like a comic book and appear more real, which the camera work of the Auschwitz scene establishes very early in the film.[35] The "reality" of the concentration camp, however, is overshadowed by the young Magneto's reaction to his mother's hysteria, as she is pulled further away from him. As the gates close, Magneto lunges forward, and the guards must restrain him, except that his power of magnetism makes its debut as more guards attempt to hold him back. It is only when Magneto manages to bend half the gate toward him that a guard jabs him in the head with the butt of his rifle, knocking the boy unconscious. At this point, the reality of the concentration camp is replaced with the clearly fictional future in which Jean addresses the senate hearing on the Mutant Registration Act, whose obvious parallels to the prior scene blur the distinction between "real/reel" horrors.

Where Jean comes across as a soft-spoken, but earnest and intelligent, scientist presenting a lecture on genetic facts, Senator Kelly, on the other hand, is presented as a sarcastic bully who turns into a tyrannical politician with an agenda similar to the Nazis of World War II. After the hearing, Professor Xavier confronts Magneto in a hallway just outside the hearing. As Professor Xavier, a telepath and the film's symbol for good, searches Magneto's head for hope, his old friend searches for a way for mutants to triumph over humans. While Magneto's tyrannical behavior is more prevalent in the second and third films, his villainy is well-established in the first installment, and his megalomania is only heightened and emphasized as the trilogy progresses, turning a Holocaust victim like Magneto into the victimizer of the future, which is suggestive of the conflicted frame rather than the classic frame.

If Magneto and Senator Kelly are emblematic of the conflicted horror frame, then Professor Xavier becomes the benevolent protector, and Wolverine represents the internal battle with the ego. The past Wolverine cannot remember haunts him in his sleep, and the lack of knowledge and certainty makes him vulnerable. However, exactly because his amnesia cripples him, Wolverine lashes out like his namesake and suppresses his vulnerability. When Rogue finds Wolverine in Canada, he survives off money raised from being the equivalent of a gladiator in a caged fighting ring, in which he always wins because of his superior strength, rapid healing, and adamantium skeleton.

The beginning of the film shows Wolverine embracing the second (rawly masculine) shadow and becoming the animal, and he does not learn how to confront his suppressed inferior (or vulnerable and feminized) shadow until he meets the X-Men. The flashes of memory that Jean resurrect in his mind allow us a glimpse of Wolverine's past as a mutant experiment at an unknown laboratory. Just as Magneto's past in Auschwitz is shot with dark camera work, so too are the flashes of Wolverine's memory, thus suggesting a "real" past filled with horror. In the memories that Jean extracts from him, dark green lighting accentuates men covered in black protective gear as they lean over a tank filled with a clear bubbling substance that holds Wolverine. A fire burns in the foreground as two similarly clothed men look on, and a man in an indiscernible military uniform watches from the background. The last shot of the brief memory sequence is a close-up of Wolverine's face, which has black lines drawn across his skull for the liquid adamantium infusion. Before the scene ends, Wolverine's eyes widen with fear.

A second memory sequence occurs that night when Wolverine is revisited by memories *à la* nightmare, roused by Jean's earlier prodding. The viewer learns nothing new here about Wolverine's mysterious past, but the scene emphasizes his victimization. Similar to the victims of unspeakable scientific experiments in Nazi concentration camps, Wolverine loses autonomy over his body and is effectively "feminized" (or at least, emasculated) in his vulnerability. The viewer moves from being a bearer of the "gaze," which is shared with the scientists, when the camera is placed in Wolverine's helpless position beneath a green-lit liquid. Momentarily, the viewer vicariously experiences Wolverine's trapped perspective in the tank. Then, the camera shifts back to the privileged gaze as it hovers over the tank and looks down at Wolverine. Government officials—more bearers of the gaze—stand in the background, and the setting is meant to evoke Nazi medical experiments, like those conducted by Dr. Josef Mengele (who was notorious for his hereditary experiments on twins) at Auschwitz. The viewer is meant not only to connect Wolverine's past with the atrocities of the Holocaust, as it summons a sense of "real" horror of what has happened and what may lie ahead, but also to recognize Wolverine's victimization and resulting vulnerability.

However, the true victim of *X-Men* is Rogue. With only the ability to borrow other mutants' powers, Rogue has no strength of her own. She cannot invade her oppressor's mind, beat him to a pulp, or throw lightning at him. In an earlier scene, Rogue borrows Wolverine's ability to heal rapidly in order to mend the damage he causes in stabbing her accidentally. She demonstrates hesitance in touching his face to gain access to his ability, but certainly she would show no such restraint in fighting Magneto. The problem, however, is that Rogue cannot get close enough to touch Magneto's skin, and she immediately falls into the role of the female victim, crying and begging for her life. Nevertheless, at the end, after her rescue, Rogue is able to return to life as normal at the X-Mansion, and unlike Wolverine, she forgets her previous subjugation, at least on the surface.

X-2: X-Men United

In *X2: X-Men United,* Magneto displays, in enhanced form, the characteristics of a conflicted frame villain when he teams up with the X-Men in an "unholy alliance"[36] to stop the formidable William Stryker. Previously set up as the archetypal "bad guy" in *X-Men,* Magneto cooperates with the X-Men, thereby problematizing our previously established notion of Magneto-as-monster. The second installment of the trilogy picks up where the first film left off—with Wolverine searching for Alkali Lake, the location of the laboratory of his past. However, the plot is further complicated when the viewer learns that Stryker controls mutants like Nightcrawler (Alan Cumming), or Deathstrike (Yuriko Oyama), with "evil fluid spawned from the spine of his son."[37] He uses this controlling agent to expedite the President's, as well as the nation's, fear of mutants, in order to push through Congress the lingering Mutant Registration Act. Thus, Magneto, who cleverly escapes the plastic cell[38] that renders him vulnerable (particularly to the will of Stryker), joins forces with the X-Men to fight a greater threat than himself. The film culminates in the foiling of Stryker's plan and Stryker himself, whom Magneto and Wolverine leave to die. Magneto's evil emerges again as he changes the order for mutant 143, Stryker's son Jason (Michael Reid MacKay) who is also telepathic and has been ordered to kill all the mutants, to instruct Professor Xavier to kill all the humans instead. Ultimately, with the death of Stryker and several of his underlings, as well as the self-sacrifice of Jean, the X-Men prevail, for a second time, against Magneto's warped need for control.

William Stryker falls easily within the conflicted frame, in that he encompasses all the qualities necessary for the Nazi-as-monster motif to be triggered. His military background lay in being part of "Black Ops" in northern Vietnam. That past explains the militant personality that he now carries within the government, and his clandestine laboratory and army accentuates his malicious plans. Earlier in the film, a military night raid on the X-Men school is suggestive of Nazi soldiers abducting people from their homes to take them to concentration camps when Stryker attempts to acquire and control more mutants. During the film's climax at Stryker's base at Alkali Lake, Stryker's monstrosity is clear with the introduction of mutant 143, or Jason, who is crippled by Stryker's experimentation. Stryker's obvious fear and revulsion of his son, on whom he blames his wife's suicide, has led him to this overwhelming compulsion either to eradicate mutants, as dark Cerebro indicates, or to control them. The one person Stryker never attempts to mentally dominate is Professor Xavier because the Professor's telepathic powers are too strong for any chemical substance to inhibit, like his strength of will and strength of self. Thus, while the Professor remains stoic, Stryker's godlike endeavors reinforce his conflicted frame characteristics.

Magneto's own attempt at godlike status is foreshadowed when Magneto called Pyro (Aaron Stanford) a "god among insects." This hubris is represented in Magneto's distorted version of "dark Cerebro,"[39] which he uses to find all the humans in his own version of genocide. Thus, Magneto has progressed in his status as a monstrous character since *X-Men*: from almost accidentally killing millions on Ellis Island and New York City to the blatantly evil villain in *X2,* in which he deliberately tries to kill all humans. In essence, he finally becomes what he had previously hated and feared most: a tyrant obsessed with control through genocide. In *X-Men,* Magneto tried to fight his darker nature by forcefully turning humans into mutants in order to achieve the world he desperately desired, but he succumbs to the second shadow in *X2* and unleashes his own tyrannical beast, which effectively smothers his inferior shadow (his vulnerable, victimized side).

Wolverine, however, does not become a monstrous personality, even though he is perhaps the only other character in the trilogy who may have some vague understanding of Magneto's past of victimization. We return to Wolverine's spotty memories of his experimentation, and unlike the flashes of memories in the first film, the viewer has a chance to discover, along with Wolverine, more of his troubled past in a slower montage sequence. Aside from the similar setting from the previous memories, which Singer explains is meant to remind the viewer of Auschwitz, the dog tags first seen in *X-Men* play a significant role here.[40] At first they dangle from a silhouetted hand and then are snapped apart after Stryker says, "Wolverine," thus assigning the former Logan a nonhuman name. Wolverine is Other-ed, and his name replacement parallels the treatment of prisoners in concentration camps during the Holocaust. Rather than animalistic names, however, Holocaust prisoners were assigned serial number tattoos, which effectively erased their human identities. In *The Last Stand,* Magneto displays his own serial number for Callisto (Dania Ramirez), who demands to see his mark (she flaunts her tattoos of the Omega-like sign of the Brotherhood), which preserves the constant parallel to Nazi concentration camps in the final film of the trilogy. In *X2,* however, Wolverine's new name probably helped determine the barbaric lifestyle he appears to lead in the beginning of *X-Men,* and over the course of the trilogy, the viewer witnesses Wolverine's slow return toward civility. He becomes more in control of himself and his emotions as he learns more about his past, and the third installment culminates in his acceptance of both his first (victimized) shadow and second (bestial) shadow, which allows him to become the hero of the conflicted frame.

X-MEN: THE LAST STAND

The final installment in the trilogy furthers the theme of control, both with Jean's return as the Phoenix, which is her alter ego fueled by passion and chaos, and the revelation of a mutant "cure" hidden within a young boy named Jimmy, who is later called Leech (Cameron Bright). Scientists unveil a vaccination that would give mutants a chance, and a choice, at a normal human life, and this constitutes the film's central dilemma. In response, Magneto assembles a small army to find the cure and eliminate Leech, as he believes the human government will forcefully use the vaccine on all mutants. The X-Men, in the wake of Professor Xavier's death, must rally to fight Magneto, his army, and Jean as the Phoenix. The film ends at Alcatraz as the war that everyone has anticipated finally erupts. In the end, Magneto receives the treatment, struck by several syringes holding the vaccine; Leech is rescued and joins the school; and Jean/the Phoenix dies again, this time at the hands/claws of Wolverine. Life as usual returns to the school in a society more integrated than before, as seen with Dr. Henry "Hank" McCoy's/Beast's (Kelsey Grammer) promotion to U.N. Ambassador. Hope dangles before Magneto as he barely moves, via his "cured" magnetic power, a metal chess piece in a park where he sits alone.

The first element of interest to us in *The Last Stand* is Professor Xavier's self-sacrifice in the face of the Phoenix's rising power. This comes immediately after Jean's alter ego takes control and refuses the Professor's attempt to restore a series of defenses that would successfully restrict the Phoenix's ability to control Jean, which he had set in place when she was younger. These defenses shatter as Jean's telepathic powers create a cocoon of telekinetic energy that surrounds her in an unconscious act of self-preservation at the end of *X2*. Although Professor Xavier tries to explain his reasons for controlling Jean to Wolverine, who vehemently disagrees with him, the Professor emerges as having a darker side. Behind the scenes, writers Zak Penn and Simon Kinberg describe the previous portrayal of the Professor as "angelic and always in the right," whereas in *The Last Stand,* he is more ambiguous.[41] After all, control is bad, isn't it? Control is the weapon of the oppressor, which the first two films emphasize (particularly *X2*); the third film confronts this idea through the disagreement over how to handle Jean and her alter ego. Therefore, the only character that has the viewer's absolute faith in being a good guy acquires a tinge of gray until his self-sacrifice. As the Professor struggles against the Phoenix's powers, Xavier constantly pleads with her, but, ultimately, he allows her to destroy him. His surrender, and not merely his defeat, is evident in two senses. First, his last statement to Jean is, "Don't let *it* [our emphasis] control you"—not "him," "me," or "them," but "it," her power. Second, his serene look, which is almost a smile, at Wolverine, who watches the scene unfold from the other room, just before he disintegrates, reveals his self-overcoming of fear, death, and the desire for control. Thus, the Professor sacrifices himself for reasons later to unfold.

Shortly after Magneto's dictatorial rallying speech, which is reminiscent of film footage we see of Hitler in the 1930s, Magneto leads the attack on Alcatraz, thus starting the war. When Magneto has been defeated and the war is coming to an end, Jean's personality is completely eclipsed by the Phoenix's rage at the slow-reacting human military. The Phoenix emerges as the third shadow, both the "feminine-as-monstrous" and the female monster. When her third shadow first appears at the lake and kills Cyclops, Jean's hair has grown much longer and is a brighter red. In short, she is more beautiful. Later, she is sexually aggressive toward Wolverine at the school when her control over the Phoenix slips again, and finally, when she kills the Professor in her old home, Jean loses all control over her alter ego. She becomes the female monster when the Phoenix fully takes over Jean; her eyes change color, her skin pales, her veins show distinctly through her skin, and her hair floats around her head on a current of her own power. She is at once beautiful and grotesque, the hybrid incarnation of the third shadow. Just like the incident with the Professor, the Phoenix unleashes her destructive power, but because Jean is fully suppressed now, there is no distinct target. The Phoenix kills anyone in her path because she can, and therefore she poses the ultimate threat. Even Magneto asks himself, "What have I done?" before turning, powerless, in retreat. Wolverine, on the other hand, who has the ability of rapid healing, fights his way toward her in order to save everyone, including Jean herself. It is only when Wolverine says to Jean that he would die for her, which is atypical of Wolverine, that Jean surfaces enough to ask him to save her. After he has confessed his love for her, Wolverine kills/saves Jean by stabbing her with his claws, releasing her from the Phoenix's control.

Since the third shadow must be eliminated, as we stated earlier, Jean must die because the Phoenix, a villain of the conflicted frame, must die. Similarly, because Professor Xavier is so innately good, he can only survive within a classic frame, and thus must die in the trilogy. Magneto, Rogue, and Wolverine, however, survive for very different reasons. First, Magneto no longer poses a threat to society. Without his only real source of dominance, his mutant power of magnetism, Magneto is a helpless old man. Rogue overcomes her own powerlessness by choosing the "proper" choice for the good woman; rather than cause others harm, she willingly accepts the vaccine and loses her mutant ability. Wolverine, however, finally reconciles the two warring shadows (the vulnerable first shadow and the hypermasculinized second shadow) inside himself. By confronting his past and confessing his love for Jean, Wolverine accepts the inferior/first shadow that his overdeveloped self/second shadow previously tried to control through animalistic instinct and behavior. His facing and embracing both shadows, through his love for Jean, transform him into the ultimate hero of the conflicted frame as order is momentarily restored in this quasi-utopian society at the end of the *X-Men* trilogy. Again, like Ofelia, it is through Wolverine's eyes that we survive the devastation of the Phoenix's destructive power and the sadness of the Fall, glimpsed in Jean Grey's death. From the science fiction and fantasy realm of the X-Men, we move into the science fiction realm of *V*, to document yet another iteration of the transmutation of the legacy of the Holocaust, and to reexamine what an ethics of spectatorship entails, within that context.

V: The Original Miniseries

Shadows of the Holocaust

This section examines how director/screenwriter Kenneth Johnson has represented the horrors of the Holocaust on television using a fantastic mode of narration like science fiction while incorporating, to some degree, the cinematic techniques of horror and documentary filmmaking, but more critically, how this more fantastic mode of narrativizing diverges from historical and cinematic depictions of the Shoah like *Schindler's List* and *Apt Pupil* that rely more heavily on the cinematic techniques of horror and documentary filmmaking. What we find is that by using the grammars of both science fiction and horror, *V* challenges the dominant or classic representation of the monstrous in Holocaust narratives, and thus arrives at a convergent way of viewing the heritage of the Holocaust as our earlier analyses of *Pan's Labyrinth* and the *X-Men*.

THE VISITOR-AS-NAZI

First, a brief sketch of *V*'s plot is beneficial. It is the 1980s, and citizens from around the world watch helplessly as 50 disc-shaped alien spacecraft, each measuring three miles across, descend upon Earth's major cities. The "Visitors," as they come to be called, emerge from the large spacecraft and appear remarkably humanoid, save for strange reverberating voices and an acute sensitivity to light. Theirs is a "mission of peace," they claim, and Earth's abundance of raw materials, vital to the survival of their home world. In exchange for some of Earth's resources, the Visitors promise knowledge, advanced technologies, and medical cures. However, in reality, they harbor a terrible agenda: they have come to rape Earth of its water and harvest human beings for food. The Visitors are actually reptilian, disguised behind suits of synthesized human flesh. Soon after their arrival, the Visitors, fearing that members of the science community on Earth will unmask their true identity, begin using various media outlets to stage a "Goebbelian" propaganda campaign. The whisper campaign alleges that scientists are secretly plotting to sabotage the Visitors' "peaceful mission," which threatens to jeopardize the exchange of technological and medicinal knowledge the Visitors have promised. The public turns a blind eye while the Visitors summarily order all scientists to register themselves and their families with Visitor officials. Some citizens obey, some go into hiding, but many more disappear, carted off *en masse* by transport ship. Much of the public believe the Visitors' ruse—that is, all but a small band of resistance fighters. They are everyday citizens, and they are humanity's only hope.

As Douglas Gomery aptly points out, "Because the turnaround time from production to presentation is so short, made-for-tv movies can deal with topical issues and even, like the immensely popular *The Day After* (1983), provoke discussion of important ideas."[42] In the director's commentary, Johnson acknowledges, "*V* was a retelling of the rise of the Third Reich" that attempted to grabble with critical issues like the horrors of the Holocaust.[43] The Visitors, like the Nazis, are fascist militants whose uniforms are laden with (or, as the director puts it, "reminiscent of") Nazi-period imagery. In summary, the Visitors' military dress—all red with black trim, and black knee-high boots—visually mirrors, and inverts, the black/red uniforms worn by the SS. The Visitor laser sidearm is patterned after the German P08 Pistol, or "Luger," Johnson notes; and even the Visitor insignia, Johnson adds, is "Nazi-esque" in design and features prominently in black on tall red draping banners that adorn publicized orations by Visitor officers. Referencing another powerful allusion, the Visitors refer to their ruler back on their home world as "our leader" or "the Leader," which bears striking resemblance to *Der Führer*.

Johnson points out in the director's commentary that his original script did not initially call for aliens, but instead considered the Chinese or the Russians to play the adversary.[44] Johnson recalls that in junior high school, he had viewed the film footage used as evidence at the Nuremberg trials, and it made "a startling impression upon [him.]"[45] He recalls further: "It [the footage] was so stunning to me that I think that's part of what shaped a lot of my work about intolerance and prejudice. I went to Auschwitz. I've stood there. It's an astonishing experience that you literally can't get your arms around. It's enormous."[46] Given the popularity of the Star Wars franchise at the time, Johnson elects a science fictional landscape to "work through"[47] the Holocaust (in specific, the registration and subsequent abduction of the scientists), which for *V* is the catalyzing event or rallying point for the resistance movement.

VISITORS AND THE GOTHIC

V's narrative operates within the conventional genre framework of science fiction. Yet, there are moments in which the film employs a Gothic vocabulary and classic horror conventions to "act out"[48] the representation of not only the perpetrators but also the victims themselves. As Johnson terms it, the film works through the Final Solution to the "scientist question"[49] (in this case, the mass abduction, and harvesting, of scientists and other undesirables). In accord with the Gothic theme, the Visitor spacecraft, for example, or "mother ships" as they are called in the film, hover ominously over Earth's major cities. At first glance, the exterior of the ships, an off-white or light gray, appears as unobtrusive as the limited interior shots to which we are given access. After a news crew is brought on board the *Los Angeles* mother ship for the first time, a reporter comments, "[F]or those of us accustomed to the likes of *Close Encounters* and Darth Vader's star destroyer, our first glimpses inside of the spacecraft of the Visitors were somewhat unexpected, even disappointing.... The docking bay looked rather like the hanger deck of one of our big aircraft carriers." However, the exterior of the mother ships, though seemingly inconsequential, deceptively masks a Gothic infrastructure. For it is only after news cameraman Mike Donovan (Mark Singer) infiltrates the interior of the *Los Angeles* mother ship by sneaking into an air duct—a labyrinthine system of dimly lit, Gothic tunnels—that we are confronted by the Visitors' macabre eating practices and true reptilian identity (Donovan captures both on camera through vents that line the air ducts), thus markedly framing these crucial plot moments within a Gothic aesthetic. The film goes on to reveal that these same Gothic elements constitute *en masse* the entire central region of the mother ship(s). Johnson uses a mixture of low-lighting, dark color palette, steam, and shadow (creating what could almost be called a chiaroscuro effect) to construct the Gothic *mise-en-scènes* that comprise the mother ship's interiority.

For the ship's interior, Johnson envisioned "a whole different feel to it... a darker feel."[50] Perhaps the most startling scene in *V* that visibly references one of the more grisly facets of the Holocaust occurs precisely within the mother ship's Gothic interior. Martin (Frank Ashmore), a seasoned Visitor lieutenant who opposes the leader's Earth initiatives, leads Donovan into an immense room containing vast stores of human bodies in suspended animation—a scene that visually gestures the footage taken at liberated concentration camps (*conzentrationslager*) in Europe (see Figure 24.1). In the director's commentary, Johnson states that he intended for this scene to convey "the immensity... the enormity of the *process* that the alien Visitors were involved with [emphasis added]."[51] The use of shadowplay and "fingernails on a blackboard... bone-chilling" music, Johnson explains, are to us recognizable conventions of horror cinema that serve to heighten the ominous feeling in this scene.[52] Another strong component of contemporary horror presented here are the connotations of vampirism and cannibalism, particularly the scene's "fixation on the use of human beings reduced to cattle, as sources of meat and leather" (see, for example, *Silence of the Lambs* [1991]), which is a "Holocaust-derived Gothic artifact,"[53] showing precisely how the American Gothic functions easily and productively as a dominant frame in American Holocaust films for "working through" some of the more macabre elements of the Shoah.

While the Gothic mode and classic horror frame can influence the way in which American Holocaust narratives represent the spectacle of the victims and their demise, these narrative elements can also restructure the ways in which Holocaust narratives configure the perpetrator as monstrous. No character in *V* is more pronouncedly monstrous than Diana (Jane Baddler), John's second in command and essentially the "real power" on Earth. Regarding the classic horror film, Picart and Frank write, "In every way, including sexual orientation, the monster

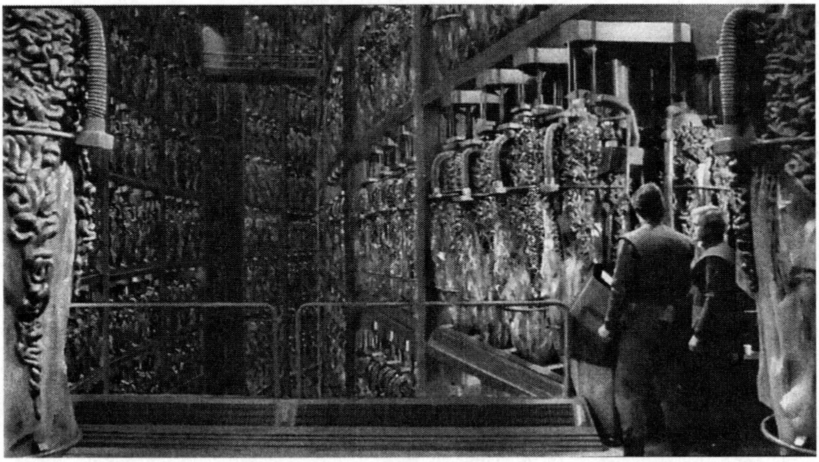

Figure 24.1 Martin (Frank Ashmore) shows Donovan (Mark Singer) the human food stores (à la death camp) aboard the mother ship in *V* (1983). (Courtesy of Kenneth Johnson Productions/Warner Brothers Television.)

is portrayed as radically different; despite some crossover into the realm of humanity, at the point at which the narrative demands that they be destroyed, they are essentially and irreducibly other."[54] Although Diana is "superficially" human, collapsing the distinction between victim and monster that is characteristic of the conflicted frame, clearly traditional concepts of the Nazi-as-monster motif inform *V*'s portrayal of Diana, ultimately "reifying stereotypic links between horror and the Holocaust."[55]

Diana's classic configuration as "other" becomes clearer as we examine specific features of her character in more detail. An amalgam of several monstrous traits, Diana is both attractive and alluring, so much so that her femininity is dangerously threatening toward men. Nevertheless, structurally, her configuration is also masculinized: she is often the bearer of "the gaze," and she is sadistically homoerotic toward women. The emphasis placed on Diana's monstrous or othered sexuality supplants an ethic of response with a more traditional Hollywood horror schematic. To borrow from Picart and Frank, Johnson, like Steven Spielberg in *Schindler's List,* "ultimately acts out, rather than works through, a representation of the Holocaust by reducing it to yet another backdrop for the unfolding of a set of perversions . . . that render Nazism monstrous."[56] One scene from *V* in particular shows Donovan and Kristine Walsh (Jenny Sullivan) in the foreground engaging in sexual foreplay, while in the background, a television (the dominant position in the room from which to overlook the couple) begins airing a press interview with Diana, before moving to a close-up on Diana's face. At this point, Diana peers eerily, and smilingly, into the camera, and by extension, into the living room, where she assumes the role of voyeur to the sexual display before her (a motif that is repeated elsewhere in the film and in subsequent installments). "Uncomfortable" moments like this one regularly occur between Kristine and Diana. In specific, two instances show Diana ambiguously placing her hand on Kristine, once on her arm, then another time on her shoulder, in a manner that, at one point, verges on the homoerotic, and at other times, on the violated. Johnson notes in the director's commentary how he intended these scenes to relate Diana's "many appetites,"[57] and that one such appetite might include a sexual attraction for Kristine.

Picart and Frank point out that the relation between the resilient nature of the "Nazi-as-sexualized-monster," the fetishization of Nazi symbology, and erotized violence continue to circulate internationally as a "visual narrative currency."[58] Diana's character is a conflation of these three formidable themes. Moreover, the tendency to concentrate several deviant "markers" within a single character (like Diana), as is common in classic horror, has the effect of elevating narratologically "the stakes of evil"[59] in the monstrous. Thus, the Nazi, or its image, as the site of Judith Halberstam's notion of a "Gothic economy" (the "ability to condense many monstrous traits into one body"[60]) has proven, in Hollywood especially, to be a lucrative enterprise. The trend in Holocaust historiography to silence or play down the atrocities committed against thousands of homosexual men, lesbians, and bisexuals under the edict of the Final Solution is clearly evidenced by the conflation of these sexual (monstrous) identities with the conception of evil. Formations of monstrous sexuality such as those we find in Holocaust narratives prove fundamentally problematic because "they rely on the same heterocentric assumptions," note Picart and Frank, "that give rise to fascist values, that is, the criminalization and extermination of individuals on the basis of sexuality."[61] In line with this method of analysis, Robin Wood contends that "The reason why patriarchal capitalist society is so reluctant to confront this aspect of Nazism is clearly that it has its own stake in the same assumptions."[62]

Yet, Diana's appropriation as Nazi-as-sexualized-monster comprises only one element of her pathology. "Diana," Johnson remarks, "is sort of my combination of Mengele, and Göring, and Himmler."[63] Later in the film, Diana figures prominently in key scenes that visibly reference narrative horror methods typically used in portrayals of Josef Mengele, which, given Mengele's relation to the Holocaust, is even more revelatory. In one such scene, Diana's terror chamber—outfitted with scalpels, a flame inducer, and a harnessing apparatus reminiscent of dentist's chair (a visual footnote to *Marathon Man* [1976] perhaps)—echoes stories Johnson had read about Nazi interrogation.[64] In another scene that is both visually striking and sexually ambiguous, Diana employs the "[fe]male gaze" during a medical experiment she authorizes and choreographs herself. Through a two-way mirror, Diana observes as Brian (Peter Nelson), a youthful Visitor lieutenant, and Robin Maxwell (Blair Tefkin), a human detainee aboard the Los Angeles mother ship, engage in coitus, the fruition of which becomes a major subplot in the next installment, *V: The Final Battle* (1984). The regendering of the fe/male gaze here invokes another crossover of Diana's with other visualizations of the monstrous.

The imbrications of power and gender in Diana place her in the realm of the "third shadow," that is, the female monster or the *feminine-as-monstrous:* a natural offshoot of Janice Rushing and Thomas Frentz's framework[65] (which, in general, does not occur in the decidedly less progressive strain of straight "Holocaust-as-horror" films, Picart and Frank point out[66]). Perhaps Diana's inclusion in *V,* a "Holocaust-as-[science fiction]" film that does not have a strict horror classification (but instead merely incorporates cinematic horror conventions), is made possible precisely because she inhabits a Mengele-type (i.e., masculinized) role, one that is firmly, and "safely," bound within the landscape of science "fiction" rather than "real/reel" horror.

Classic and Conflicted Frames: Redux

To close our analysis of *V,* it is necessary to review some of the complex interrelationships that bind the classic and conflicted frame in the film. By the end of the next installment, *V: The Final Battle,* and in the opening episodes of *V: The Series* (1984–1985), in which Diana is tried for crimes against humanity (a media spectacle the humans liken to Nuremberg), we begin to see her vulnerable side. Diana, like the exterior of the mother ship(s), or like the Visitors themselves even, has many faces that blend seamlessly into the natural order.

In addition to classic elements of horror, *V* simultaneously invokes the conflicted frame, where: (1) the Visitors' "natural" façade, (2) the humans who, during the course of the film, "look the other way" in exchange for power, and (3) Visitor factionists (like Martin and others) who oppose the Leader's initiatives on Earth, all actively "interrogat[e] the binaries (e.g., normality-abnormality, active monster-passive victim) at the base of traditional conceptualizations of evil and mass murder."[67] Johnson intended the Visitor faction (the "Fifth Column," as it comes to be known in *V: The Final Battle*) "to show good Nazis and bad Nazis."[68] He goes on to say, "The aliens, just as, indeed, all the members of the *Wehrmacht* in World War II, were not out to kill everybody. They were people just like us."[69] In short, while other Holocaust narratives that appropriate the conflicted frame in isolation often resort to merely questioning dominant portrayals of the monstrous as "abnormal," *V* challenges, to some extent, the culturally dominant mode often used to simplistically narrativize the monstrous in the Holocaust. In so doing, *V* forms complex cross-fertilizations between the classic and conflicted frames, and thus, like *Pan's Labyrinth* and the *X-Men Trilogy,* resists easy binaries.

Conclusion

In *Imagining the Holocaust,* Daniel R. Schwarz writes, on the work of memory, that "If ever a past needs a human shape, it is the Holocaust; yet as we shall see, putting a human face upon inhuman behavior challenges our ability to imagine evil and to represent it linguistically."[70] *Pan's Labyrinth,* the *X-Men* trilogy, and *V: The Original Miniseries* all, in their own ways, offer different ways in which to revisualize the face of evil, using the grammars and narrative techniques of fantasy, science fiction, and horror to move across the classic as well as the conflicted frames—to visualize stories of monsters and heroes. In *Pan's Labyrinth,* the use of contrasting color palettes infused with mythic, as well as Holocaust references, creates a delicate balance between fantasy and history. In *X-Men,* the visual translations of graphic novels into science fiction film create a look that maintains a memory of the nightmare of the Holocaust within the dream of a possible futuristic utopia. In *V,* the strategic use of handheld shots frequently invokes the "docudramatic" or "authentic look" of the Holocaust, albeit within the more fluid structure of a science-fictionalized narrative. The result, in all three, is the collision of "real/reel" worlds, which allows for a much more complex narrative capable of breaching the realm of fiction to address "real" concerns. All three oeuvres work through the numerous horrors of the Holocaust and imaginatively rework them into visions of brave new worlds, thus inviting us, as imaginative spectator-participants, to critically examine our enjoyment of and identification with these worlds of conflicted frames. As such, this chapter converges with Dominick LaCapra's aspiration for an "ethic of response"[71] to those who have suffered and continue to suffer from the trauma of the Holocaust. The methods employed by this chapter thus shift the focus to critical practices of viewership and interpretation, and ultimately inquire whether there is any kind of responsibility that accompanies our enjoyment of films that draw from, and yet imaginatively diverge from, the traumatic heritage of the Holocaust.[72] In thus deploying these tools, we ask, drawing from Daniel Schwarz, whether "the intelligibility of history, even the place of evil in history, depends on reconfiguring its imaginative and aesthetic terms."[73] Much like the heroes of the conflicted frame, we know there are no easy binaries, both aesthetically and morally. Although we know that the notion of what is "heroic" can no longer be recaptured as "classic" or "pure," we know that such heroism, however conflicted, can be glimpsed and lived.

Notes

1. Caroline Joan (Kay) S. Picart and David A. Frank, *Frames of Evil: The Holocaust as Horror in American Film,* foreword Dominick LaCapra, introduction Edward J. Ingebretsen (Carbondale, IL: Southern Illinois University Press, 2006).
2. Caroline Joan (Kay) Picart and Cecil Greek, *Monsters in and Among Us: Toward a Gothic Criminology* (Madison, NJ: Fairleigh Dickinson University Press, 2007), 12.

3. For a concise exposition of this argument, see Caroline J. S. Picart and David Frank, "Horror and the Holocaust: Genre Elements in *Schindler's List* and *Psycho,*" in *The Horror Film,* ed. Stephen Prince (New Brunswick, NJ: Rutgers University Press, 2003), 206–223.
4. Picart and Frank, "Horror and the Holocaust," 5–8.
5. Isabel Christina Pinedo, "Postmodern Elements of the Contemporary Horror Film," in *The Horror Film,* ed. Steven Prince (New Brunswick: Rutgers University Press, 2004), 85–117.
6. Pinedo contrasts "postmodern" to "classic," but given the many rhetorical valences that freight the word "postmodern," we prefer to use "conflicted."
7. Pinedo, "Postmodern Elements of the Contemporary Horror Film," 89.
8. Noël Carroll, *Philosophy of Horror, or Paradoxes of the Heart* (New York: Routledge, 1990), 16.
9. Steffen Hantke, "The Kingdom of the Unimaginable: The Construction of Social Space and the Fantasy of Privacy in Serial Killer Narratives," *Literature/Film Quarterly* 26 (1998): 179–195.
10. Ruthe Stein writes, "Whether intentional or not, 'Labyrinth' bears a resemblance to Picasso's 'Guernica.' Del Toro uses a similar palette—the color is so faded that some scenes appear to be in black and white with shades of gray—and his eerie mythical characters sport multiple eyes in unusual locations as on the famous mural." See Ruthe Stein, "The Horror of the Underworld (and This World)," *San Francisco Chronicle,* December 29, 2006, accessed February 27, 2007, http://www.sfgate.com.
11. In the director's commentary, Del Toro mentions that this scene is inspired by both a real incident from the civil war and his own personal experiences that unlike Hollywood movies, where bottles constantly break, in real life, the base of bottles prove extremely sturdy as instruments of violence. Guillermo Del Toro, "Feature Audio Commentary by Writer/Director," *Pan's Labyrinth* (*El laberinto del fauno*), Disc One, New Line 2-Disc Platinum Series (MMVII New Line Entertainment, Inc., 2007).
12. Guillermo Del Toro, "Pan and the Fairies (El Fauno y Las Hadas)," *Pan's Labyrinth* (*El laberinto del fauno*), Disc Two, DVD (New Line Entertainment, Inc., 2007).
13. Del Toro, "Feature Audio Commentary by Writer/Director," Disc One.
14. Rudolf Otto, *The Idea of the Holy* (Oxford: Oxford University Press, 1923).
15. For a review of this perspective, see A. D. Moses, "Structure and Agency in the Holocaust: Daniel J. Goldhagen and His Critics," *History and Theory* 37 (1998): 194–220, especially 204. See also Daniel Goldhagen, *Hitler's Willing Executioners: Ordinary Germans and the Holocaust* (New York: Knopf, 1996) and Bruno Chaouat, "In the Image of Auschwitz," *diacritics* 36, no. 1 (Spring 2006): 86–96.
16. Del Toro, "Feature Audio Commentary by Writer/Director," Disc One.
17. Del Toro, "Feature Audio Commentary by Writer/Director," Disc One.
18. Del Toro, "Feature Audio Commentary by Writer/Director," Disc One.
19. Del Toro, "Feature Audio Commentary by Writer/Director," Disc One.
20. Del Toro, "Feature Audio Commentary by Writer/Director," Disc One.
21. Del Toro, "Feature Audio Commentary by Writer/Director," Disc One.
22. Del Toro, "Feature Audio Commentary by Writer/Director," Disc One.
23. Del Toro, "Feature Audio Commentary by Writer/Director," Disc One.
24. Del Toro, "Feature Audio Commentary by Writer/Director," Disc One.
25. Notably, Bryan Singer also directed *Apt Pupil,* a Holocaust film that portrays the Nazi-as-monster motif and utilizes the Holocaust as horror.
26. Bryan Singer, "Fox Special: 'The Mutant Watch,' " *X-Men,* DVD (Twentieth Century Fox Home Entertainment, 2005).
27. Dr. Ferdinand Sauerbruch used the term "megalomaniac" to describe Adolf Hitler's personality and mentioned that he would not be surprised if Hitler became "the craziest criminal" the world had ever seen, in Richard Breitman, "Adolf Hitler," *Historical Analysis of 20 Name Files from CIA Records,* April 2001, The U.S. National Archives and Records Administration, accessed October 2009, http://www.archives.gov/iwg/declassified-records/rg-263-cia-records/rg-263-report.html?template=print
28. Janice Hocker Rushing and Thomas J. Frentz, *Projecting the Shadow: The Cyborg Hero in American Film* (Chicago: University of Chicago Press, 1995), 39.
29. Rushing and Frentz, *Projecting the Shadow,* 40.
30. Rushing and Frentz, *Projecting the Shadow,* 40.
31. Rushing and Frentz, *Projecting the Shadow,* 76.

32. Caroline Joan (Kay) Picart, *The Cinematic Rebirths of Frankenstein: Universal, Hammer, and Beyond* (Westport, CT: Praeger, 2002), 19.
33. Picart, *The Cinematic Rebirths of Frankenstein,* 19.
34. Picart, *The Cinematic Rebirths of Frankenstein,* 19.
35. Bryan Singer, "Bryan Singer Interview," *X-Men,* DVD (Twentieth Century Fox Home Entertainment, 2005).
36. Bryan Singer, "Full-Length Audio Commentary (Director Bryan Singer and Cinematographer Newton Thomas Sigel, ASC)," *X2: X-Men United,* DVD (Twentieth Century Fox Home Entertainment, 2006).
37. Singer, "Full-Length Audio Commentary."
38. It is noteworthy to mention that Bryan Singer was a big fan of *The Silence of the Lambs* and used the idea of Hannibal Lecter's cell to construct Magneto's, particularly the circles through which noxious gas filters in, thus adding to the horror element of the film. Singer, "Full-Length Audio Commentary."
39. Singer, "Full-Length Audio Commentary."
40. Singer, "Full-Length Audio Commentary."
41. Simon Kinberg and Zak Penn, "Full-Length Audio Commentary by Director Brett Ratner and Screenwriters Simon Kinberg and Zak Penn," *X-Men: The Last Stand,* DVD (Twentieth Century Fox Home Entertainment, 2006).
42. Douglas Gomery, "The Economics of the Horror Film," in *Horror Films: Current Research on Audience Preferences and Reactions,* ed. James B. Weaver, III and Ron Tamborini (Mahwah, NY: Lawrence Erlbaum Associates, 1996), 46–62.
43. Kenneth Johnson, "Feature-Length Commentary by Writer/Director," *V: The Original Miniseries,* Side A, DVD (Warner Home Video, 2001).
44. Johnson, "Feature-Length Commentary by Writer/Director," Side A.
45. Johnson, "Feature-Length Commentary by Writer/Director," Side A.
46. Johnson, "Feature-Length Commentary by Writer/Director," Side A.
47. For further discussion, see Dominick LaCapra, *Writing History, Writing Trauma* (Baltimore, MD: Johns Hopkins University Press, 2001); Dominick LaCapra, *Representing the Holocaust: History, Theory, Trauma* (Ithaca, NY: Cornell University Press, 1994); Dominick LaCapra, *History and Memory after Auschwitz* (Ithaca, NY: Cornell University Press, 1998).
48. For further discussion, see LaCapra's, *Writing History, Writing Trauma*; *Representing the Holocaust;* and *History and Memory after Auschwitz.*
49. Johnson, "Feature-Length Commentary by Writer/Director," Side A.
50. Johnson, "Feature-Length Commentary by Writer/Director," Side A.
51. Johnson, "Feature-Length Commentary by Writer/Director," Side A.
52. Johnson, "Feature-Length Commentary by Writer/Director," Side A.
53. Picart and Frank, *Frames of Evil,* 28.
54. Picart and Frank, *Frames of Evil,* 7.
55. Picart and Frank, *Frames of Evil,* 125.
56. Picart and Frank, *Frames of Evil,* 102.
57. Johnson, "Feature-Length Commentary by Writer/Director," Side A.
58. Picart and Frank, *Frames of Evil,* 133.
59. Picart and Frank, *Frames of Evil,* 124.
60. Judith Halberstam, *Skin Shows: Gothic Horror and the Technology of Monsters* (Durham, NC: Duke University Press, 1995/2006), 88, 102–105.
61. Picart and Frank, *Frames of Evil,* 124.
62. Robin Wood, "Nuit Brouillard," in *International Dictionary of Films and Filmmakers 1,* ed. Christopher Lyon (Chicago: St. James Press, 1984), 332.
63. Johnson, "Feature-Length Commentary by Writer/Director," Side A.
64. Johnson, "Feature-Length Commentary by Writer/Director," Side A.
65. See Rushing and Frentz, *Projecting the Shadow.* For further discussion on the "third shadow," see Caroline Joan (Kay) Picart, *The Cinematic Rebirths of Frankenstein.*
66. Picart and Frank, *Frames of Evil,* 131.

67. Picart and Frank, *Frames of Evil,* 127.
68. Johnson, "Feature-Length Commentary by Writer/Director," Side A.
69. Johnson, "Feature-Length Commentary by Writer/Director," Side A.
70. Daniel R. Schwarz, *Imagining the Holocaust* (New York: St. Martin's, 1999), 6.
71. LaCapra, *Writing History, Writing Trauma,* 86–112.
72. For a detailed examination of an "ethics of spectatorship" in relation to the cross pollination of horror and documentary film conventions and historical narrative, see Picart and Frank, *Frames of Evil,* 126–146.
73. Schwarz, *Imagining the Holocaust,* 37.

BIBLIOGRAPHY

Abley, Sean. "Arts and Entertainment: Scary!" *The Advocate*, November 8, 2005.

Abraham, Karl. "The Spider as a Dream Symbol." In *Selected Papers*. Trans. Douglas Bryand and Alix Strachey (London: Hogarth Press, 1927).

Adams, Carol. *Neither Man Nor Beast* (New York: Continuum, 1995).

Adams, Henry E. et al. "Is Homophobia Associated with Homosexual Arousal?" *Journal of Abnormal Psychology* 105, no. 3 (1996) 440–445.

Aho, James. *This Thing of Darkness: A Sociology of the Enemy* (Seattle, WA: University of Washington Press, 1995).

Aja, Alexandre. "Audio Commentary by Director." *Switchblade Romance*. DVD (Lions Gate Films Home Entertainment, 2004).

Al-Rawi, Ahmed K. "The Arabic Ghoul and Its Western Transformation." *Folklore* 120, no. 3 (2009) 291–306.

Anon. "*Dead of Night* Pressbook" (Universal, 1946): no pagination.

——. "Oliver Twist." *Variety*, June 30, 1948: 10.

——. "The Red Shoes." *Variety*, August 4, 1948: 11.

ApolloBoy109. "I Just Never Stopped Laughing. I Loved It." *IMDb* User Comments for *Leeches!* December 1, 2004, http://www.imdb.com/title/tt0339288/usercomments?start=20 (accessed July 20, 2010).

Aristotle. *The Complete Works of Aristotle*. Ed. Jonathan Barnes (Princeton, NJ: Princeton University Press, 1984a).

——. *Generation of Animals*. In *The Complete Works of Aristotle*. Ed. Jonathan Barnes (Princeton, NJ: Princeton University Press, 1984b).

Auerbach, Nina. *Our Vampires, Ourselves* (Chicago: University of Chicago Press, 1995).

Augustine of Hippo. *The City of God Against the Pagans*. Ed. R.W. Dyson (Cambridge: Cambridge University Press, 1998/2010).

A.W. "At the Winter Garden." *New York Times*, December 23, 1946: 19.

Baldick, Chris. *In Frankenstein's Shadow: Myth, Monstrosity, and Nineteenth-Century Writing* (Oxford: Oxford University Press, 1990).

Baldwin, James. *The Evidence of Things Not Seen* (New York: Henry Holt and Co., LLC, 1985).

Barkun, Michael. *Religion and the Racist Right: The Origins of the Christian Identity Movement* (Chapel Hill, NC: University of North Carolina Press, 1997).

Bates, James. "No Credits Where Credit Due." *The Los Angeles Times*, October 30, 1995.

Baynton, Doug. "Disability and the Justification of Inequality in American History." In *Race, Class, and Gender, in the United States: An Integrated Study* (7th ed.). Ed. Paula S. Rothenberg (New York: Worth Publishers, 1998/2007), 92–101.

Beal, Timothy K. *Religion and Its Monsters* (London and New York: Routledge, 2002).

Bell, Catherine. *Ritual Theory, Ritual Practice* (Rev. ed.). (New York: Oxford University Press, 2009).

Bennett, David. *The Party of Fear* (Chapel Hill, NC: University of North Carolina Press, 1988).

Benshoff, Harry M. "The Monster and the Homosexual." In *Horror: The Film Reader*. Ed. Mark Jancovich (London: Routledge, 2002).

——. *Monsters in the Closet: Homosexuality and the Horror Film* (Manchester: Manchester University Press, 1997).

Bercovitch, Sacvan. *The Puritan Origins of the American Self* (New Haven, CT: Yale University Press, 1975).

Birrell, Anne (Trans.) *The Classics of Mountains and Seas* (Harmondsworth: Penguin, 1999).

Bivins, Jason. *Religion of Fear: The Politics of Horror in Conservative Evangelicalism* (New York: Oxford University Press, 2008).

Block, Dorothy. *"So the Witch Won't Eat Me"* (Boston: Houghton Mifflin Co, 1978).

Bloss, Lowell W. "The Buddha and the Nāga: A Study in Buddhist Folk Religiosity." *History of Religions* 13, no. 1 (1973) 36–53.

Bogdan, Robert. *Introduction to Freak Show: Presenting Human Oddities for Amusement and Profit* (Chicago: University of Chicago Press, 1988), 1–21.

Borntreger, Andrew. "Review of Leeches!" June 8, 2009. *BadMovies.org* Comments for *Leeches!* July 20, 2010, http://www.badmovies.org/movies/leeches/index.html?start=0.

Bourdieu, Pierre. *Outline of a Theory of Practice* (Cambridge: Cambridge University Press, 1977).

"Box Office/Business for *Alien Resurrection* (1997)." *IMDb*, http://www.imdb.com/title/tt0118583/business (accessed July 20, 2010).

Boyce, Brandon. "'Apt Pupil,' Based on the Novel by Stephen King." Shooting script, February 3-March 14, 1997. From The Academy of Motion Picture Arts and Sciences script section.

Boyer, Pascal. *Religion Explained: The Evolutionary Origins of Religious Thought* (New York: Basic Books, 2001).

Boyer, Paul. *When Time Shall Be No More: Prophecy Belief in Modern American Culture* (Cambridge, MA: Belknap Press of Harvard University Press, 1994).

Braidotti, Rosi. *Metamorphoses: Towards a Materialist Theory of Becoming* (Malden: Blackwell Publishers, 2002).

——. *Transpositions* (Cambridge: Polity, 2006).

Breitman, Richard. "Adolf Hitler." *Historical Analysis of 20 Name Files from CIA Records*, April 2001. The U.S. National Archives and Records Administration, http://www.archives.gov/iwg/declassified-records/rg-263-cia-records/rg-263-report.html?template=print (accessed October 2009).

Breslin, Jimmy and Dick Schaap. *.44* (New York: The Viking Press, 1978).

Bronfen, Elisabeth. *The Knotted Subject: Hysteria and Its Discontents* (Princeton, NJ: Princeton University Press, 1998).

Brown, Lyn Mikel. *Raising Their Voices: The Politics of Girls Anger* (Cambridge, MA: Harvard University Press, 1998).

——. *Girlfighting: Betrayal and Rejection Among Girls* (New York: New York University Press, 2003).

Brownmiller, Susan. *Femininity* (New York: Ballantine, 1984).

Brumberg, Joan. *The Body Project: An Intimate History of American Girls* (New York: Random, 1997).

Bulfinch, Thomas. *Mythology* (New York: Dell Publishing Co, 1959).

Burke, Edmund. *A Philosophical Enquiry Into the Origin of Our Ideas of the Sublime and the Beautiful*. Ed. James Boulton (Notre Dame, IN: University of Notre Dame Press, 1968).

Buscombe, Edward. "The Idea of Genre in the American Cinema." In *Film Genre Reader III*. Ed. Barry Keith Grant (Austin, TX: University of Texas Press, 2003).

Butler, Judith. *Gender Trouble: Feminism and the Subversion of Identity* (New York: Routledge, 1990).

Butler, Ivan. *The Horror Film* (London: Zwemmer, 1967).

Buzard, James. *Disorienting Fiction: The Autoethnographic Work of Nineteenth-Century British Novels* (Princeton, NJ: Princeton University Press, 2005).

Byron, Glennis. "'Where Meaning Collapses': Tunku Halim's *Dark Demon Rising* as Global Gothic." In *Asian Gothic: Essays on Literature, Film and Anime*. Ed. Andrew Hock Soon Ng (Jefferson, NC: McFarland Press, 2008), 32–45.

"The Cagots." *All the Year Round* 21, no. 518 (1878): 416–420.

"The Cagots of the Pyrenees." *Illustrated London News* 96, no. 2662 (April 12, 1890): 535.

Calhoun, John. "Childhood's End: *Let the Right One In* and Other Deaths of Innocence." *Cineaste* (Winter 2009).

Cameron, Kate. "'Lost Weekend' Daring Film of Drunk's Orgy." In *New York Motion Picture Critics' Reviews 1945* (New York: Critics' Theatre Reviews, Inc., 1945).

Campany, Rob. "Demons, Gods, and Pilgrims: The Demonology of His-yu Chi." *Chinese Literatures: Essays, Articles, Reviews (CLEAR)* 7, no. 1/2 (1989) 95–115.
Cane. "Black Narcissus." *Variety*, May 7, 1947: 18.
——. "Stairway to Heaven." *Variety*, November 13, 1946: 16.
Carroll, Noël. *Philosophy of Horror, or Paradoxes of the Heart* (New York: Routledge, 1990).
Cart. "[Review of] *Clownhouse.*" *Variety*, February 1, 1989.
Céard, Jean. *La Nature Et Les Prodiges* (Geneva: Droz, 1977).
Chaouat, Bruno. "In the Image of Auschwitz." *Diacritics* 36, no. 1 (Spring 2006): 86–96.
Chehade, Carol. *Big Little White Lies: Our Attempt to White-Out America* (Kearney, NE Nehmarche Publishing, Inc., 2001/2003).
Clark, Anni. "Lightning Strikes *Powder* with Pedophilia Theme." *The Northeastern News*, November 1, 1995: 20.
Clarke, James W. *The Lineaments of Wrath: Race, Violent Crime and American Culture* (New Brunswick, NJ: Transaction Publishers, 1998).
"CNN Documentary: The Atlanta Child Murders." *CNN*, June 1, 2010.
"CNN Viewers: Williams 'Guilty' in Atlanta Child Murders." *CNN Justice*, June 11, 2010, http://articles.cnn.com/2010-06-11/justice/atlanta.murders.poll.ireport_1_atlanta-child-murders-two-life-sentences-killings/2?_s=PM:CRIME.
Cohen, Carl and Tom Regan. *The Animal Rights Debate* (Lanham, MD and Oxford: Rowman & Littlefield, 2001).
Cohen, Jeffrey Jerome. *Preface to Monster Theory*. Ed. Jeffrey Jerome Cohen (Minneapolis, MN: University of Minnesota Press, 1996).
Colebrook, Claire. "How Queer Can You Go?" In *Queering the Non-Human.* Ed. Noreen Giffney and Myra J. Hird (Surrey, England: Ashgate, 2008).
Corrigan, John (Ed.). *Religion and Emotion: Approaches and Interpretations* (New York: Oxford University Press, 2004).
du Coudray, Chantal Bourgault. *The Curse of the Werewolf: Fantasy, Horror and the Beast Within* (London: I.B. Tauris, 2006).
Cozad, Laurie. "Reeling in the Demon: An Exploration into the Category of the Demonized Other as Portrayed in 'The Journey to the West.'" *Journal of the American Academy of Religion* 66, no. 1 (1998) 117–145.
Creed, Barbara. "Dark Desires: Male Masochism in the Horror Film." In *Screening the Male: Exploring Masculinities in Hollywood Cinema.* Ed. Steven Cohan and Ina Rae Hark (London: Routledge, 1993).
——. "Horror and the Monstrous-Feminine: An Imaginary Abjection." In *The Dread of Difference: Gender and the Horror Film*, Ed. Barry Keith Grant (Austin, TX: University of Texas Press, 1996).
Crenshaw, Kimberlé. "Mapping the Margins: Intersectionality, Identity Politics, and Violence Against Women of Color." In *Critical Race Theory: The Key Writings That Formed the Movement.* Ed. Kimberlé Crenshaw, Neil Gotanda, Gary Peller, and Kendall Thomas (New York: The New Press, 1995).
Crowther, Bosley. "'Jane Eyre,' A Sombre Version of the Bronte Novel, with Joan Fontaine and Orson Welles, Opens at the Music Hall." *New York Times*, February 4, 1944a: 12.
——. "'Phantom Lady,' a Melodrama of Weird Effects, with Ella Raines and Franchot Tone, Has Premiere at Loew's State." *New York Times*, February 18, 1944b: 15.
——. "'The Lost Week-End,' in Which Ray Milland Presents a Study in Dipsomania, Makes Its Appearance at the Rivoli." *New York Times*, December 3, 1945a: 28.
——. "The Screen: A Costume Picture." *New York Times*, November 30, 1945b: 18.
——. "Screen in Review: Six New Films Arrive on the Holiday in Midtown Houses—Gene Tierney Appears in 'Leave Her to Heaven' at Roxy Cornered with Dick Powell, at Palace—'Seventh Veil,' a British Picture, Makes Its Debut at Winter Garden." *New York Times,* December 26, 1945c: 15.
——. "THE SCREEN: 'Dead of Night,' a British-Made Film, Is Premiere at Winter Garden—Rialto Offers New Melodrama by Fox Studios." *New York Times*, June 29, 1946a: 22.
——. "Screen in Review: 'Stairway to Heaven,' a British Production at Park Avenue, Proves Holiday Delight." *New York Times*, December 26, 1946b: 28.
——. "'Great Expectations,' in Which British Producers Do Very Well by Charles Dickens, Makes Its Bow at Radio City." *New York Times*, May 23, 1947a: 31.

——. "The 'Ten Best'—Five Foreign Films Among the 1946 Leaders." *New York Times*, December 29, 1947b: 11.

——. "Lawrence Olivier's 'Hamlet' Bows at the Park Avenue Theatre—'Saxon Charm' Seen." *New York Times*, September 30, 1948a: 32.

——. "The Screen in Review: 'The Red Shoes' a British Film About the Ballet, Stars Moira Shearer at Bijou." *New York Times*, October 23, 1948b: 9.

——. "The Screen in Review: 'Oliver Twist,' Rank Film Based on Charles Dickens Novel, at Park Avenue Theatre." *New York Times*, July 31, 1951: 17.

Cuneo, Andrew. *American Exorcism: Expelling Demons in the Land of Plenty* (New York: Broadway Books, 2002).

Cunningham, Jim. "Creepy Pix Cleaning Up: Studios Cash in on Cycle." *Variety*, March 31, 1943: 46.

Curtis, L. Perry. *Apes and Angels: The Irishman in Victorian Caricature* (Washington, DC: Smithsonian Institution Press, 1997).

Daniels, F.J. "Snake and Dragon Lore of Japan." *Folklore* 71, no. 3 (1960) 145–164.

Dargis, Manohla. "[Review of] *Powder*." *LA Weekly*, November 3, 1995.

Daston, Lorraine. "Marvelous Facts and Miraculous Evidence in Early Modern Europe." *Critical Inquiry* 18 (1991): 93–124.

Daston, Lorraine and Katharine Park. *Wonders and the Order of Nature: 1150–1750* (New York: Zone Books, 1998).

Davies, Ama Lee. "Priest." *Sight and Sound*. July 2011 74.

Davis, Lennard J. "Constructing Normalcy: The Bell Curve, the Novel, and the Invention of the Disabled Body in the Nineteenth Century." In *The Disability Studies Reader*. Ed. Lennard J. Davis (New York: Routledge, 2006), 3–16.

DeCecco, John P. (Ed.). *Bashers, Baiters, and Bigots: Homophobia in American Society* (New York: Harrington Park Press, 1999).

Deleuze, Gilles. *Difference and Repetition*. Trans. Paul Patton (New York: Columbia University Press, 1994).

——. *Spinoza: Practical Philosophy*. Trans. Robert Hurley (San Francisco: City Lights Books, 1988).

Deleuze, Gilles and Félix Guattari. *A Thousand Plateaus*. Trans. Brian Massumi (Minneapolis, MN: University of Minnesota Press, 1987).

——. *What Is Philosophy?* Trans. Hugh Tomlinson and Graham Burchill (London: Verso, 1994).

——. *Anti-Oedipus: Capitalism and Schizophrenia*. Trans. Robert Hurley (Minneapolis, MN: University of Minnesota Press, 1996).

Demos, John Putnam. *Entertaining Satan: Witchcraft and the Culture of Early New England* (New York: Oxford University Press, 1982).

Derrida, Jacques and Derek Attridge. *Acts of Literature* (London: Routledge, 1992).

Dervin, Daniel. "The Primal Scene and the Technology of Perception in Theater and Films: A Historical Perspective with a Look at *Potemkin* and *Psycho*." *Psychoanalytic Review* 62, no. 2 (1975) 269–304.

DeVun, Leah. "The Jesus Hermaphrodite: Science and Sex Difference in Premodern Europe." *Journal of the History of Ideas* 69, no. 2 (2008): 193–218.

Dickstein, Morris. "The Aesthetics of Fright." In *Planks of Reason: Essays on the Horror Film*. Ed. Barry K. Grant (Metuchen, NJ: Scarecrow, 1984), 65–78.

Doniger, Wendy "Hanuman." In *Encyclopedia Britannica*, http://www.britannica.com/EBchecked/topic/254649/Hanuman.

Douglas, Mary. *Purity and Danger* (London: Routledge, 2007).

Dowling, Colette. *The Frailty Myth: Redefining the Physical Potential of Women and Girls* (New York: Random House, 2000).

Dreger, Alice Domurat. *One of Us: Conjoined Twins and the Future of Normal* (Cambridge, MA: Harvard University Press, 2004).

Dubuisson, Daniel. *The Western Construction of Religion: Myths, Knowledge, and Ideology* (Baltimore, MD: Johns Hopkins University Press, 2007).

Ebert, Roger. "High Tension." *Chicago Sun Times*, June 9, 2005, http://rogerebert.suntimes.com/apps/pbcs.dll/article?AID=/20050609/REVIEWS/50601001/102 (accessed August 20, 2009).

——. "Why Movie Audiences Aren't Safe Anymore." *American Film* 6, no. 5 (March 1981) 54–56.

Edelman, Lee. *No Future: Queer Theory and the Death Drive* (Durham, NC: Duke University Press, 2005).

Edmonson, G. "Rice Defends Bush on Terrorism Policy." *Rocky Mount Telegram*, April 9, 2004, http://www.rockymounttelegram.com/news/content/shared/news/rice/09rice.html (accessed June 13, 2004).

Edmundson, Mark. *Nightmare on Main Street: Angels, Sadomasochism, and the Culture of the Gothic* (Cambridge, MA: Harvard University Press, 1999).

El Rico. "Reply # 5." *BadMovies.org* Comments for *Leeches!* June 9, 2009, http://www.badmovies.org/movies/leeches/index.html?start=0 (accessed July 20, 2010).

Emmons, Paul. "Apt Pupil." *BigScreen Cinema Guide*, 1998, http://www.bigscreen.com/ReaderReview?movie=AptPupil.

Englade, Ken. *Cellar of Horror* (New York: St. Martin's Press, 1988).

Evans, Walter. "Monster Movies: A Sexual Theory." *Journal of Popular Film* 2 (1973) 353–365.

Faludi, Susan. *Backlash* (New York: Doubleday, 1991).

al-Fārūkī, Ismail. "Islam and Art." *Studia Islamica* 37 (1973) 81–109.

Fessenden, Tracy. *Culture and Redemption: Religion, the Secular, and American Literature* (Princeton: Princeton University Press, 2006).

Fonseca, Anthony and June Michele Pulliam. *Hooked on Horror III: A Guide to Reading Interests* (Westport, CT: Libraries Unlimited, 2009).

Foucault, Michel. *The Order of Things*. Trans. Unknown (London: Routledge, 1970/2002).

——. "What Is an Author?" In *The Foucault Reader.* Ed. Paul Rabinow (Harmondsworth: Penguin, 1977/1984).

——. "For an Ethics of Discomfort." In *Power*. Ed. James D. Faubion and Trans. Robert Hurley (London: Penguin, 1994).

——. *Abnormal: Lectures at the College De France, 1974–1975* (New York: Picador, 2003).

——. *Abnormal: Lectures at the Collège De France 1974–1975*. Trans. Graham Burchell (New York: Picador, 2004).

Foundas, Scott. "[Review of] *Powder*." *LA Weekly*, August 29, 2003.

Franchot, Jenny. *Roads to Rome: The Antebellum Protestant Encounter with Catholicism* (Berkeley, CA: University of California Press, 1994).

Frankfurter, David. *Evil Incarnate: Rumors of Demonic Conspiracy and Satanic Abuse in History* (Princeton, NJ: Princeton University Press, 2008).

Franklin, Sarah. "The Cyborg Embryo: Our Path to Transbiology." In *Theory, Culture and Society Annual Review* 1, no. 1 (Autumn 2006): 167–188.

Freud, Sigmund. *Civilisation and Its Discontents*. Trans. James Strachey (New York: W.W. Norton & Company, Inc., 1962a).

——. *Totem and Taboo* (New York: Norton, 1962b).

——. *The Future of an Illusion* (New York: Norton, 1989).

Friedan, Betty. *The Feminine Mystique* (Harmondsworth, UK: Penguin, 1963).

Friedman, John Block. *The Monstrous Races in Medieval Art and Thought* (Syracuse, NY: Syracuse University Press, 2000).

Gallup, George et al. "ARI Report 163, Princeton 25th July." In *Gallup Looks at the Movies: Audience Research Reports 1940–1950* (Delaware: Scholarly Resources, 1979).

Gardell, Matthias. *In the Name of Elijah Muhammad: Louis Farrakhan and the Nation of Islam* (Durham, NC: Duke University Press, 1996).

Gaskell, Elizabeth. "An Accursed Race." In *Household Words* 12, no. 83 (1855): 73–78.

Gelder, Peter Van. *That's Hollywood: A Behind the Scenes Look at 60 of the Greatest Films of All Times* (New York: Harper Perennial, 1990).

Gigante, Denise. "Facing the Ugly." *ELH* 67 (2000) 565–587.

Gilman, Sander. *Difference and Pathology: Stereotypes of Sexuality, Race, and Madness* (Ithaca, NY: Cornell University Press, 1985).

Girard, René. *The Scapegoat* (Baltimore, MD: Johns Hopkins University Press, 1989).

Glassner, Barry. *The Culture of Fear: Why Americans Are Afraid of the Wrong Things* (New York: Basic Books, 1999).

Goldberg, Herb. *The New Male: From Macho to Sensitive But Still All Male* (New York: Signet, 1975/1979).

Goldhagen, Daniel. *Hitler's Willing Executioners: Ordinary Germans and the Holocaust* (New York: Knopf, 1996).

Gomery, Douglas. "The Economics of the Horror Film." In *Horror Films: Current Research on Audience Preferences and Reactions.* Ed. James B. Weaver, III and Ron Tamborini (Mahwah, NY: Lawrence Erlbaum Associates, 1996), 46–62.

Grattan, Thomas. *The Cagot's Hut.* In *Highways and by-Ways; or, Tales of the Roadside, Picked up in the French Provinces by a Walking Gentleman,* Third series, Vol. 1 (London: Henry Colburn, 1823/1827).

Griffin, Susan. *Pornography and Silence: Culture's Revenge Against Nature* (New York: Harper and Row, 1981).

Grosrichard, Alain. "The Case of Polyphemus or, A Monster and Its Mother." *Cogito and the Unconscious.* Ed. Slavoj Žižek and Trans. Marina Harss and Sina Nafaji (Durham, NC: Duke University Press, 1998).

Guattari, Fèlix. *Soft Subversions.* Trans. David L. Sweet (New York: Semiotext[e], 1996).

gypsywitch84. "Roman vs Victor War of the Pedos." *IMDb* Message Board for Victor Salva, April 18, 2004, http://www.imdb.com/name/nm0759207/board/nest/7889805 (accessed October 26, 2004).

Halberstam, Judith. "Technologies of Monstrosity: Bram Stoker's 'Dracula.'" *Victorian Studies* 36, no. 3 (Spring 1993) 333–352.

——. *Skin Shows: Gothic Horror and the Technology of Monsters* (Durham, NC: Duke University Press, 1995/2006).

——. "F2M: The Making of Female Masculinity." In *Feminist Theory and the Body: A Reader.* Ed. Janet Price and Margrit Shildrick (Edinburgh: Edinburgh University Press, 1999).

Hantke, Steffen. "The Kingdom of the Unimaginable: The Construction of Social Space and the Fantasy of Privacy in Serial Killer Narratives." *Literature/Film Quarterly* 26 (1998): 179–195.

Hayward, Susan. *Cinema Studies: The Key Concepts* (London: Taylor and Francis, 2006).

Headley, Bernard. *The Atlanta Youth Murders and the Politics of Race* (Carbondale, IL: Southern Illinois University Press, 1998).

Herr, Richard. "Flow and Ebb 1700–1833." In *Spain: A History.* Ed. Raymond Carr (Oxford: Oxford University Press, 2000), 191–204.

Heyrman, Christine Leigh. *Southern Cross: The Beginnings of the Bible Belt* (Chapel Hill, NC: University of North Carolina Press, 1997).

Hickey, Eric W. *Serial Murderers and Their Victims* (Pacific Grove, CA: Brooks/Cole Publishing Company, 1991.

——. *Serial Murderers and Their Victims* (5th ed.). (Florence, KY: Carnegie Learning, 2010).

"Highways and Byways." *Monthly Review* 6, no. 25 (September 1827): 105–116.

Hillblad, Thorolf. *Twilight of the Gods: A Swedish Waffen-SS Volunteer's Experiences with the 11th Panzergrendier Division "Nordland", Eastern Front 1944–45* (Solihull, England: Helion & Company Limited, 2004).

Hoberman, J. "Nazi Business." *Village Voice,* December 21, 1993 135.

Hochschild, Arlie Russell. *The Managed Heart: Commercialization of Human Feeling* (2nd ed.). (Berkeley, CA: University of California Press, 2003).

Hoeveler, Diane Long. "Objectifying Anxieties: Scientific Ideologies in Bram Stoker's *Dracula* and *The Lair of the White Worm.*" *Romanticism on the Net* 44 (2006), http://www.erudit.org/revue/ron/2006/v/n44/014003ar.html.

Hollings, K. "Review of the Motion Picture *The Siege.*" *British Film Institute,* February 1999. http://www.bfi.org.uk/sightandsound/reviews/details.php?id=41 (accessed June 17, 2006).

Holmes, Ronald M. and Stephen T. Holmes. *Serial Murder* (3rd ed.). (Thousand Oaks, CA: SAGE Publications, Inc., 2010).

Huddy, Leonie. "Fear and How It Works: Science and the Social Sciences." *Social Research* 71, no. 4 (Winter 2004) 801–805.

Huffman, H.A. "WOW, Giant Leeches... Attacking Pretty Boys?" December 14, 2003, Amazon.com Customer Reviews of *Leeches!* http://www.amazon.com/review/R1RNOGGT0WG2UU (accessed October 26, 2004).

Hume, David. *The Natural History of Religion* (New York: Oxford University Press, 1998).

Hutchings, Peter. *Hammer and Beyond: The British Horror Film* (Manchester: Manchester University Press, 1993).

——. "High Tension." In *100 European Horror Films*. Ed. Steven Jay Schneider (London: BFI, 2007).

Ide, Wendy. "Switchblade Romance." *The Times* [London], September 23, 2004, http://entertainment.timesonline.co.uk/tol/arts_and_entertainment/film/article1076058.ece (accessed August 20, 2009).

Ingebretsen, Edward J. *At Stake: Monsters and the Rhetoric of Fear in Public Culture* (Chicago: University of Chicago Press, 2003).

Irigaray, Luce. "Sexual Difference." In *The Irigaray Reader*. Ed. Margaret Whitford and Trans. Sèan Hand (London: Blackwell, 1992), 175.

——. *An Ethics of Sexual Difference*. Trans. Carolyn Burke and Gillian C. Gill (Ithaca, NY: Cornell University Press, 1993).

Jaher, Frederic. *A Scapegoat in the New Wilderness: The Origins and Rise of Anti-Semitism in America* (Cambridge, MA: Harvard University Press, 1996).

Jancovich, Mark. "Female Monsters: Horror, the 'Femme Fatale' and World War II." *European Journal of American Culture* 27 (2008): 133–149.

——. " 'Thrills and Chills': Horror, the Woman's Film and the Origins of Film Noir." *The New Review of Film and Television* 7, no. 2 (June 2009): 157–171.

——. "Two Ways of Looking': The Critical Reception of 1940s Horror." *Cinema Journal* 49, no. 3 (2010): 45–66.

——. " 'An Italianmade Spectacle Film Dubbed in English': Cultural Distinctions, National Cinema and the Critical Reception of the Postwar Historical Epic." In *The Epic Film in World Culture*. Ed. Robert Burgoyne (New York: Routledge/American Film Institute, 2012), 161–175.

Jātaka: or, Stories of the Buddha's Former Births. Ed. E.B. Cowell, et al. (Cambridge: Cambridge University Press, 1895–1913).

Jenkins, Philip. "African-Americans and Serial Homicide." In *Contemporary Perspectives on Serial Murder*. Ed. Ronald M. Holmes and Stephen T. Holmes (Thousand Oaks, CA: SAGE Publications, Inc., 1998).

Jensen, Robert. *The Heart of Whiteness: Confronting Race, Racism, and White Privilege* (San Francisco, CA: City Lights Books, 2005).

Jian, Ma. *Beijing Coma*. Trans. Flora Dew (London: Chatto & Windus, 2008).

jk90. "Is This Guy Gay?" *IMDb* Message Board for Victor Salva, January 27, 2004, http://www.imdb.com/name/nm0759207/board/flat/5877131?d+6531609#6531609 (accessed October 26, 2004).

Johnson, Kenneth. "Feature-Length Commentary by Writer/Director." *V: The Original Miniseries*. Side A. DVD (Warner Home Video, 2001).

Johnson, Ted. "*Powder* Rolls $7 Mil Amid Flap." *Variety*, October 30, 1995.

Johnson, T.W. "Far-Eastern Fox Lore." *Asian Folklore Studies* 33, no. 1 (1974) 35–68.

Johnson, T.W. "Salva Salvos Continue." *Variety*, October 26, 1995.

Juergensmeyer, Mark. *Terror in the Mind of God: The Global Mind of Religious Violence* (3rd ed.). (Berkeley, CA: University of California Press, 2003).

Kaagaard. "Is This Guy Gay?" *IMDb* Message Boar for Victor Salva, March 5, 2004, http://www.imdb.com/name/nm0759207/board/flat/5877131?d+6531609#6531609 (accessed October 26, 2004).

Kahn, Jeffrey. *The Cult of Kean* (Aldershot, UK: Ashgate, 2006).

Kamen, Henry. *A Concise History of Spain* (New York: Scribener's, 1973).

Kāmîr, Ôrît. *Every Breath You Take: Stalking Narratives and the Law* (Ann Arbor, MI: Michigan University Press, 1991).

Kao, Karl S.Y. "Projection, Displacement, Introjection: The Strangeness of *Liaozhai zhiyi*." In *Paradoxes of Traditional Chinese Literature*. Ed. Eva Hung (Hong Kong: The Chinese University Press, 1994).

Kearney, Richard. *Strangers, Gods and Monsters* (London and New York: Routledge, 2003).

Kegley, Charles W. *The New Global Terrorism: Characteristics, Causes, Controls* (Saddle River, NJ: Prentice Hall, 2003).

Kendrick, Walter. *The Thrill of Fear: 250 Years of Scary Entertainment* (New York: Grove Weidenfield, 1991).

Kimmel, Michael S. "Masculinity as Homophobia: Fear, Shame, Silence in the Construction of Gender Identity." In *Theorizing Masculinities*. Ed. Harry Brod and Michael Kaufman (Thousand Oaks, CA: Sage Publications, 1994).

Kinberg, Simon and Zak Penn. "Full-Length Audio Commentary by Director Brett Ratner and Screenwriters Simon Kinberg and Zak Penn." *X-Men: The Last Stand*. DVD (Twentieth Century Fox Home Entertainment, 2006).

Kincaid, James R. *Erotic Innocence: The Culture of Child Molesting* (Durham, NC: Duke University Press, 1998).

King, Stephen. *Apt Pupil*. In *Different Seasons* (New York: Signet, 1982).

Klause, Annette Curtis. *Blood and Chocolate* (New York: Delacourt Press, 1997).

Klawans, Stuart. "*Scream* 4: The Holocaust?" *Nation* 267, no. 14 (November 2, 2002) 34–35.

Klinger, Barbara. *Melodrama and Meaning: History, Culture, and the Films of Douglas Sirk* (Bloomington, IN: Indiana University Press, 1994).

The Koran. Trans N.J. Dawood (Harmondsworth: Penguin, 1997).

Kracauer, Siegfried. "Hollywood's Terror Films: Do They Reflect an American State of Mind." *New German Critique* 89 (2003): 107.

Kristeva, Julia. *Pouvoirs De L'horreur. Essai Sur L'abjection* (Paris: Seuil, 1980).

——. *Powers of Horror: An Essay on Abjection*. Trans. Leon S. Roudiez (New York: Columbia University Press, 1982).

Lacapra, Dominick. *Representing the Holocaust: History, Theory, Trauma* (Ithaca, NY: Cornell University Press, 1994).

——. *History and Memory After Auschwitz* (Ithaca, NY: Cornell University Press, 1998).

——. *Writing History, Writing Trauma* (Baltimore, MD: Johns Hopkins University Press, 2001).

Lahr, Angela M. *Millennial Dreams and Apocalyptic Nightmares: The Cold War Origins of Political Evangelicalism* (New York: Oxford University Press, 2007).

Lal, P. (Ed.). *The Bhagavadgita* (New Delhi: Roli Books, 1994).

Lang, Andrew. (Trans. and Ed.). *Tales from the Arabian Nights* (Hertfordshire: Wordsworth Classics, 1993).

Leach, Edmund. "Anthropological Aspects of Language: Animal Categories and Verbal Abuse." In *New Directions in the Study of Language*. Ed. Eric H. Lenneberg (Cambridge, MA: Massachusetts Institute of Technology Press, 1967).

Leydon, Joe. "[Review of] *Powder*." *Variety*, October 30, 1995: 72.

Lindqvist, John Ajvide. *Let the Right One in* (Melbourne: Text Publishing Company, 2007).

Lindsay, Paul. "Anthony Sowell, Alleged 'Cleveland Strangler': Is Race a Factor in Serial Killer Probe?" *Crimesider*, April 14, 2010, http://www.cbsnews.com/8301-504083_162-20002361-504083.html.

Little, Ralph. "Oral Aggression in Spider Legends." *American Imago* 23 (1966): 169–180.

——. "Umbilical Cord Symbolism of the Spider's Dropline." *Psychoanalytic Quarterly* 35 (1966): 587–590.

Lorber, Judith. *Paradoxes of Gender* (New Haven, CT: Yale University Press, 1994).

Lucas, Tim. "Under the Influence." *Sight and Sound*, February 2011.

Lutz, William D. "The Rhetoric of Fear." *NY Newsday*, September 7, 2003, http://www.commondreams.org/views03/0907-06.htm (accessed June 11, 2004).

Lyman, Stanford M. "Rereading Robert E. Park: Toward a Gothic Perspective on Capitalism and Imperialism." In *Explorations: The Age of Enlightenment*. Ed. M.W. duQuesnay (Lafayette, LA: University of Southwestern Louisiana Foundation, 1990), 29–108.

——. *The Seven Deadly Sins: Society and Evil* (New York: St. Martin's Press, 1978).

Lyotard, Jean-Françoise. *Driftworks*. Trans. Richard Lockwood (New York: Semiotext[e], 1984).

——. *The Inhuman*. Trans. Geoffrey Bennington and Rachel Bowlby (Palo Alto, CA: Stanford University Press, 1988).

——. *Libidinal Economy*. Trans. Iain Hamilton Grant (Bloomington, IN: Indiana University Press, 1993).

Mackenzie, Donald A. *China and Japan: Myths and Legends* (London: Senate, 1923/1994).

MacNab, Geoffrey. *J. Arthur Rank and the British Film Industry* (London: Routledge, 1993).

Madden, Edward. "Some Characteristics of Islamic Art." *The Journal of Aesthetics and Art Criticism* 33, no. 4 (1975).
Malchow, H.L. "Frankenstein's Monster and Images of Race in Nineteenth-Century Britain." *Past & Present* no. 139 (May 1993): 90–130.
Mallard, Jack. *The Atlanta Child Murders: The Night Stalker* (Charleston, SC: BookSurge Publishing, 2009).
Margolis, Harriet. "A Childe in Love, or Is It Just Fantasy? The Values of Women's Genres." *Paradoxa: Studies in World Literary Genres* 3, nos. 1–2 (1997).
Marsden, George. *Fundamentalism in American Culture: The Shaping of Twentieth-Century Evangelicalism, 1870–1925* (New York: Oxford University Press, 1980).
Martin, Jay. *Who Am I This Time?: Uncovering the Fictive Personality* (New York: W.W. Norton & Co, 1988).
Masuzawa, Tomoko. *The Invention of World Religions: Or, How European Universalism Was Preserved in the Language of Pluralism* (Chicago: University of Chicago Press, 2005).
Mauss, Marcel. *The Gift: The Form and Reason for Exchange in Archaic Societies* (New York: Norton, 2000).
McClintock, Anne. *Imperial Leather: Race, Gender, and Sexuality in the Colonial Contest* (New York: Routledge, 1995).
McCutcheon, Russell. *Manufacturing Religion: The Discourse on Sui Generis Religion and the Politics of Nostalgia* (New York: Oxford University Press, 1997).
McDonald, Fred. "Apt Pupil" (Abingdon College and District Film Society Program Note, November 2, 1998), http://homepage.ntlworld.com/holtnet/abcdfs/prognote/apt_pupil.pdf.
Merari, Ariel. "The Readiness to Kill and Die." In *Origins of Terrorism: Psychologies, Ideologies, Theologies, States of Mind*. Ed. Walter Reich (Baltimore, MD: Johns Hopkins University Press, 1998), 192–209.
Michel, Francisque. *Histoire des Races Maudites de la France et de L'Espange*, 2 vols (Paris, 1847).
Michie, Elsie. *Outside the Pale: Cultural Exclusion, Gender Difference, and the Victorian Woman Writer* (Ithaca, NY: Cornell University Press, 1993).
Midnight. "Reply #10." *BadMovies.org* Comments for *Leeches!* June 11, 2009, http://www.badmovies.org/movies/leeches/index.html?start=8 (accessed July 20, 2010).
Mirken, Harris. "The Pattern of Sexual Politics: Feminism, Homosexuality and Pedophilia." *Journal of Homosexuality* 37, no. 2 (1999): 1–24.
Modleski, Tania. *Loving with a Vengeance: Mass-Produced Fantasies for Women* (New York: Methuen, 1982).
Moers, Ellen. *Literary Women* (Garden City, NY: Anchor, 1977).
Molan, Peter D. "Sinbad the Sailor: A Commentary on the Ethics of Violence." *Journal of the American Oriental Society* 98, no. 3 (1978).
Monkkonen, Eric. "Racial Factors in New York City Homicides, 1800–1874." In *Ethnicity, Race and Crime: Perspectives Across Time and Place*. Ed. Darnell F. Hawkins (Albany, NY: State University Press of New York, 1995).
de Montaigne, Michel. *Essais*. Ed. Pierre Villey (Paris: Presses Universitaires de France, 1978).
Moore, Michael. *Fahrenheit 9/11* (Hollywood: CA: Miramax Films, 2004).
Moore, R. Laurence. *Selling God: American Religion in the Marketplace of Culture* (New York: Oxford University Press, 1994).
Morell, Virginia. "Minds of Their Own: Animals Are Smarter Than You Think." *National Geographic* 213, no. 3 (March 2008): 37–61.
Morgenstern, Joe. "[Review of] *Powder*." *The Wall Street Journal*, October 27, 1995.
Morton, Samuel George. *Crania Americana; or, a Comparative View of the Skulls of Various Aboriginal Nations of North and South America: To Which Is Prefixed an Essay on the Varieties of the Human Species* (Philadelphia: J. Dobson, 1839).
Moses, A.D. "Structure and Agency in the Holocaust: Daniel J. Goldhagen and His Critics." *History and Theory* 37 (1998): 194–220.
Mulvey, Laura. "Visual Pleasure and Narrative Cinema." In *Feminism and Film Theory*. Ed. Constance Penley (New York: Routledge, 1988).
Murphy, Robert. *Realism and Tinsel: Cinema and Society in Britain 1939–1949* (London: Routledge, 1989).
Nancy, Jean-Luc. *Being Singular Plural*. Trans. Robert D. Richardson and Anne E. O'Byrne (Palo Alto, CA: Stanford University Press, 2000).

Narayan, R.K. *Gods, Demons and Others* (London: Heinemann, 1965).

——. *The Ramayana: A Shortened Modern Prose Version of the Indian Epic* (London: Penguin, 1972).

Nathan, Debbie and Michael Snedeker. *Satan's Silence: Ritual Abuse and the Making of a Modern American Witch Hunt* (New York: Basic Books, 1995).

Newton, Michael and Judy Ann Newton. *Racial and Religious Violence in America: A Chronology* (New York: Garland, 1991).

Ng, Andrew Hock Soon. *Interrogating Interstices: Gothic Aesthetics in Postcolonial Asian and Asian American Literature* (New York and Bern: Peter Lang, 2007).

Nicol, Bran. " 'Police Thy Neighbour': Crime Culture and the *Rear Window* Paradigm." In *Crime Culture: Figuring Criminality in Fiction and Film*. Ed. Bran Nicol, Eugene McNulty, and Patricia Pulham (London: Continuum, 2011).

Nik. "Reply #7." *BadMovies.org* Comments for *Leeches!* June 9, 2009, http://www.badmovies.org/movies/leeches/index.html?start=0 (accessed July 20, 2010).

Nix. "High Tension (2003) Movie Review." *BeyondHollywood.com*, February 16, 2004, http://www.beyondhollywood.com/high-tension-2003-movie-review/ (accessed August 20, 2009).

Nussbaum, Felicity. *The Limits of the Human: Fictions of Anomaly, Race, and Gender in the Long Eighteenth Century* (Cambridge: Cambridge University Press, 2003).

"On Location." *The Hollywood Reporter*, July 18, 2001.

O' Sullivan, Tim and Alan Burton . *The Cinema of Basil Dearden and Michael Relph* (Edinburgh: Edinburgh University Press, 2009).

Otto, Rudolf. *The Idea of the Holy* (Oxford: Oxford University Press, 1923).

——. "*The Idea of the Holy*." In *Theory and Method in the Study of Religion: A Selection of Critical Readings*. Ed. Carl Olson (Belmont, CA: Wadsworth Publishing, 2002).

Owenson, Sydney. *The Wild Irish Girl*. Ed. Kathryn Kirkpatrick (Oxford: Oxford University Press, 1806/1999).

Paré, Ambroise. *Des Monstres Et Prodiges*. Ed. Jean Céard (Geneva: Droz, 1971).

——. *On Monsters and Marvels*. Trans. Janis Pallister (Chicago: University of Chicago Press, 1982).

Parikka, Jussi. *Insect Media: An Archaeology of Animals and Technology* (Minneapolis, MN: University of Minnesota Press, 2010).

Perazzo, John. *The Myths That Divide Us: How Lies Have Poisoned American Race Relations* (2nd ed.). (Briarcliff Manor, NY: World Studies Books, 1999).

Petley, Julian. "The Lost Continent." In *All Our Yesterdays: 90 Years of British Cinema*. Ed. Charles Barr. (London: British Film Institute, 1986), 98–119.

Phillips, Lynn M. *Flirting with Danger: Young Women's Reflections on Sexuality and Domination* (New York: New York University Press, 2000).

Picart, Caroline Joan ("Kay"). *The Cinematic Rebirths of Frankenstein: Universal, Hammer, and Beyond* (Westport, CT: Praeger, 2002).

Picart, Caroline Joan and Cecil E. Greek. "Introduction: Toward a Gothic Criminology." In *Monsters in and Among Us* (Madison, NJ: Fairleigh Dickinson University Press, 2007a).

——. *Monsters in and Among Us: Toward a Gothic Criminology* (Madison, NJ: Fairleigh Dickinson University Press, 2007b).

——. "When Women Kill: Undead Imagery in the Cinematic Portrait of Aileen Wuornos." In *Draculas, Vampires & Other Undead Forms: Essays on Gender, Race and Culture*. Ed. John Edgar Browning and Caroline Joan (Kay) Picart (Lanham, MD: Scarecrow Press, 2009).

Picart, Caroline Joan ("Kay") and David A. Frank. "Horror and the Holocaust: Genre Elements in *Schindler's List* and *Psycho*." In *The Horror Film*. Ed. Stephen Prince (New Brunswick, NJ: Rutgers University Press, 2003), 206–223.

——. *Frames of Evil: The Holocaust as Horror in American Film* (Carbondale, IL: Southern Illinois University Press, 2006).

Picart, Caroline J.S. and Jason G. McKahan. "Sadomasochism, Sexual Torture, and the Holocaust Film: From Misogyny to Homoeroticism and Homophobia in *Apt Pupil*." *Jump Cut* 45 (September 2002), http://www.ejumpcut.org/archive/jc45.2002/picart/index.html.

Pinedo, Isabel Christina. *Recreational Terror: Women and the Pleasures of Horror Film Viewing* (Albany, NY: State University of New York Press, 1997).
——. "Postmodern Elements of the Contemporary Horror Film." In *The Horror Film*. Ed. St even Prince (New Brunswick, NJ: Rutgers University Press, 2004), 85–117.
Pirie, David. *A Heritage of Horror: The English Gothic Cinema, 1946–1972* (London: Equinox, 1973).
Pliny. *Natural History* (Cambridge, MA: Harvard University Press, Loeb Classical Library, 2006).
Pollock, Sheldon. "The Divine King in the Indian Epic." *Journal of the American Oriental Society* 104, no. 3 (1984): 505–528.
Porter, Vincent. "Methodism versus the Market-Place: The Rank Organisation and British Cinema." In *The British Cinema Book*. Ed. Robert Murphy (London: British Film Institute, 1997), 122–132.
Posiedon-3. "The Leeches Aren't the Only Things That Suck!" October 17, 2007, *IMDb* User Comments for *Leeches!* http://www.imdb.com/title/tt0339288/usercomments?start=10 (accessed 20 July 2010).
Pryor, Thomas M. "Black Narcissus." *New York Times*, August 14, 1947: 29.
Pu, Songling. *Selected Tales of Liaozhai*. Trans. Yang Xianyi and Gladys Yang (Beijing: Panda Books, 1981).
Radat, Iva. "Haute Tension: Lesbian Audience and the Slasher Film" (Presentation, Transgressing Gender Conference: Two is not enough for gender (e)quality, Zagreb, Croatia, October 7–9, 2005).
Raiderofthelastfries. "Re: Some New (?) Thoughts on the Meaning of the Movie." *IMDb* User Comments for *Jeepers Creepers* (2001), April 3, 2004, http://www.imdb.com/title/tt0263488/board/nest/3334638 (accessed October 26, 2004).
Ramsdell, Kristin. *Romance Fiction: A Guide to the Genre* (Englewood, CO: Libraries Unlimited, 1999).
Raphael, Ray. *The Men from the Boys: Rites of Passage in Male America* (Lincoln: University of Nebraska Press, 1988).
Regan, Tom. *The Case for Animal Rights* (Berkeley, CA: University of California Press, 1983).
Rembrandt36. "Reply #9." *BadMovies.org* Comments for *Leeches!* June 10, 2009, http://www.badmovies.org/movies/leeches/index.html?start=8 (accessed July 20, 2010).
Rigby, Jonathan. *English Gothic: A Century of Horror Cinema* (London: Reynolds and Hearn, 2000).
Robertson, Theo. "Re: Ok SHUT UP." *IMDb* Message Board for Victor Salva, April 28, 2004, http://www.imdb.com/name/nm0759207/board/nest/7987155 (accessed October 26, 2004).
Robert, Ulysse. *Les Signes D'infamie Au Moyen Age: Juifs, Sarrasins, Hérétiques, Lépreux, Cagots Et Filles Publiques* (Paris: Honoré Champion Librarie, 1891).
Robin, Corey. *Fear: The History of a Political Idea* (New York: Oxford University Press, 2004).
Rogers, Robert. *A Psychoanalytic Study of the Double in Literature* (Detroit: Wayne State University Press, 1970).
Rogin, Michael. *Ronald Reagan: The Movie, and Other Essays in Political Demonology* (Berkeley, CA: University of California Press, 1988).
Rushdie, Salman. *Shame* (London: Picador, 1983).
Rushing, Janice Hocker and Thomas J. Frentz. *Projecting the Shadow: The Cyborg Hero in American Film* (Chicago: University of Chicago Press, 1995).
Russell-Brown, Katheryn. *Protecting Our Own: Race, Crime and African Americans* (Lanham, MD: Rowman & Littlefield Publishing, 2006).
——. *The Color of Crime* (2nd ed.). (New York: New York University Press), 2008/2009.
Russo, Mary. *The Female Grotesque* (New York: Routledge, 1995).
Ryan, Michael and Douglas Kellner. *Camera Politica: The Politics and Ideology of Contemporary Hollywood Film* (Bloomington, IN: Indiana University Press, 1990).
Sahlins, Peter. *Boundaries: The Making of France and Spain in the Pyrenees* (Berkeley, CA: University of California Press, 1989).
Santner, Eric L. "Miracles Happen: Benjamin, Rosenweig, Freud, and the Matter of the Neighbour." In *The Neighbour: Three Inquiries in Political Theology*. Ed. Slavoj Zizek, Eric L. Santner, and Kenneth Reinhard (Chicago: University of Chicago Press, 2005).
——. *On Creaturely Life: Rilke/Benjamin/Sebald* (Chicago: University of Chicago Press, 2006).
——*On the Psychotheology of Everyday Life: Reflections on Freud and Rosenzweig* (Chicago: University of Chicago Press, 2001).

Scapperotti, Dan. "Stephen King's *Apt Pupil*: *Unusual Suspects* Auteur Bryan Singer on Adapting King's Timely Shocker." *Cinefantastique* 30, no. 9 (1998).

Schallert, E. "New British Psycho Opus Fantastic." *Los Angeles Times*, August 8, 1946: A3.

Schiebinger, Londa. *Nature's Body: Gender in the Making of Modern Science* (2nd ed.). (Piscataway, NJ: Rutgers University Press, 2004).

Scheib, Richard. "Apt Pupil." *Science Fiction, Horror and Fantasy Film Review*, 1998, http://members.fortunecity.com/roogulator/horror/aptpupil.htm.

Schwarz, Daniel R. *Imaging the Holocaust* (New York: St. Martin's, 1999).

Sedgwick, Eve Kosofsky. *Between Men: English Literature and Male Homosocial Desire* (New York: Columbia University Press, 1985).

Seggelin, C. "Ack!! The Badness!!! The Aching Badness!!" *Amazon.com* Customer Reviews of *Leeches!* November 12, 2003a, http://www.amazon.com/Leeches-Julie-Briggs-II/product reviews/B0001IXU6W/ref=cm_cr_pr_link_next_3?ie=UTF8&showViewpoints=0&pageNumber=3&sortBy=bySubmissionDateDescending (accessed October 26, 2004).

——. "Plastereddragon." *Amazon.com* Customer Reviews of *Leeches!* November 12, 2003b, http://www.amazon.com/Leeches-Julie-Briggs-II/productreviews/B0001IXU6W/ref=cm_cr_pr_link_next_3?ie=UTF8&showViewpoints=0&pageNumber=3&sortBy=bySubmissionDateDescending (accessed October 26, 2004).

Serres, Michel. *Genesis*. Trans. Genevieve James and James Nielson (Ann Arbor, MI: University of Michigan Press, 1995).

——. *The Birth of Physics*. Trans. Jack Hawkes (Manchester, UK: Clinamen Press, 2000).

——. *The Five Senses: A Philosophy of Mingled Bodies*. Trans. Margaret Sankey and Peter Cowley (London: Athlone, 2008).

Sharpe, Andrew. *Foucault's Monsters and the Challenge of the Law* (New York: Routledge, 2010).

Sharpe, Ella Freeman. "Cautionary Tales." *International Journal of Psychoanalysis* 24 (1945).

Shea, Christian Leopold. "[Review of] Apt Pupil." *Jaundiced Eye*, 1998, http://www.geocities.com/Hollywood/Hills/1670/aptpupil.html.

Shelley, Mary. *Frankenstein, or the Modern Prometheus* (London: Penguin, 1817/1992).

ShifterCat. "Reply #19." *BadMovies.org* Comments for *Leeches!* June 25, 2009, http://www.badmovies.org/movies/leeches/index.html?start=16? (accessed July 20, 2010).

Shildrick, Margrit. *Embodying the Monster: Encounters with the Vulnerable Self* (London: Sage, 2002).

Shinkle, Peter. "Serial Killer Caught by His Own Internet Footprint." *St. Louis Post-Dispatch*, June 17, 1992, http://www.rense.com/general26/serial.htm.

Showalter, Elaine. *Hystories: Hysterical Epidemics and Modern Media* (New York: Columbia University Press, 1998).

Singer, Bryan. "Bryan Singer Interview." *X-Men*. DVD (Twentieth Century Fox Home Entertainment, 2005a).

——. "Fox Special: 'The Mutant Watch.'" *X-Men*. DVD (Twentieth Century Fox Home Entertainment, 2005b).

——. "Full-Length Audio Commentary (Director Bryan Singer and Cinematographer Newton Thomas Sigel)." *X2: X-Men United*. DVD (Twentieth Century Fox Home Entertainment, 2006).

Singer, Peter. *Animal Liberation: A New Ethics for Our Treatment of Animals* (New York: Avon Books, 1975).

Singer, Peter (Ed.). *In Defense of Animals* (Oxford: Blackwell, 1985).

Skal, David J. *The Monster Show: A Cultural History of Horror* (Rev ed.). (New York: Faber & Faber, 2001).

Smith, Barbara Hernstein. "Belief and Resistance: A Symmetrical Account." *Critical Inquiry* 18 (Autumn 1991).

Sorabji, Richard. *Animal Minds and Human Morals: The Origins of the Western Debate* (Ithaca, NY: Cornell University Press, 1995).

"Stanford Psychologist Questions Over-Use of the Word 'Evil'." *Business Journal*, November 28, 2001, http://sanjose.bizjournals.com/sanjose/stories/2001/11/26/daily22.html (accessed June 17, 2004).

Stanley, Fred. "Hollywood Shivers: The Studios Are Busily Stirring Up a Grade A Witches Brew—Other Items." *New York Times* 48, May 1944: X3.

Stein, Ruthe . "The Horror of the Underworld (and This World)." *San Francisco Chronicle*, December 29, 2006, http://www.sfgate.com (accessed February 27, 2007).

Stephens, Elizabeth. "Queer Monsters: Technologies of Self-Transformation in Bulwer's *Anthropometamorphosis* and Braidotti's *Metamorphosis*." In *Somatechnics: Queering the Technologisation of Bodies*. Ed. Nikki Sullivan and Samantha Murray (Surrey: Ashgate Publishing, 2009), 171–186.

Sterba, Richard. "On Spiders, Hanging and Oral Sadism." *American Imago* 7 (1950): 21–28.

Street, Sarah. *British National Cinema: 2* (London: Routledge, 2008).

——. *Transatlantic Crossings: British Feature Films in the USA* (London: Continuum, 2002).

Surette, Raymond. "Gothic Criminology and Criminal Justice Policy." In *Monsters in and Among Us*. Ed. Caroline Joan (Kay) Picart and Cecil E. Greek (Madison, NJ: Fairleigh Dickinson University Press, 2007).

Talb. "Dead of Night." *Variety*, September 19, 1945: 12.

——. "The Seventh Veil." *Variety*, October 31, 1945: 17.

——. "The Wicked Lady." *Variety*, November 28, 1945: 10.

Taves, Ann. *Fits, Trances, & Visions: Experiencing Religion and Explaining Experience from Wesley to James* (Princeton, NJ: Princeton University Press, 1999).

Taylor, Jared. *Paved with Good Intentions: The Failure of Race Relations in Contemporary America* (New York: Carroll and Graf Publishers, Inc., 1992/1993).

Thernstrom, Stephan and Abigail Thernstrom. *America in Black and White: One Nation, Indivisible* (New York: Touchstone, 1997/1999).

T.M.P. " 'Madonna of the Seven Moons,' British Importation Starring Phyllis Calvert in Two Roles, Is New Bill at Winter Garden." *New York Times*, May 23, 1946: 18.

Tobin-McClain, Lee. "Paranormal Romance." *Journal of the Fantastic in the Arts* 11 (2000).

Del Toro, Guillermo. "Feature Audio Commentary by Writer/Director." *Pan's Labyrinth*. Disc One. New Line 2-Disc Platinum Series (MMVII New Line Entertainment, Inc., 2007).

Totaro, Donato. "The Final Girl: A Few Thoughts on Feminism and Horror." *Offscreen*, January 31, 2002, http://www.horschamp.qc.ca/new_offscreen/final_girl.html (accessed August 20, 2009).

Traveshamockery. "Campy/Homoerotic Classic." *IMDb* User Comments for *Leeches!* August 27, 2007, http://www.imdb.com/title/tt0339288/usercomments?start=10 (accessed July 20, 2010).

Tweed, Thomas A. *Crossing and Dwelling: A Theory of Religion* (Cambridge: Harvard University Press, 2006).

Verner, Lisa. *The Epistemology of the Monstrous in the Middle Ages* (New York: Routledge, 2005).

de Waal, Frans. *Primates and Philosophers: How Morality Evolved* (Princeton, NJ: Princeton University Press, 2006).

Walsh, Anthony. "African Americans and Serial Killing in the Media: The Myth and the Reality." *Homicide Studies* 9, no. 4 (2005).

——. *Race and Crime: A Biosocial Analysis* (Hauppauge, NJ: Nova Science Publishers, Inc., 2004).

Wang, Ban. *The Sublime Figure of History: Aesthetics and Politics in Twentieth-Century China* (Palo Alto, CA: Stanford University Press, 1997).

Wang, David Der-Wei. *The Monster That Is History: History, Violence, and Fictional Writing in Twentieth-Century China* (Berkeley: University of California Press, 2004).

Warner, Marina. *No Go the Bogeyman: Scaring, Lulling, and Making Mock* (New York: Farrar, Straus and Giroux, 1998).

Weber, Eugen. *Apocalypses: Prophecies, Cults, and Millennial Beliefs Through the Ages* (Cambridge, MA: Harvard University Press, 1999).

White, Jonathan Randall. *Terrorism: An Introduction* (4th ed.). (Belmont, CA: Wadsworth Publishing, 2003).

Whitehouse, Harvey. "Rites of Terror: Emotion, Metaphor, and Memory in Melanese Initiation Cults." In *Religion and Emotion*. Ed. John Corrigan (New York: Oxford University Press, 2004), 133–148.

William, David. *Deformed Discourses: The Function of the Monster in Mediaeval Thought and Literature* (Montreal-Kingston and London: McGill-Queen's University Press, 1996).

Williams, Linda Ruth. *The Erotic Thriller in Contemporary Cinema* (Bloomington, IN: Indiana University Press, 2005).

Williams, Linda. "When Women Look: A Sequel." *Senses of Cinema* 15 (2001), http://archive.sensesofcinema.com/contents/01/15/horror_women.html (accessed August 20, 2009).

Wilson, Jake. "Apt Pupil." *Urban Cinefile*, November 9, 2001, http://www.urbancinefile.com/home/view.asp?a=2242&s=mVideo_files.

Wolf, Naomi. *The Beauty Myth: How Images of Beauty Are Used Against Women* (New York: Harper Perennial, 2002).

Wolfgang, Marvin E. and Franco Ferracuti. *The Subculture of Violence* (London: Travistock, 1967).

Wood, Gary. "Whatever Happened to *Apt Pupil*?" *Cinefantastique* 21, no. 4 (February 1991).

Wood, Robin. "Nuit Brouillard." In *International Dictionary of Films and Filmmakers*, Vol. 1. Ed. Christopher Lyon (Chicago: St. James Press, 1984).

——. *Hollywood: From Vietnam to Reagan* (New York: Columbia University Press, 1986).

Wynne, Clive D.L. *Do Animals Think?* (Princeton, NJ: Princeton University Press, 2004).

Youngquist, Paul. *Monstrosities: Bodies and British Romanticism* (Minneapolis, MN: University of Minnesota Press, 2003).

Young, Robert. *The Idea of English Ethnicity* (Oxford: Blackwell Publishing, 2008).

Zanger, Jules. "Metaphor into Metonymy: The Vampire Next Door." In *Blood Read: The Vampire as Metaphor in Contemporary Culture*. Ed. Veronica Hollinger (Philadelphia: University of Pennsylvania Press, 1997).

Zinn, Howard. *A People's History of the United States* (New York: Harper Perennial, 2001).

Žižek, Slavoj. *The Sublime Object of Ideology* (New York: Verso, 1989).

——. "Afterword: Lenin's Choice." In Vladimir Lenin. *Revolution at the Gates: A Selection of Writings from February to October 1917*. Ed. Slavoj Zizek (London: Verso, 2004).

Žižek, Slavoj, Eric L. Santner, and Kenneth Reinhard. *The Neighbor: Three Inquiries in Political Theology* (Chicago: University of Chicago Press, 2005).

Zvelebil, K.V. "Ravana the Great in Modern Tamil Fiction." *Journal of the Royal Asiatic Society of Great Britain and Ireland* 1 (1998): 126–134.

Notes on Contributors

Editors

John Edgar Browning (B.A., Florida State University; M.A., University of Central Oklahoma; Ph.D. Candidate 2013, State University of New York at Buffalo) completed coursework for the Ph.D. in English at Louisiana State University (2008–2011) before transferring to the doctoral program in American Studies at the State University of New York at Buffalo, where currently he is an Arthur A. Schomburg Fellow in the Department of Transnational Studies and a member of the adjunct faculty in the Department of English. He has contracted and co-written nine books, including (with Caroline Joan (Kay) S. Picart) *Draculas, Vampires, and Other Undead Forms: Essays on Gender, Race, and Culture* (2009); (also with Picart) *Dracula in Visual Media: Film, Television, Comic Book and Electronic Game Appearances, 1921–2010* (2010) – winner of the Lord Ruthven Award for Nonfiction *The Vampire, His Kith and Kin: A Critical Edition* (2011), *Bram Stoker's Dracula: The Critical Feast, An Annotated Reference of Reviews and Reactions, 1897–1913* (2012); and *The Forgotten Writings of Bram Stoker* (Palgrave, forthcoming). His work on horror and the fantastic has appeared in several books, including *Asian Gothic: Essays on Literature, Film, and Anime* (2008), *The Encyclopedia of the Vampire* (2010), *Nyx in the House of Night: Mythology, Folklore and Religion in the PC and Kristin Cast Vampyre Series* (2011), and *Fear and Learning: Essays on the Pedagogy of Horror* (forthcoming); and in various journals, including *Film & History*, *Horror Studies*, *Studies in the Fantastic*, and *Dead Reckonings: A Review Magazine for the Horror Field.* John has taught vampire- and monster-themed coursework at various universities across the southeastern and southwestern United States, and during that time he has also presented and been asked to speak on these subjects at various national conferences, festivals, and universities. Additionally, John spent two years conducting an ethnographic study of persons living in New Orleans who self-identify as vampire, a project that has become the focal point of his doctoral dissertation.

Caroline Joan (Kay) S. Picart (M.Phil, Cambridge University, Sir Run Run Shaw Scholar & Wolfson Prize Winner; Ph.D., Pennsylvania State University; Postdoctoral Scholar, Cornell School of Criticism and Theory), formely a tenured associate professor of English and Humanities at Florida State University, is a joint Juris Doctor-MA Candidate (WST) at the University of Florida Levin College of Law and an adjunct professor of Humanities at Santa Fe College. A scholar and critic, she is author/co-author of 15 published and forthcoming scholarly books; numerous refereed and edited articles, published or forthcoming in research journals, inclusive of the *East Asia Law Review, Cardozo Journal of Law and Gender, Florida Journal of International Law, California Western Law Review, Arizona State Law Journal, Journal of Criminal Justice and Popular Culture, Film & History, Qualitative Inquiry, The Long Term View, Women and Performance, Scope, Communication and Critical/Cultural Studies, Rhetoric & Public Affairs, Film and History, p.o.v., A Danish Journal of Film Studies, Jump Cut, Pacific Coast Philology, Critical Studies in Media Communication, Journal of Aesthetics and Art Criticism, Human Studies: A Journal for Philosophy and the Social Sciences, Philosophy Today, Social Studies of Science, Journal of Nietzsche Studies, Journal of Speculative Philosophy, ACME: An International E-Journal for Critical Geographies, Southern Journal of Communication*; and 87 print publications as a columnist or invited writer in newspapers and magazines in Seoul South Korea and in various parts of the United States, such as *The Korea Times*, *The Korea Herald*, *Center Daily Times*, *Voices of Central Pennsylvania*, *Boca Raton News*, *Filipinas Magazine*, *Asia Trend Magazine*, and the *Tallahassee Democrat*. Picart has served as a manuscript referee or reader for 21 journals and presses, such as *Science, Technology, & Human Values*, *Critical Studies in Media Communication*, State University of New York Press, *Journal of Nietzsche Studies*, *Kaleidoscope: A Graduate Journal of Qualitative Communication Research*, University of Wisconsin Press, *Rhetoric and Public Affairs*, *Social Studies of Science*, *Kenneth Burke Journal*, *Journal of Contemporary Ethnography*, *Journal of Criminal Justice and Popular Culture*, *Review of Communication*, *American Ethnologist*, W.W. Norton and Company, Prentice Hall, *Critical and Cultural Studies*, *Florida Historical Quarterly*, Fairleigh Dickinson University Press, *Men and Masculinities*, *Qualitative Inquiry*, and the *International Journal of Qualitative Studies in Education*, among others. Currently, she serves as Editor-in-Chief of the *Florida Journal of International Law* and Communications Executive and former Articles Editor and Research Editor of the *Journal of Technology Law & Policy*. She has taught courses in Philosophy, Biology, English, and Film and Law, across the Philippines, South Korea, and various parts of the United States for 21 years, prior to proceeding on to law school at the University of Florida Levin College of Law, where she is currently a full-time law student while serving as Adjunct Professor of Humanities at Santa Fe College. From August 2008 to April 2009, she produced and hosted her own radio show, available through www.drpicart.com; market research showed that when she closed the radio show, en route to law school, the show, in a mere nine months, was carried by 59 national and international affiliates, which amounts to an estimated listenership of over two million monthly listeners, nationally and internationally.

CONTRIBUTORS

Lonnie H. Athens, a full professor in the Department of Criminal Justice at Seton Hall University, is the author of three books on violence. In addition to writing *The Creation of Dangerous Violent Criminals* (1992) and *Violent Criminal Acts and Actors Revisited* (1997), he co-edited and contributed to *Violent Acts and Violentization: Assessing, Applying and Developing Lonnie Athens' Theories* (2003). His latest work on violence is an article "Violent Encounters: Violent Engagements, Skirmishes, and Tiffs," which appeared in *The Contemporary Journal of Ethnography* (2005). He has had the good fortune of having two books written about him: *Why They Kill: The Discoveries of a Maverick Criminologists*, by Richard Rhodes and *La Cosmoligia Degli Attori Violenti: L' inedita prospecti Di Lonnie Athens* [*The Cosmology of Violent Actors: The Unknown Perspective of Lonnie Athens*], by Adolfo Cerretti and Lorenzo Natali. Athens is a past president of the Society for the Study of Symbolic Interaction and a recipient of the society's highest honor, the *George Herbert Mead Award*.

Harry M. Benshoff is Associate Professor of Radio, Television, and Film at the University of North Texas. His research interests include topics in film genres, film history, film theory, and multiculturalism. He has published essays on blaxploitation horror films, Hollywood LSD films, *The Talented Mr. Ripley* (1999), and *Brokeback Mountain* (2005). He is the author of *Monsters in the Closet: Homosexuality and the Horror Film* (Manchester University Press, 1997) and *Dark Shadows* (Wayne State University Press, 2011). With Sean Griffin, he co-authored *America on Film: Representing Race, Class, Gender and Sexuality at the Movies* (Blackwell Publishers, 2004) and *Queer Images: A History of Gay and Lesbian Film in America* (Rowman & Littlefield, 2006).

Jason C. Bivins, Associate Professor and Associate Department Head in the Department of Philosophy and Religious Studies at North Carolina State University, is a specialist in religion and American culture, focusing particularly on the intersection between religions and politics since 1900. He is the author of *The Fracture of Good Order: Christian Antiliberalism and the Challenge to American Politics* (University of North Carolina Press, 2003) and *Religion of Fear: The Politics of Horror in Conservative Evangelicalism* (Oxford University Press, 2008), in addition to multiple articles, review essays, and occasional pieces on religion, politics, and culture in the United States. He is currently working on two book-length research projects. The first is *Spirits Rejoice!: Improvising New Religious Communities*, a study of the intersections of jazz and American religions. The second is *Embattled Majority*, a genealogy of the rhetoric of "religious bigotry" in conservative Christian politics since the 1960s.

Noël Carroll is Distinguished Professor of Philosophy at the Graduate Center of the City University of New York and one of the leading philosophers of art and aesthetics in the United States. He is the author of eleven monographs, including *The Philosophy of Motion Pictures*, *Beyond Aesthetics*, and *The Philosophy of Horror*; three edited collections; and over 200 academic articles and reviews. His work also encompasses the philosophy of literature, the philosophy of visual arts, and social and cultural theory, and he has served as president of the American Society for Aesthetics. Carroll has been a regular contributor of journalistic reviews of dance, theater, and film in publications such as *Artforum* and the *Village Voice*. His new book *On Criticism* was published in Fall 2008, and he is currently working on a book on the philosophy of humor for Oxford University Press.

Reading *Dracula* (1897) at the age of 12 ignited **Margaret L. Carter**'s interest in a wide range of horror, fantasy, and science fiction. Vampires, however, have always remained close to Carter's heart, beginning with her first published book *Curse of the Undead*, an anthology of vampire fiction. Her dissertation for the University of California, Irvine, contained a chapter on *Dracula*, and its publication in book form was shortly followed by *Dracula: The Vampire and the Critics* and *The Vampire in Literature: A Critical Bibliography*. Her fiction includes stories in small press magazines and in anthologies such as Marion Zimmer Bradley's *Darkover* and *Sword and Sorceress* volumes; a werewolf novel, *Shadow of the Beast*; a vampire novel, *Dark Changeling*, which won an Eppie Award (presented by EPIC, an e-published authors' organization) in 2000 in the horror category; *Child of Twilight*, its sequel, an Eppie finalist in horror in 2004; and other horror and paranormal romance novels. Her first mass-market novel, a vampire romance entitled *Embracing Darkness*, was published in March 2005 by Silhouette Intimate Moments. Her monograph *Different Blood: The Vampire as Alien* was a 2005 Eppie finalist in nonfiction. She has had several erotic paranormal romances released in the thriving e-publishing market. For more information, visit Carter's Crypt: www.margaretlcarter.com.

Jeffrey Jerome Cohen (http://www.jeffreyjeromecohen.com) is Professor of English and Director of the Medieval and Early Modern Studies Institute (MEMSI) (http://www.gwmemsi.com) at the George Washington University. His research explores what monsters promise; how postcolonial studies, queer theory, postmodernism, and posthumanism might help us to better understand the literatures and cultures of the Middle Ages (and might be transformed by that encounter); the limits and the creativity of our taxonomic impulses; the complexities of time when thought outside of progress narratives; and ecotheory. He is the author of three books: *Of Giants: Sex, Monsters and the Middle Ages*; *Medieval Identity Machines*; and *Hybridity, Identity and Monstrosity in Medieval Britain: On Difficult Middles* and the editor of four more books. He blogs at: In the Middle (http://www.inthemedievalmiddle.com).

Ian Conrich is a Fellow in the Department of Literature, Film, and Theatre at the University of Essex. He is an editor of the *Journal of British Cinema and Television*, associate editor of *Film and Philosophy*, and an advisory board member of *Interactive Media*, and *Studies in Australasian Cinema*. He has been a guest editor of *Post Script*, *Asian Cinema*, the *Harvard Review*, and *Studies in Travel Writing*, and he is the author or editor of 14 books, including *The Cinema of John Carpenter: The Technique of Terror* (2004) and *Horror Zone: The Cultural Experience of Contemporary Horror Cinema* (2009). His work on the horror genre has appeared in many books, including *The Modern Fantastic: The Films of David Cronenberg* (2000), *The Horror Film Reader* (2001), *British Horror Cinema* (2001), *The Horror Film* (2004), *Horror International* (2005), *Japanese Horror Cinema* (2005), and *Seventies British Cinema* (2008).

David A. Frank, Professor of Rhetoric at the University of Oregon and Academic Dean of the Robert D. Clark Honors College, is the author of 6 books and 23 articles in the leading journals in his field. His most recent publication, *Frames of Evil: The Holocaust as Horror in American Film*, co-authored with Caroline J. S. Picart, critiques the use of visual rhetoric and narrative devices in *Schindler's List* and other popular films to explain evil in the world. In February 2008, during the height of the Democratic election primaries, Frank, who is also the director of the UO forensics program, was interviewed on National Public Radio about Barack Obama's rhetoric of consilience.

Ken Gelder is Professor of English at the University of Melbourne. His books include *Reading the Vampire* (1994), *Uncanny Australia: Sacredness and Identity in a Postcolonial Nation* (1998, with Jane M. Jacobs), *Popular Fiction: The Logics and Practices of a Literary Field* (2004), and *Subcultures: Cultural Histories and Social Practice* (2007).

Cecil E. Greek was born in Latrobe, PA. He attended Eastern College and the New School for Social Research, earning the Ph.D. in sociology in 1983. His doctoral dissertation, *The Religious Roots of American Sociology*, was later published by Garland Press. Greek continues to be interested in the social construction of social problems. His research interests focus on media coverage of crime and criminal justice, consumer culture, and sociological theory. He has written on antipornography crusading, the use of forfeiture penalties, and cybercrime. He is currently Associate Professor of Sociology at University of South Florida Polytechnic.

Judith (Jack) Halberstam is Professor of English, American Studies and Ethnicity, and Gender Studies at the University of Southern California. Halberstam works in the areas of popular, visual, and queer culture with an emphasis on subcultures. Halberstam's first book, *Skin Shows: Gothic Horror and the Technology of Monsters* (1995), was a study of popular gothic cultures of the nineteenth and twentieth centuries and it stretched from Frankenstein to contemporary horror film. Her book *Female Masculinity* (1998) made a groundbreaking argument about nonmale masculinity and tracked the impact of female masculinity upon hegemonic genders. Halberstam's last book, *In a Queer Time and Place: Transgender Bodies, Subcultural Lives* (2005), described and theorized queer reconfigurations of time and space in relation to subcultural scenes and the emergence of transgender visibility. This book devotes several chapters to the topic of visual representation of gender ambiguity. Halberstam was also the co-author with Del LaGrace Volcano of a photo/essay book, *The Drag King Book* (1999), and with Ira Livingston of the anthology *Posthuman Bodies* (1995). Halberstam regularly speaks on visual culture and publishes journalism in venues like *BITCH* Magazine and *The Nation*; Halberstam has a new book from Duke University Press titled *The Queer Art of Failure* (2011) and another forthcoming titled *Gaga Feminism*.

Mark Jancovich is Professor of Film and Television Studies at the University of East Anglia, UK. He is the author of several books: *Horror* (Batsford, 1992); *The Cultural Politics of the New Criticism* (CUP, 1993); *Rational Fears: American Horror in the 1950s* (MUP, 1996); and *The Place of the Audience: Cultural Geographies of Film Consumption* (with Lucy Faire and Sarah Stubbings, BFI, 2003). He is also the editor of several anthologies: *Approaches to Popular Film* (with Joanne Hollows, MUP, 1995); *The Film Studies Reader* (with Joanne Hollows and Peter Hutchings, Arnold/OUP, 2000); *Horror, The Film Reader* (Routledge, 2001); *Quality Popular Television: Cult TV, the Industry and Fans* (with James Lyons, BFI, 2003); *Defining Cult Movies: The Cultural Politics of Oppositional Taste* (with Antonio Lazaro-Reboll, Julian Stringer and Andrew Willis, MUP, 2003); *Film Histories: An Introduction and Reader* (with Paul Grainge, and Sharon Monteith, EUP, 2006); *Film and Comic Books* (with Ian Gordon and Matthew P. McAllister, University Press of Mississippi, 2007); and *The Shifting Definitions of Genre: Essays on Labeling Films, Television Shows and Media* (with Lincoln Geraghty, McFarland, 2008). He was also the founder of *Scope: An Online Journal of Film Studies*; is series editor (with Eric Schaefer) of the MUP book series *Inside Popular Film*; and is series editor (with Charles Acland) of the Berg book series *Film Genres*. He is currently writing a history of horror in the 1940s.

Ôrît Kāmîr is Professor of Law, Culture and Gender at the Peres Law School in Israel. She received her LL.M. and S.J.D. at the University of Michigan Law School, and her publications (including six books), in both Hebrew and English, offer interdisciplinary analyses of law, society, and culture, often focusing on film and on the construction of gender. Her first book, *Every Breath You Take: Stalking Narratives and the Law*, offers an interdisciplinary analysis of the sociocultural conception of stalking, including the role played by cinema in the contemporary construction of stalking. Her most recent book in English *Framed: Women in Law and Film* (Duke University Press, 2006) develops a feminist theory of law and film, reading films from around the world, and examining the social implications of fundamental, underlying values such as honor and dignity.

Dominick LaCapra, Bryce & Edith M. Bowmar Professor in Humanistic Studies, began teaching in the History Department at Cornell in 1969. He also holds a joint appointment in the Department of Comparative Literature and is a member of the graduate field of Romance Studies and the program in Jewish Studies. He served for ten years as director of Cornell's Society for the Humanities and for four years as Associate Director and for eight years as director of the School of Criticism and Theory. In the course of his career, LaCapra's own principal contributions have been to intellectual and cultural history and to critical theory, which he sees as closely related fields of inquiry. His teaching interests range widely in the areas of modern European intellectual and cultural history, historiography, trauma studies, history and literature, and critical theory. His publications include 13 individually authored books and two edited or co-edited volumes: *Emile Durkheim: Sociologist and Philosopher* (1972); *A Preface to Sartre* (1978); *"Madame Bovar" on Trial* (1982); *Rethinking Intellectual History: Texts, Contexts, Language* (1983); *History & Criticism* (1985); *History, Politics, and the Novel* (1987); *Soundings in Critical Theory* (1989); *Representing the Holocaust: History, Theory, Trauma* (1994); *History and Memory after Auschwitz* (1998); *History and Reading: Tocqueville, Foucault, French Studies* (2000); *Writing History, Writing Trauma* (2001); *History in Transit: Experience, Identity, Critical Theory* (2004); *History and Its Limits: Human, Animal, Violence* (2009); edited [with S. L. Kaplan]: *Modern European Intellectual History: Reappraisals and New Perspectives* (1982); edited: *The Bounds of Race: Perspectives on Hegemony and Resistance* (1991).

Kathleen Long is Professor of French in the Department of Romance Studies at Cornell University. Her recent publications include *Hermaphrodites in Renaissance Europe* (Ashgate, 2006) and *Religious Differences in France, Past and Present* (Sixteenth Century Essays and Studies, 2006), as well as an edited volume on *Gender and Scientific Discourse in Early Modern Culture* (Ashgate, 2010). Current projects include a book-length study of the representation of the body in alchemic treatises, *Odd Bodies: Reviewing Corporeal Difference in Early Modern Alchemy*, and a study on *Monsters A-X (Aristotle to the X-Files).*

Patricia MacCormack is Reader in English, Communication, Film and Media at Anglia Ruskin University, Cambridge. She has published extensively on Guattari, Blanchot, Serres, Irigaray, queer theory, teratology, body modification, posthuman theory, animal rights, and horror film. Patricia's articles have appeared in journals such as *Women: A Cultural Review*, *Theory, Culture and Society*, *New Formations* and *Body and Society*. She has published chapters in anthologies such as *Queering the Non/Human*, *Deleuze and Queer Theory*, *Caligari's Heirs* and *Zombie Culture*, which include work on masochism, cinesexuality, horror film, and continental theory. She is the author of *Cinesexuality* and the co-editor of *The Schizoanalysis of Cinema*. She is currently writing on posthuman ethics.

Andrew Hock-Soon Ng obtained his Ph.D. from the University of Western Australia. His research interest includes the Gothic and postcolonial literature. He is the author of *Dimensions of Monstrosity in Contemporary Narratives: Theory, Psychoanalysis, Postmodernism* (2004), *Interrogating Interstices: Gothic Aesthetics in Postcolonial Asian and Asian American Literature* (2007), and *Intimating the Sacred: Religion in English Language Malaysian Fiction* (2011). He is also the editor of *Asian Gothic: Essays in Literature, Film and Anime* (2008) and *The Poetics of Shadows: The Double in Literature and Philosophy*

(2008). Currently, he is Senior Lecturer in Literature at Monash University, Malaysia, where he teaches contemporary fiction and postcolonial writing.

Daniel A. Novak is Associate Professor of English at Louisiana State University. He is author of *Realism, Photography and Nineteenth-Century Fiction* (Cambridge, 2008) and co-editor of *Masculinity Lessons: Rethinking Men's and Women's Studies* (The Johns Hopkins University Press, forthcoming). He current book project, *Victoria's Accursed Race,* analyzes nineteenth-century representations of the Cagots—an ethnic group of mysterious origins and indeterminate race.

Dejan Ognjanović has contributed to several books, including Steven Jay Schneider's *BFI's 100 European Horror Films, 501 Film Directors,* and *101 Sci-fi and Horror Films.* Ognjanović has also published three books (in Serbian) that deal with horror in cinema and literature: *Faustian Screen: The Devil in Cinema* (2006), *In the Hills, the Horrors: Serbian Horror Film* (2007), and *A Study in Terror: Essays on the Horror Genre* (2008). He also co-edited *New Frames: Neglected Tendencies in Serbian Cinema* (2008). Ognjanović is an alumnus of *Junior Faculty Development Program* (JFDP) through *American Councils for International Education*; and in 2004, he was a Fulbright Scholar at the University of California, Berkeley. He got his Ph.D. (with a thesis on "Historical Poetics of Horror Genre in Anglo-American Literature") at the University of Belgrade in 2012. He writes film and book reviews for websites, including *Beyond Hollywood* and *Twitch*, and for his own blog, *The Temple of Ghoul.*

Stephen Prince, Professor of Theatre and Cinema, has taught film history, criticism, and theory at Virginia Tech for 22 years. His work has appeared in *Film Quarterly, Cinema Journal, Quarterly Review of Film and Video*, and *The Chronicle of Higher Education.* He is a former president of the Society for Cinema and Media Studies, the world's largest organization of film scholars, academics, students, and professionals. His books include: *Digital Visual Effects: The Seduction of Reality* (2011), *Firestorm: American Film in the Age of Terrorism* (2009), *American Cinema of the 1980s: Themes and Variations* (2007), *Movies and Meaning: An Introduction to Film* (2007), *Classical Film Violence: Designing and Regulating Brutality in Hollywood Cinema, 1930–1968* (2003), *The Horror Film* (2004), *The Warrior's Camera: The Cinema of Akira Kurosawa* (1999, Chinese-language edition 1995), *A New Pot of Gold: Hollywood Under the Electronic Rainbow* (2000), *Screening Violence* (2000), *Savage Cinema: Sam Peckinpah and the Rise of Ultraviolent Movies* (1998), *Sam Peckinpah's The Wild Bunch* (1999), *Visions of Empire: Political Imagery in Contemporary American Film* (1992).

June Pulliam teaches courses in horror and adolescent literature at Louisiana State University. She is also the author of several articles on horror, including "The Zombie," in *Icons of Horror and the Supernatural* and "Gothic, Romantic, or Just Sado-Masochistic? Gender and Manipulation in Stephenie Meyer's Twilight Saga," in *21st Century Gothic: Great Gothic Novels Since 2000*, as well as works on adolescent literature including "Charlie's Evolving Moral Universe: Filmic Interpretations of Roald Dahl's Charlie and the Chocolate Factory," in *Fantasy Fiction into Film.* She has co-authored (with Anthony Fonseca) volumes 1, 2, and 3 of *Hooked on Horror: A Guide to Reading Interests in the Genre and Read On . . . Horror Fiction.*

Laurence A. Rickels moved to the Coast in 1981 upon completing his graduate training in German philology at Princeton University. While in California, he established his reputation as theorist and earned his license in psychotherapy. He has published numerous studies of the phenomenon he calls "unmourning," a term that became the title of his trilogy *Aberrations of Mourning, The Case of California*, and *Nazi Psychoanalysis.* His more recent publications include *The Devil Notebooks* and *I Think I Am: Philip K. Dick.* In April 2011, Rickels followed the call or "Ruf" to the Academy of Fine Arts in Karlsruhe, where he is Klaus Theweleit's successor as the professor of art and theory.

David J. Skal has appeared on the *Today Show, Charlie Rose*, and ABC's *20/20*, to name just a few. His widely published and read work has been featured in A&E's *Biography*, Disney Home Video, Warner Home Video, and Universal Studios. His publications on the horror genre in general, and on Dracula and vampires in particular, remain some of the most highly regarded works in the field. Among them include *Hollywood Gothic: The Tangled Web of Dracula from Novel to Stage to Screen* and *The Monster Show*, in addition to many other books on horror and monsters in popular culture, including *Dracula: The Ultimate, Illustrated Edition of the World-Famous Vampire Play*, *Dark Carnival: The Secret World of Tod Browning*, *V Is for Vampire: The A-Z Guide to Everything Undead*, *Screams of Reason: Mad Science and Modern Culture*, *Dracula* (Norton Critical Editions), *Vampires: Encounters with the Undead*, *Death Makes a Holiday: A Cultural History of Halloween*, and *Romancing the Vampire: Collectors Vault*. He is presently completing a new "cultural biography," *Bram Stoker: The Final Curtain*, and is an annual visiting lecturer in popular literature at Trinity College, Dublin.

Carla María Thomas (B.A. with Honors, Florida State University 2006; M.A., 2008; Ph.D. Candidate 2014, New York University) is currently a Henry M. MacCracken Fellow at New York University, where she also teaches courses on Medieval and Early Modern English literature. Her first publication was an edition and translation of the early Middle English versified homily "Poema Morale" in the third edition of *Old and Middle English c.890-c.1400: An Anthology*, edited by Elaine Treharne in 2009. Recently, she was accepted to study at the New York University London Study Center under the Provost's Global Research Initiative in Fall 2012 to research and write her dissertation, which will focus on specific themes, such as the Virgin Mary as the "sea star," within the evolution of the moralisée in the early Middle English period (ca.1100–1300). The International Society of Anglo-Saxonists awarded her with a competitive travel grant for the biennial conference and pre-conference graduate student manuscript workshop in Madison, Wisconsin, July-August 2011, which will culminate in a presentation on the manuscript of the late twelfth-century gospel harmony *Ormulum*. Carla is active in the Graduate English Organization and is a co-organizer for the graduate student Medieval Forum at NYU. She has presented and responded at numerous conferences, organized the first annual medieval manuscripts workshop at New York University in October 2010, and organized, and will preside over, a special session ("Vernacular Religious Writing in Twelfth- and Thirteenth-Century England") sponsored by the Early Middle English Society at the 47th International Congress on Medieval Studies at Western Michigan University in May 2012.

INDEX

NOTE: Locators in bold refer figures and locators followed by 'n' refer notes.